The Surgical Neonate: Anaesthesia and Intensive Care

David Hatch
Portex Department of Paediatric Anaesthesia, Institute of
Child Health, University of London, London, UK

Edward Sumner
The Hospital for Sick Children Trust, Great Ormond Street,
London, UK

and

Johnathan Hellmann
The Neonatal Intensive Care Unit, The Hospital for Sick
Children, Toronto, Ontario, Canada

Edward Arnold
A member of the Hodder Headline Group
LONDON   BOSTON   MELBOURNE   AUCKLAND

© 1995 Edward Arnold

First published in Great Britain 1981 as *Neonatal Anaesthesia*
Second edition 1986 entitled *Neonatal Anaesthesia and Perioperative
Care*
Third edition 1995 entitled *The Surgical Neonate: Anaesthesia
and Intensive Care*

Distributed in the Americas by Little, Brown and Company,
34 Beacon Street, Boston, MA 02108

British Library Cataloguing in Publication Data

Hatch, David J.
  Surgical Neonate: Anaesthesia and
  Intensive care
  I. Title
617.96798

  ISBN 0–340–55305–7

Typeset in 10/11 Plantin by Anneset, Weston-super-Mare, Avon, UK.
Printed and bound in Great Britain for Edward Arnold, a division
of Hodder Headline PLC, 338 Euston Road, London NW1 3BH by
Butler & Tanner Ltd., Frome and London.

ANAESTHETIC DEPT
Phone 01483 464116
Fax   01483 453135

Contents

Preface

This book is the third in an evolving series. The first, published in 1981, concentrated almost exclusively on neonatal anaesthesia, whilst the second, 1986 edition, recognised the need to include a section on immediate perioperative care. It has now become clear that those involved in the management of the surgical neonate need to keep abreast of the rapid advances in neonatal intensive care that have taken place in recent years, many of which have come from neonatal paediatrics. For this reason, the original authors have recruited Dr Jonathan Hellmann, Clinical Director of the Neonatal Intensive Care Unit at the Hospital for Sick Children, Toronto, Canada, to take responsibility for a major new section on this important topic. This section covers all the main aspects of the intensive care of the surgical neonate, including not only clinical management but also organisational matters and ethical considerations. The addition of Dr Hellmann to the authorship brings to the book the expertise of a highly respected neonatologist and adds a welcome international flavour to balance those sections which are based on the extensive clinical experience of the original authors at the Hospital for Sick Children, Great Ormond Street, London, England, where more than 500 anaesthetics are administered each year to neonates for all types of surgery.

The book is intended to help all those involved in the perioperative management of the surgical neonate, including not only paediatric anaesthetists but also neonatologists and neonatal surgeons. It includes essential new information on drugs and techniques, and incorporates the improved understanding of neonatal physiology and pathology which has emerged from the increasing survival of babies with gestational ages as low as 23 weeks. Because of this increased survival of babies of low gestational age, the application of the term 'neonatal' has broadened and much of the information in this volume is relevant to infants beyond the first month of extra-uterine life.

Although the whole book has been radically revised, with the addition of a more comprehensive reference list for those who wish to delve even further into the subject, the general layout remains similar to the previous editions. The first section is devoted to perinatal physiology, where the differences between the neonate and adult have major implications for clinical management, but has been expanded under Dr Hellmann's guidance to provide a detailed description of relevant perinatal medical disorders. Modern advances in antenatal diagnosis have been encompassed, and improved methods of patient care are described. A system-based approach has been adopted, which we hope will help the reader find relevant sections within the text more easily. The clinical approach is based on concepts and techniques which have proved safe over many years. Where appropriate, however, new techniques have been described, and this is particularly noticeable in the sections on pain control and regional analgesia, where there have been major improvements in management in recent years.

Acknowledgements

We gladly acknowledge the help and encouragement which we have received from colleagues at the Hospitals for Sick Children both in London and Toronto. We are particularly grateful for the substantial contribution made to the section on ethics by Dr Abbyann Lynch, PhD, Director of Bio-Ethics, Hospital for Sick Children, Toronto and Associate Professor of Pediatrics, University of Toronto.

We also thank Dorothy Duranti, Leigh Stanger, Joy Lowe and Katy Andrews for help with the preparation of the manuscript, the Departments of Diagnostic Imaging at both hospitals for providing X-rays and the Departments of Medical Illustration for producing many beautiful photographs. We are also grateful to those authors and publishers who have kindly allowed us to use certain figures and tables from their original publications.

Finally, we gratefully acknowledge the major contribution made by Mrs Diana Newlands by improving the grammar and style of the writing throughout the book. We are convinced that this will be appreciated by our readers.

1 Perinatal physiology and medicine

Respiratory physiology

Intrauterine development

A working knowledge of the intrauterine and postnatal development of the lungs and the factors which may impede that development is important for all those who are involved in the care of the surgical neonate before, during and after anaesthesia. A clear understanding of the pathophysiology of disorders of the lung in the newborn helps the practitioner not only to minimize any iatrogenic lung damage but also to instigate the optimum therapy.

Although prenatal gas exchange and acid base balance are functions of the placenta, irregular breathing movements are a normal feature in the fetus and may well be essential for normal lung development. Infants with spinal muscular atrophy which begins *in utero* tend to have hypoplastic lungs compared to those whose disease begins postnatally. Recent studies conducted both in fetal lambs and in humans have demonstrated that these intrauterine breathing movements occur between 30 and 40 per cent of the time and only during rapid eye movement (REM) sleep.[1] Although there is evidence to indicate that the respiratory centre and chemoreceptors are functional *in utero*, the fetal breathing movements are not affected by fluctuations in fetal PaO_2 and $PaCO_2$ and the chemical control of breathing is much less pronounced than after birth. Hypoxaemia in the fetus abolishes fetal breathing movements possibly as a result of a reduction in REM sleep.[2] Maternal alcohol ingestion and cigarette smoking also abolish fetal breathing movements, possibly as a result of hypoxaemia secondary to placental insufficiency.[3]

Recent reports of survival of infants born as early as 23 weeks postconceptional age indicate that lung development is at least in some instances adequate to support gas exchange even at this early stage. The bronchial tree is fully developed by week 16 as are the preacinar blood vessels, whose development follows that of the airways. Between the 16th and 24th weeks the airways change from blind-ending tubules lined by non-respiratory cuboidal epithelium to contain clearly delineated respiratory portions in which blood vessels grow beneath this cuboidal epithelium, thinning it whilst new branches also with thin-walled epithelium develop. By week 28 the preacinar pattern of airways, arteries and veins is complete, the blood/gas barrier is thin and capillary vessels are present within the alveolar wall. Muscularization of the intra-acinar arteries does not, however, keep pace with the appearance of new vessels.

Specialized type II pneumonocytes of the alveolar epithelial lining become discernible by electron microscopy during the sixth month of gestation. Differentiation of the type II alveolar cell, the pneumonocyte, the sole site of surfactant synthesis, is usually complete by about 32 weeks gestation. Timing of this differentiation is, in part, under genetic control and regulated by both endocrine and paracrine hormones. The lipoprotein complex, surfactant, is stored in type II cells as lamellar bodies. The type II cell secretes surfactant as vesicles which spread and line the alveolar surface; at the air–liquid interface surfactant enables the alveolar lining layer to alter surface tension with changes in surface area and thereby promote alveolar stability and prevent atelectasis at end–expiration. Without surfactant, the lungs would be unable to retain gas within them and would be unstable because the pressure within them required to prevent collapse due to surface tension is inversely proportional to their radius (Laplace formula). As areas of lung collapse, the collapsing forces increase and thus a state of unstable equilibrium exists. Although surfactant can be detected in lung extracts from human fetuses from week 23 onwards, the quantity which can be detected increases greatly towards term and this is one of the main reasons why the older fetus has a greater chance of surviving in air than those delivered very prematurely.

Optimal activity of lung surfactant depends on the presence of surfactant proteins A, B and C in the alveolar fluid which are thought to modify surfactant phospholipid function and metabolism. Glucocorticoids have been shown to accelerate the morphological and biochemical maturation of the lung and cause accumulation of messenger RNAs in coding surfactant proteins B and C in cultures of fetal lung. The effect of glucocorticoids on the synthesis of surfactant protein A is, however, still uncertain. Work on human fetal lung tissue from second trimester abortions demonstrated that dexamethasone had a biphasic effect, initially stimulating and later inhibiting surfactant protein A. Whether or not a similar biphasic response occurs in later second trimester or early third trimester fetal lungs is uncertain but, if demonstrated, would suggest that glucocorticoids should not be used for more than a week in women in premature labour.[4]

The surfactant protein A content of the amniotic fluid has been used to assess the maturity of the fetal lung. A level of less than 0.6 μg.ml^{-1} predicted the development of respiratory distress syndrome (RDS) reasonably accurately in one study whilst a level[5] greater than 3.0 μg.ml^{-1} was seldom associated with RDS[5]. The overall predictability of RDS using this method was similar to the lecithin/sphingomyelin (L/S) ratio and phosphatidyl glycerol (PG). A L/S ratio of more than 2 is normally present by 35–36 weeks and is seldom associated with the development of RDS. Low L/S ratios (less than 1.4) are less reliable predictors of lung development. PG appears by week 35 and peaks at birth. Combining all three tests increases the ability to predict RDS from 52 per cent to 74 per cent.

During the third trimester there is further differentiation of the respiratory region of the lung with additional respiratory bronchioles developing whose terminal saccules are capable of acting as gas exchanging areas. New alveoli continue to grow for several years after birth.

Gas transport in fetal life

The oxygen tension of fetal blood is considerably lower than that of the mother, fluctuating between 2.5 and 3.5 kPa (20–25 mmHg). Raising the maternal PO_2 by 20 kPa (150 mmHg) increases fetal PO_2 by only 1.1 kPa (8 mmHg) and falls in maternal PO_2 will also have relatively less effect on the fetus. Fetal blood has a greater affinity for oxygen than adult blood, which enables it to carry more oxygen in the presence of a relatively low PO_2; the oxygen/haemoglobin dissociation curve is shifted to the left.

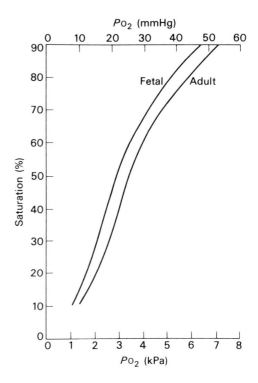

Fig. 1.1 Oxygen dissociation curves for fetal and adult blood. (Reproduced with permission from [6])

This is due to the fact that fetal haemoglobin (HbF) is relatively insensitive to 2,3-diphospho–glycerate (2,3-DPG), which in itself lowers the oxygen affinity of the haemoglobin molecule. A decrease in pH and a rise in body temperature will move the dissociation curve to the right; conversely, a rise in pH or fall in body temperature will have the reverse effect.

It might be thought that the increased affinity of fetal blood for oxygen would hinder the release of oxygen at the tissues but the simultaneous uptake of carbon dioxide shifts the dissociation curve to the right. Because the tissue oxygen tension is so low – about 2 kPa (15 mmHg) – and because the dissociation curve is so steep, adequate oxygen delivery to the tissues is ensured.

One method of expressing the position of the dissociation curve is to measure the oxygen tension at which the blood is 50 per cent saturated. This is known as the P50. For adult blood the P50 is about 3.6 kPa (27 mmHg) whilst at birth it is around 2.7 kPa (20 mmHg). It rises slowly, reaching the adult value by six months of age. At birth approximately 70 per cent of the haemoglobin is HbF and total replacement of this by HbA does not occur until

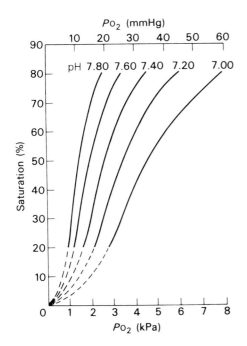

Fig. 1.2 Oxygen/haemoglobin dissociation curves for fetal blood at various pH levels. (Reproduced with permission from [7]).

about three months after birth. The steepness and position of the fetal oxygen/haemoglobin dissociation curve are advantageous for normal fetal gas exchange. After birth, however, severe tissue hypoxia can occur if arterial oxygen tension is allowed to fall substantially, since the AV oxygen content or 'unloading capacity' of HbF is considerably less than that of HbA.

Adaptation to extrauterine life

The normal fetus undergoes extraordinary physiological changes at the moment of birth in order to adapt to extrauterine life. During vaginal delivery the baby's thorax is squeezed as it passes through the birth canal and up to 35 ml of fluid drains out of the mouth. As the thoracic cage re-expands at birth, this volume of fluid is replaced by the entry of an equivalent volume of air into the trachea and main air passages. At birth the type II pneumonocytes rapidly discharge their surface active phospholipids into the alveolar space and are then seen to be vacuolated rather than containing dense inclusion bodies.

There appears to be no simple explanation for the onset of continuous breathing at birth, which probably results from a combination of events.

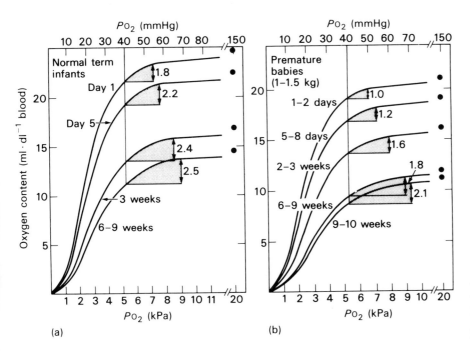

(a)   (b)

Fig. 1.3 The blood oxygen-releasing capacity at various ages from birth. (a) Term infants. (b) Preterm infants. The shaded areas represent AV oxygen content in ml O_2.dl^{-1} blood. (Reproduced with permission from [8]).

Removal of the placental circulation decreases the concentration of prostaglandin E2, a known inhibitor of fetal breathing.[9] However, cord clamping alone is not sufficient to initiate continuous breathing. Oxygenation is almost certainly an important factor though immature fetuses do not respond to oxygenation alone. Studies in fetal sheep have shown that lung distension without an increase in fetal PO_2 does not stimulate the onset of regular breathing at any gestational age though a combination of oxygenation and lung distension results in a significant increase in breathing in relatively mature fetuses.[10] Both lung distension and oxygenation alter the distribution of fetal blood flow and may initiate other effects that contribute to the onset of regular breathing. During normal vaginal delivery the fetus sustains a considerable degree of hypoxia and in term fetal lambs this itself stimulates ventilation even after denervation of the peripheral chemoreceptors.

After the onset of the first breath, which may require inspiratory pressures of 7 kPa (70 cmH$_2$O) or more, a functional residual capacity (FRC) of 30–35 ml.kg^{-1} is rapidly established.

Remaining lung fluid is removed by the pulmonary lymphatics and lung capillaries which open up with lung expansion. A normal FRC is usually established within 60 minutes of birth. The onset of regular respiration and rapid rise in arterial oxygen tension lead to a dramatic fall in pulmonary vascular resistance and an uptake of up to 100 ml of blood into the pulmonary circulation.[11] Prostaglandin inhibition prevents this fall.[12] Combined ventricular output increases markedly at birth, partly in response to the β-adrenergic surge that occurs during delivery.[13] The fall in pulmonary vascular resistance with increased pulmonary blood flow, together with a reduction in inferior vena caval return due to clamping of the umbilical cord, causes left atrial pressure to exceed right

Table 1.1 Respiratory and cardiovascular effects of birth-related manipulations in the fetus. (Reproduced with permission from[2])

	PCO$_2$	PO$_2$	Breathing	Cardiac function	Circulatory changes
Static distension	NC	NC	NC	Unknown	Unknown
Plus oxygen	NC	I	I	Unknown	Unknown
	1		Continuous†††	Unknown	Unknown
Plus oxygen and cord occlusion	I	I	I	Unknown	Unknown
			Continuous	Unknown	Unknown
Rhythmic distension	NC	NC	Unknown	I left ventricle output	I pulmonary flow
				I P left atrium	D pulmonary resistance
				D foramen R–L Shunt	
				D ductus R–L shunt	
Plus oxygen	NC	I	Unknown	D right ventricle output	D umbilical flow
				D foramen R–L shunt	D cerebral flow
				D ductus R–L shunt	I pulmonary flow
				D P descending aorta	D pulmonary resistance
				D P pulmonary artery	
Plus oxygen and cord occlusion	NC	I	Unknown	D right ventricle output	
				D ductus R–L shunt	
Plus cord occlusion	NC	NC	I	Unknown	
			Continuous†††	Unknown	Unknown
Oxygen	NC	I	NC	Unknown	Unknown
Plus cord occlusion	I	I	I	I P axillary artery	Unknown
			Continuous	I heart rate	Unknown
External cooling	NC	D	I	NC combined ventricular output	I adrenal flow
			Continuous	I P arterial	I brown fat flow
				I heart rate	D skin flow

†††Variable present under some conditions.
D–decreased; I–increased; NC–no change; P–pressure; R–L–right to left.

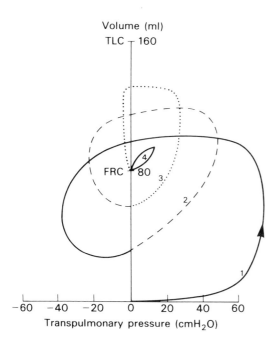

Volume (ml)

Transpulmonary pressure (cmH$_2$O)

Fig. 1.4 The first four breaths. Each successive breath requires less pressure and adds increasing volume to the lungs. (Based on data from [10])

atrial pressure with closure of the foramen ovale. As the arterial oxygen tension rises, the smooth muscle in the ductus arteriosus constricts and closure is usually physiologically complete within 1–15 hours. These cardiac and pulmonary changes are obviously inter-related; ventilation improves both pulmonary perfusion and surfactant release, which in turn help further improve ventilation. Surfactant synthesis is dependent upon satisfactory oxygenation and acid-base state.

Respiratory function in the newborn

The adaptation of the neonatal lung to extrauterine life takes several weeks to complete and the lungs continue to develop well beyond infancy. However, the most rapid changes occur immediately after birth.

Assessment of lung size at birth is usually made by measurement of lung volume at or near end-expiration, referred to as functional residual capacity (FRC). Measurements using gas dilution or washout techniques assume that all units within the lung equilibrate within a relatively short period of time. Studies in healthy infants indicate that there is considerable maldistribution of gas within the lungs which may lead to significant under-estimation of lung volume using these methods. Plethysmographic measurements of lung volume depend on the assumption that uniform pressure changes exist within the lung during airway occlusion and also that only gas contained within the thorax contributes to the measured change in volume. Studies in infants have suggested that pressure changes measured at the airway opening may not reflect changes within the lung as a whole and again care must be taken in interpreting results of these measurements, particularly in the first few hours of life.

However, despite these methodological reservations, the evidence suggests that lung volume in the neonate is relatively small in relation to body size. Since the neonate's metabolic rate when expressed in relation to body size is nearly twice that of the adult, the resting alveolar ventilation per unit of lung volume is extremely high. Since the horizontal ribs limit the tidal volume to approximately 6 ml.kg^{-1}, this high resting alveolar ventilation is achieved largely by a rapid breathing frequency. Over the first few hours of life the newborn infant normally establishes a breathing frequency of between 30 and 40 breaths per minute though preterm infants may breathe at considerably higher frequencies. The deadspace/tidal volume ratio is about 0.3 which is similar to the adult. Changes in inspired oxygen concentration will rapidly affect arterial oxygen tension and the neonate can be seen to have far less reserve of lung function than older infants. In premature infants with reduced amounts of surfactant in the alveolar lining layer FRC is likely to be even further reduced.

The act of breathing must overcome the elastic and resistive properties of the respiratory system. The water content of the lungs is relatively high at birth and airway pressures of up to 7 kPa (70 cmH$_2$O) may be required to expand them initially in asphyxiated babies.[14] Once the baby has taken a breath, much lower pressures are likely to be required. The initial period of neonatal adaptation leads to an increase in compliance (volume change per unit pressure change) over the first few hours.

Classic studies in animals have shown the chest wall of the very young to be much more compliant than that of the older animal.[15] These studies have been widely extrapolated to human newborns and have largely been confirmed by measurements made in anaesthetized infants during surgery. The deformable nature of the chest wall in the newborn undoubtedly enables it to change shape dramatically during passage through the birth canal and means that very little work is required to move the chest after birth. The markedly reduced outward recoil of the chest wall in the newborn compared to the only slightly reduced inward recoil of the lung may be the main reason for the reduction in FRC described above.

Absolute pleural pressure will be less negative with respect to atmosphere than in older infants or adults causing an increased tendency to closure of small airways. In the paralysed state if positive end expiratory pressure (PEEP) is not applied the lungs will collapse to a point where the opposing recoil forces are balanced and this may lead to reduction in ventilation/perfusion ratio, increase in intrapulmonary shunting and hypoxia, especially when breathing air. In the awake spontaneously breathing neonate, however, laryngeal braking during expiration causes a dynamic elevation of FRC which minimizes this problem. In addition there is some evidence to suggest that expiration is not entirely passive in the newborn[16] and that muscular tone both in the diaphragm and intercostal muscles may help maintain a higher FRC. The change from non-REM to REM sleep has been shown to be associated with a decrease in FRC of approximately 30 per cent, possibly due to loss of tonic activity of the respiratory muscles and reduction in laryngeal braking. A significant reduction in FRC has also been demonstrated during anaesthesia in children as it has in adults.[17]

The resistance to the flow of gases through the airways decreases from about 90 $cmH_2O.l^{-1}.s$ in the first minute to about 25 $cmH_2O.l^{-1}$ by the end of the first day, by which time an intrathoracic pressure change of only 5 cmH_2O is needed for normal tidal breathing. The resistance of the nasal passages in the newborn is approximately 50 per cent of the total resistance for Caucasians and 30 per cent of the total for black infants.[18] These values are lower than the figure of 63 per cent commonly quoted for adults, which is important as neonates are obligatory nose breathers. Nasal resistance can be significantly increased by the presence of an indwelling nasogastric tube, particularly if placed in the larger nostril.

In adults most of the airway resistance occurs in the large central airways, peripheral airways contributing only about 10 per cent to the total resistance despite their smaller calibre.

This apparent anomaly arises because of the large total cross–sectional area of the peripheral airways. Studies both in anaesthetized and sleeping infants suggest that peripheral airway resistance contributes even less to the total resistance in the early postnatal years. Few measurements have been made of lung tissue resistance in infants though at the relatively high breathing frequencies seen in the newborn this is likely to be less significant than in adults. Resistance of the chest wall accounts for about 25 per cent of the total respiratory resistance during spontaneous breathing in unanaesthetized newborns.[19]

Gas exchange in the newborn

Oxygen consumption in the newborn at neutral environmental temperature is approximately 7 $ml.kg^{-1}$. min, which is about twice that of the adult on a weight basis. Measurements made below neutral environmental temperature will be misleadingly high because of the increase in metabolic rate in response to cold. The respiratory quotient is low in the immediate postnatal period at about 0.7, increasing to 0.8 by the end of the first week.

Studies of arterial blood gas tensions in the newborn show that the relative hypoxia of the fetus is largely corrected by 5 minutes after birth, the hypercapnia by 20 minutes and the acidosis by 24 hours. The arterial oxygen tension in the neonate remains lower than the adult value, at about 10–10.7 kPa (75–80 mmHg) and the arterial carbon dioxide tension is also a little low at about 4.7 kPa (35 mmHg). This reduced oxygen tension is thought to be due to persistent amounts of right-to-left shunting through remaining fetal channels, or to intrapulmonary shunting through poorly ventilated or unventilated areas of lung, or to the draining of small amounts of systemic blood into the left side of the heart from the bronchial circulation. It should be remembered when taking samples from the umbilical artery that umbilical arterial blood is distal to the ductus arteriosus, and will be contaminated by any blood that has been shunted from right to left through this. Radial to umbilical arterial oxygen tension differences of up to 1.3 kPa (10 mmHg) have been demonstrated. Oxygen tension rises rapidly in the first months of life.

Although the newborn appears somewhat hypoxic by adult standards, it must be remem-

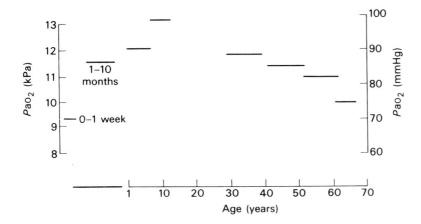

Fig. 1.5 Oxygen tensions in the newborn and at various subsequent ages. (Data from [20] and [21]).

bered that the oxygen dissociation curve is shifted to the left and therefore arterial oxygen saturation is probably over 95 per cent; moreover, because of the higher haemoglobin level in the newborn period the actual volume of oxygen transported in the arterial blood tends to offset the reduced unloading capacity described above.

Control of breathing in the newborn

Although term neonates establish regular continuous breathing at birth, preterm infants have frequent apnoeic pauses. The pathophysiology of apnoea in the preterm infant is not, however, fully understood. Most research has focused on the relationship between breathing pattern and carbon dioxide responsiveness, oxygenation, sleep state and thermoregulation.

The term newborn infant has an easily measurable ventilatory response to an increase in inspired carbon dioxide concentration. The slope of this response when corrected for the smaller ventilatory capacity of the newborn is similar to that of the adult. At birth, however, the chemoreceptors are functioning at a lower arterial carbon dioxide tension and thus the CO_2 response curve is shifted to the left. Although preterm infants have previously been shown to have a flatter response curve than term infants, recent studies using endogenous changes in end tidal CO_2 during spontaneous variations in breathing produced a significantly steeper slope than did testing with steady state increases. Thus preterm infants may be more responsive to CO_2 than has previously been shown. Because the respiratory centre normally responds to changes in endogenous CO_2 this response may be more physiologically correct than challenging the infant with exogenous CO_2.[22] Another recent study[23] using normoxic rebreathing to obviate the effect of hyperoxia on the ventilatory response showed a lower and more variable response to CO_2 challenge during active REM sleep than during quiet sleep. Tidal and minute volume increased in both sleep states but frequency only increased consistently during quiet sleep. Sleep state must therefore be taken into account when testing respiratory responsiveness to carbon dioxide.

Increasing the concentration of oxygen in the inspired gas depresses respiration, and giving low concentrations of oxygen stimulates it. Unlike the effects of carbon dioxide, however, change in inspired oxygen concentration has only a transient effect on ventilation in the immediate postnatal period, passing off after about two minutes. This transient response develops into a fully sustained adult response by the tenth day of life. In a cool environment the newborn infant does not respond to hypoxia by an increase in ventilation, and respiratory depression is seen as the only response. After the first week of life, however, hypoxia invariably increases ventilation.

Hypercapnia potentiates the ventilatory response to hypoxia in the neonate as in the adult, although the converse effect is less certain. Hypoxia in term infants in one recent study caused periodic breathing in both active and quiet sleep.[25] In a study of preterm infants with bronchopulmonary dysplasia[26] oxygen supplementation significantly decreased the rate of periodic breathing, the number of episodes of central apnoea and the incidence of arterial desaturation.

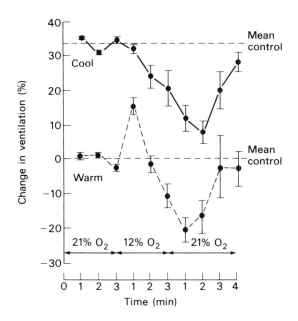

Fig. 1.6 Percentage change in ventilation while breathing air and 12 per cent oxygen in normal term infants in cool and warm environments. (Reproduced with permission from [24]).

Pauses of up to five seconds occurring five or six times an hour in infants at sea level, and more frequently at high altitudes, are normal. They also occur more often in premature infants, especially during REM sleep. These episodes of periodic breathing may develop into frank spells of apnoea, defined as 15 or more seconds of cessation of airflow with either 10 per cent fall in saturation or 20 per cent decrease in heart rate. The peak incidence of these occurs between days 3 and 10 of life. Most episodes of apnoea also occur during REM sleep.[27] Periodically breathing babies have a lower arterial oxygen tension than those breathing normally, although still within the normal range. Periodic breathing may be abolished by increasing lung volume (e.g. constant distending pressure) or by increasing the inspired oxygen or carbon dioxide concentrations.

No constant changes in heart rate occur during periodic breathing, which appears to have no serious consequences and usually ceases by 4–6 weeks of age. When apnoea occurs in association with periodic breathing, the incidence and severity of arterial hypoxaemia increases.[28]

Research into the relationship between respiratory control and thermoregulation has been stimu-

lated by suggestions that sudden infant death is more common in infants wearing excessive clothing.[29]

There are two pulmonary reflexes which may be important in the control of respiration in the newborn:

1. Head's paradoxical inflation reflex. When the lungs are inflated the infant makes an extra inspiratory effort before exhaling. This reflex can be demonstrated even during deep anaesthesia. Although it has been suggested that it is important in the initiation of respiration, the newborn rabbit has been shown to be capable of initiating respiration after all the pulmonary reflexes have been abolished by vagotomy.
2. Hering–Breuer reflex. This reflex is invoked by a more gradual inflation of the lungs than Head's reflex and consists of transient apnoea following inflation. Weakness of this reflex may lead to apnoeic spells. Recent work has demonstrated the persistence of this reflex beyond the neonatal period.[30]

The work of breathing

The work of breathing can be calculated from the area of a pressure/volume loop for an individual breath and may be subdivided into elastic work and flow-resistive work, as illustrated in Fig.1.7. Work can also be calculated from formulae based on the measured compliance and resistance or from the oesophageal pressure required to produce a given tidal volume.

Calculations of the work of breathing in the newborn suggest that its value is about 0.004 J (40 g.cm) per breath or 0.14 J (1400 g.cm) per minute. About 75 per cent of this work is elastic work and the rest is flow resistive. Quiet breathing in healthy babies requires little work and calculations based on the time constant obtained from normal data for compliance and resistance suggest that a respiratory rate of 35–40 per minute is the most efficient with regard to energy consumption for the healthy neonate. In respiratory disease, increased pulmonary stiffness (reduced compliance) or increased airway resistance may lead to a significant increase in work, and this in turn will lead to an increase in oxygen consumption by the respiratory muscles. The work of breathing may then represent a substantial proportion of metabolic rate.

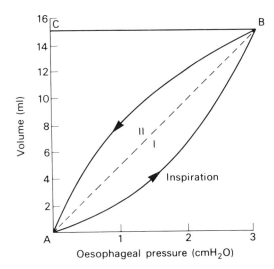

Fig. 1.7 A pressure/volume respiratory loop. Elastic work = the area of the triangle ABC. Inspiratory and expiratory flow-resistive work are represented by areas I and II respectively. Total pulmonary work = area ABC + area I. (Data from [31]).

Anatomy of the airway

The neonate has a relatively large head because of the advanced development of the brain, but the neck is short and the shoulders and chest are narrow.

Various anatomical differences can make the neonate difficult to intubate. The tongue is large in relation to the size of the oropharynx and this may interfere with visibility and the easy positioning of a laryngoscope blade.

The vocal cords lie opposite the lower border of the C4 vertebra and at about the fourth year of life are found at the adult level of C5 or C6. Thus, the infant glottis lies higher and more anteriorly than in the older child and is behind a soft and often 'folded' epiglottis. The infant epiglottis inclines to the posterior pharyngeal wall at an angle of 45 degrees and the vocal cords are angled more forward and downwards than in the adult. During growth the epiglottis reaches the adult position closely approximated to the base of the tongue.

The anatomical differences mean that a straight–bladed laryngoscope is usually required for intubation in this age group.

The trachea is approximately 4 cm in length and between 6 and 8 mm in diameter in a term baby and bronchial intubation is more likely than in older children. The right main bronchus is intubated more easily than the left, as the latter crosses the midline from the right side at a sharper angle than the right. The right main bronchus is also wider than the left and this ratio is unchanged from birth to adult life.

The narrowest part of a child's airway is at the level of the cricoid ring, which is easily damaged by the inadvertent use of a tracheal tube which is too large but which may have passed through the glottis. Because there is a complete ring of cartilage at this level, any oedema will narrow the airway: 1 mm of mucosal oedema at the cricoid level may reduce the area of the airway by as much as 60 per cent in a newborn infant.

Clinical presentation of respiratory disorders

History

A review of the maternal history and the events of labour and delivery is essential in the differentiation of the various causes of respiratory distress in the newborn.

Estimated gestational age
The mother's estimated date of confinement and other indices of dating the pregnancy help determine the maturity of the infant because a premature infant, regardless of birthweight, is likely to have respiratory distress syndrome (RDS). Postmaturity is strongly associated with meconium aspiration. Polycythaemia may also complicate small for gestational age (SGA) infants and give rise to respiratory distress.

Maternal history of oligohydramnios/ polyhydramnios
A history of chronic amniotic leak or the detection of oligohydramnios during pregnancy suggests the possibility of pulmonary hypoplasia. Polyhydramnios may be associated with fetal anomalies (e.g. tracheo–oesophageal fistula) and is a feature of non-immune hydrops with pleural effusions, and myotonic dystrophy.

Labour and delivery
A history of peripartum maternal fever, premature or prolonged rupture of membranes, foul smelling amniotic fluid or excessive obstetric manipulation all suggest pneumonia. Placenta previa or abruption

increase the likelihood of hypovolaemia with acute respiratory distress. The passage of meconium is highly suggestive of meconium aspiration syndrome and perinatal asphyxia with transient myocardial ischaemia. Traumatic or breech delivery suggests an intracerebral haemorrhage or phrenic nerve palsy, which may manifest with respiratory distress. Delivery by caesarean section raises the suspicion of transient tachypnoea of the newborn (TTN) or RDS.

Time of onset of respiratory distress

Infants with RDS and TTN usually have acute respiratory distress in the first few hours, although these signs may be subtle and consist only of tachypnoea. When signs and symptoms develop in a newborn infant who has been normal for hours to days, bacterial and viral sepsis, cardiac disorders, inborn errors of metabolism and intracranial haemorrhage may all be suspected. Choking or difficulty with the first feed suggests tracheo–oesophageal fistula.

Physical examination

Respiratory disorders in the newborn present with one or more of the following signs: respiratory distress, cyanosis, stridor/upper airway obstruction or apnoea.

Respiratory Distress:

The clinical signs of tachypnoea, retractions, nasal flaring and cyanosis are common to many respiratory disorders of the newborn. Respiratory distress does not constitute a specific diagnosis *per se* and a definitive cause for the distress must be sought in all infants.

Physical examination should include an assessment of all of the following:

Tachypnoea   The normal respiratory rate after the first 24 hours of life is approximately 40 breaths per minute in the term and 50–55 breaths per minute in the premature infant: a sustained respiratory rate greater than 60 breaths per minute is therefore regarded as tachypnoea. A persistently elevated respiratory rate is one of the most easily detectable signs of distress and may also be the only sign of respiratory difficulty. As the infant starts to tire from the increased work of breathing, the respiratory rate may decrease; this is an ominous, often unrecognized sign of imminent respiratory failure.

Retractions   With the respiratory effort required to increase negative intrathoracic pressure, and because of the stiff (poorly compliant) lung but pliable chest wall, the softest parts of the thorax are pulled inwards on inspiration. This gives rise to retraction of the intercostal, suprasternal and infrasternal spaces, as well as the sternum itself. The degree of retraction is proportional to the negative pressure generated within the thorax and correlates with the severity of disease in RDS. Retractions are accompanied by the use of accessory respiratory muscles, as well as with flaring or widening of the alae nasi on inspiration.

Central Cyanosis   Central cyanosis (cyanosis of the mucous membranes) is a common and important sign of respiratory distress. It may be difficult to appreciate clinically in the newborn and may only be detected when the haemoglobin oxygen saturation declines below 80 per cent or the PaO_2 to 4–5.5 kPa (30–40 mmHg). Cyanosis is evidence of severe distress, and if progressive, may be a grave prognostic sign. The differentiation of respiratory from cardiac or other causes of cyanosis is discussed on p. 24

Grunting   This is an expiratory sound often heard in the first few minutes of life. It is produced with each expiration in an effort to increase alveolar volume. If the grunt is intermittent and not accompanied by other signs of distress, it may be insignificant; if it is loud or persistent, it indicates the presence of moderate to severe lung disease. It is particularly audible in RDS, but occasionally occurs in other lung disorders of the newborn as well.

Air entry   is subjectively assessed by auscultation to 'quantify' alveolar ventilation; poor air entry is a useful means of gauging the severity of RDS. A unilateral decrease in breath sounds suggests a pneumothorax, diaphragmatic hernia or other thoracic mass lesion. Clinical examination must therefore include palpation of the position of the trachea in the suprasternal notch and auscultation for the position of maximal intensity of the heart sounds. Deviation in the position of these signs indicates mediastinal shift secondary to one of the above disorders.

In any infant with respiratory difficulty associated signs may aid in determining the underlying cause, as well as the severity of the respiratory distress; these include temperature, heart rate, BP, muscle tone, activity and lability in oxygenation with handling.

Table 1.2 Differential diagnosis of respiratory distress in the newborn period

Pulmonary disorders

Common	Less common	Surgical
Respiratory distress syndrome	Pulmonary haemorrhage	Congenital diaphragmatic hernia
Transient tachypnoea of the newborn	Pulmonary hypoplasia	Cystic adenomatoid malformation
Meconium aspiration	Pleural effusion Chylothorax	Congenital lobar emphysema
Pneumonia		Less common congenital anomalies
Pneumothorax/air leaks		
Persistent pulmonary hypertension of the newborn		

Extrapulmonary disorders

Cardiac	Haematological	Metabolic	Neurological
Congenital heart disease	Anaemia	Acidosis	Meningitis
Hypovolaemia	Polycythaemia	Hypoglycaemia	Cerebral haemorrhage
		Hypothermia	Neuromuscular disorders
		Sepsis	Spinal cord injury Phrenic nerve palsy
			Drugs (morphine, phenobarbitone)

Common respiratory disorders

Respiratory distress syndrome (RDS)

RDS implies respiratory distress in preterm infants with surfactant deficiency, but with no other identifiable cause for the respiratory disease. The older term, hyaline membrane disease (HMD), was first used by pathologists who noted widespread atelectasis and eosinophilic material lining the overdistended terminal bronchioles. While there is clear evidence that lack of surfactant in the air spaces produces the clinical picture of RDS, the designation of this clinical condition as *surfactant deficiency* is generally not used for a number of reasons: it is not known to what degree structural aspects of lung immaturity (e.g. airway development, alveolarization, development of the pulmonary vasculature) also play a role in the pathogenesis of RDS; specific assays of surfactant phospholipid are seldom made in clinical practice; and the role of *relative* surfactant deficiency in the pathogenesis of other clinical forms of neonatal lung disease is not known.

Important risk factors that affect the incidence and severity of RDS include:

1. *Gestational age*: the risk is inversely proportional to gestational age. RDS affects 60 per cent of infants at 29 weeks and approximately 30 per cent of infants at less than 34 weeks gestational age
2. *Mode of delivery and effect of labour*: at any given gestational age the incidence is higher for caesarean section without labour than for

vaginal delivery. There is also good evidence that the mode of delivery itself is a potent risk factor for RDS in preterm infants and for other forms of respiratory distress in mature infants.[32,33]

3. *Sex/race*: male infants are at higher risk than females, as are Caucasian infants as compared with black infants.
4. *Asphyxia*: a compromised condition at birth with low Apgar scores is an independent risk factor for RDS.
5. *Maternal diabetes*: maternal diabetes increases the risk of RDS independent of gestational age and mode of delivery.[34]
6. *Twin pregnancy*: the non–presenting twin is at greater risk than the first. This has been assumed to be due to the second twin's predisposition to asphyxia; however, it may be more a reflection of the second twin not benefiting from the salutary effects of labour to the same degree as the first.[35]
7. *Maternal corticosteroids*: antenatal treatment with dexamethasone decreases the incidence of RDS,[36] probably not only by altering surfactant synthetic enzymes, but by multiple effects on developing systems, including alterations of lung structure.[37]
8. *Pregnancy related conditions*: earlier reports documented the effect of chronic maternal hypertension, intrauterine growth retardation and prolonged rupture of membranes in decreasing the incidence of RDS by 'stressing' the fetus and enhancing lung maturation. More recent studies have questioned whether these conditions do in fact protect against RDS;[38,39] in pregnancies complicated by maternal hypertension for example, the incidence of RDS may be increased, due more to the absence of labour prior to delivery via caesarean section than to the potential 'sparing' effect of maternal hypertension.[40]

Pathophysiology of RDS

The limited capacity of the premature infant to synthesize pulmonary surfactant has already been discussed (p. 1). Absence of surfactant at the gas–liquid interface leads to decreased pulmonary compliance, increased work of breathing, increased right to left shunting and decreased alveolar ventilation, thus setting up a worsening cycle of hypoxia and acidosis (see below). Lack of surfactant or inhibition of its action also leads to increased capillary permeability and pulmonary oedema and contributes to the development of acute lung injury.

Clinical Course

Respiratory distress usually appears at birth or soon thereafter. It generally worsens over the first few hours, as tachypnoea, retractions and expiratory grunting increase in severity. Right to left intrapulmonary shunting across poorly ventilated regions of the lung (and to a lesser extent extrapulmonary shunting through PDA and PFO)[41], results in hypoxaemia. Ventilation/perfusion (Va/Q) imbalance also contributes to the venous admixture, although pulmonary circulation vasoconstriction in response to hypoxia, with resultant reduction of perfusion to poorly ventilated alveoli, may decrease the degree of the V/Q mismatch.[42]

Oxygen requirements usually increase over the first 24–48 hours. (This sign could formerly be used as an indication of the severity of RDS; however, the advent of surfactant replacement therapy has

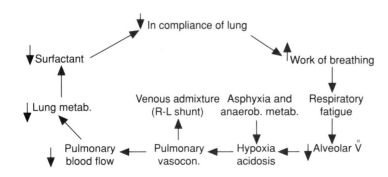

Fig. 1.8 Pathophysiology of the respiratory distress syndrome.

rendered the degree of oxygen requirements less clinically useful when surfactant has been administered.) Urine output is low for the first 24–48 hours; soon thereafter a diuresis usually ensues.

The diagnosis of RDS is essentially clinical; it is based on the clinical descriptive variables as above, the chest radiographic appearance and the natural history of the disease process. The chest radiograph in typical RDS consists of a diffuse, fine reticulogranular pattern developing over the first few hours, air bronchograms, low lung volumes and an indistinct heart border. Positive pressure ventilation may limit these radiographic findings. Blood gases show a moderate to severe oxygenation defect, hypercarbia due to decreased alveolar ventilation, and a mild metabolic acidosis.

RDS generally persists for 3–5 days in larger infants; in infants > 1500 gm with an uncomplicated course it tends to resolve by 7–10 days. The course in VLBW infants is usually more protracted, particularly when complicated by pulmonary or systemic disorders, e.g. air leaks, pulmonary haemorrhage, sepsis, patent ductus arteriosus, necrotizing enterocolitis or intraventricular haemorrhage.

Transient tachypneoa of the newborn (TTNB)

TTNB or 'wet lung' disease is a very common respiratory disorder in the newborn. It tends to occur in term or close to term infants, in whom there is delayed resorption of fetal lung fluid from the air spaces and interstitial tissues via the pulmonary capillaries and lymphatics. It is seen following elective caesarean section, birth asphyxia, excess maternal fluid administration and delayed cord clamping.

Distress manifests at birth or within the first 2–6 hours of life and is characterized by marked tachypnoea up to 120 breaths/min and minimal retractions, (implying relatively normal lung compliance). The tachypnoea usually peaks by 6–12 hours and resolves over 24–48 hours. More severe forms of the condition are encountered and TTNB may precipitate the development of PPHN in infants who become hypoxic, hypercarbic or acidotic.

As the clinical signs are non-specific and no applicable means of measuring lung water content exists, the condition is diagnosed by exclusion of other causes, the radiographic findings and the natural course of the disease process. Radiologically the lungs are generally hyperinflated with fluid in the lung fissures, increased vascular markings and mild cardiomegaly. The radiographic appearance is often difficult to distinguish from RDS; the two conditions may coexist, as infants may have an element of pulmonary oedema from retained fetal lung liquid complicating their surfactant deficiency. It is also often not possible to exclude pneumonia and, where pulmonary vascular engorgement and mild cardiomegaly persist, CHD, particularly TAPVD, must also be considered.

Meconium aspiration

Meconium staining of amniotic fluid occurs in approximately 10 per cent of all deliveries; it is a marker of fetal distress and is seen predominantly in term or post–term pregnancies. Fetal hypoxia is thought to result in relaxation of the anal sphincter with the passage of meconium into the amniotic fluid; fetal gasping respiration may result in subsequent aspiration of the meconium *in utero*. Meconium enters the trachea and airways and produces mechanical obstruction of the airways. It is not clear to what degree meconium migrates peripherally to affect smaller, distal airways prior to delivery; respiration after birth may lead to distal migration of meconium into the smaller airways with plugging, air trapping and atelectasis. This potential postnatal distal aspiration of meconium is the basis for the delivery room recommendation that, in pregnancies complicated by the passage of thick meconium, the infant's mouth be carefully aspirated with crowning of the head and prior to delivery of the shoulders. Subsequent intubation and suctioning of the upper and lower airways in those infants with respiratory depression or perinatal asphyxia is also recommended.

The pathophysiology of meconium aspiration syndrome is related to the mechanical obstructions in the airways (with areas of hyperinflation and patchy atelectasis), the chemical effects of meconium on the lung (chemical pneumonitis), as well as the effect of the asphyxia which accompanies meconium aspiration (increasing pulmonary vascular resistance (PVR) and potentiating PPHN). Pulmonary hypertension may also be the result of a more chronic *in utero* hypoxic vasoconstriction of the pulmonary arterioles, secondary to the extension of vascular smooth muscle to the walls of normally non-muscular intra-acinar arterioles.

Furthermore, there is evidence that meconium may contribute to functional surfactant deficiency by inhibiting surfactant surface tension lowering properties, thereby compounding the atelectasis in the meconium aspiration syndrome (MAS).[43]

Respiratory distress is evident at birth and is often accompanied by features of perinatal asphyxia, metabolic acidosis and/or hypoglycaemia. The respiratory distress may increase in severity over the subsequent few hours with marked tachypnoea, cyanosis and lability in oxygenation with handling. The chest is usually hyperinflated with diffuse rales and rhonchi. The chest radiograph is one of overexpansion with wide–spread coarse infiltrates and possibly signs of air leak, particularly pneumomediastinum. Pneumothorax may complicate the course in about 20 per cent of cases and fullblown PPHN and respiratory failure are seen in a significant number of the most severely affected infants.

The distress in mildly affected infants usually resolves within 2–3 days, whereas in severely affected infants respiratory distress with tachypnoea and increased O_2 requirements may persist for days or even weeks.

Pneumonia

Pneumonia is suspected in any infant with respiratory distress in whom there is a history of maternal fever, premature labour and premature or prolonged rupture of the membranes prior to delivery. There may be a history of fetal tachycardia or distress with low Apgar scores and perinatal asphyxia.

Respiratory distress usually develops at or soon after birth; findings include tachypnoea, tachycardia and generalized signs of infection, including temperature instability, lethargy, poor peripheral perfusion, apnoea, metabolic acidosis and early onset jaundice. The course in a number of infants evolves rapidly from early mild respiratory distress to a state of septic shock with PPHN and occasionally pulmonary haemorrhage and DIC.

The presence of white blood cells or bacteria in the gastric or tracheal aspirate collected within hours of delivery may be suggestive of pneumonia; more commonly, however, neutropaenia and/or a bacteraemia are required to make a definitive diagnosis. In pneumonia due to group B streptococci, the rapid latex agglutination test for capsular polysaccharide antigen performed on a clean catch urine sample may be helpful, as well as culture of the CSF where appropriate. The chest radiograph may be indistinguishable from RDS or show more coarse, diffuse densities. Pleural effusions may be seen and occasionally the radiological picture may be one of lobar or segmental consolidation.

Pneumothorax/air leaks

Spontaneous pneumothorax occurs in 1 per cent of all newborn infants, presumably due to the high transpulmonary pressures exerted at birth. Pneumothorax occurs with far greater frequency in infants with underlying lung disease, particularly RDS and meconium aspiration, and with the use of positive pressure ventilation. Pneumothorax is also particularly common in infants with pulmonary hypoplasia.

Alveolar air leaks appear to track through the perivascular and peribronchial sheaths to the hilum, with rupture into the mediastinum. Pneumomediastinum alone does not cause circulatory compromise. From the mediastinum air can enter the pleural space to produce a pneumothorax. With a unilateral pneumothorax there may be mediastinal shift away from the side of the air leak, with decreased breath sounds, hyperresonance, increased transillumination on the affected side and abdominal distension. Tension pneumothorax results in high intrapleural pressures collapsing the lung on the ipsilateral side, impeding venous return and producing acute cardiac tamponade.

Radiologically, the lung on the affected side is separated from the chest wall by a radiolucent stripe of free pleural air. Air can also collect along the inferior margin of the lung and in the various interlobar fissures. With a tension pneumothorax there is a greater degree of collapse of the lung with mediastinal shift to the opposite side, flattening or even inversion of the ipsilateral diaphragm leaflets, and bulging of the intercostal spaces between the separated ribs. If the pneumothorax is substantial there is no difficulty identifying the abnormality on chest radiograph; however, AP and cross table lateral radiographs should be taken as small pneumothoraces may be missed on AP films alone.

Occasionally interstitial air may track along the great vessels into the pericardial sac producing a pneumopericardium, with resultant poor cardiac output. Infants demonstrate acute cyanosis, distant heart sounds and hypotension; acute needle aspiration and definitive treatment with continuous pericardial tube drainage are required.

Pneumoperitoneum results from dissection of air from the mediastinum along the sheaths of the aorta and vena cava, with rupture into the peritoneal cavity and acute abdominal distension.

Persistent pulmonary hypertension of the newborn (PPHN)

This condition, which is associated with several respiratory problems in the newborn such as respiratory distress syndrome and meconium aspiration syndrome, is discussed on p. 22.

Less common pulmonary disorders

Pulmonary haemorrhage

Pulmonary haemorrhage is considered a form of haemorrhagic pulmonary oedema occurring secondary to left ventricular failure and damage to pulmonary capillaries.[44] It may occur in infants with a wide variety of predisposing factors. These include prematurity, intrauterine growth retardation, asphyxia, overwhelming sepsis, aspiration, severe hypothermia, hypoglycaemia, acidosis, CHD and coagulopathies. The haemorrhage tends to occur between days 2–4 in sick infants who are being mechanically ventilated and who show acute clinical deterioration with cyanosis, bradycardia, hypotension and the appearance of pink or red frothy fluid from the tracheal tube. The chest radiograph reveals areas of diffuse consolidation and opacification.

Pulmonary haemorrhage has been described with increased frequency in infants with RDS treated with surfactant replacement. It is possible that improved oxygenation of pulmonary blood leads to haemorrhagic pulmonary oedema; the clinical consequences of pulmonary haemorrhage in this clinical scenario, however, appear to be less severe than with pulmonary haemorrhage that occurs in extremely sick SGA or premature infants with other associated factors, as described above.

Pulmonary hypoplasia

Conditions causing oligohydramnios and fetal compression are associated with pulmonary hypoplasia; pathologically the condition is characterized by low lung weight, volume and DNA and reduced radial alveolar counts.

The common clinical associations are with renal agenesis or dysplasia (Potter's syndrome), obstructive uropathy and prolonged leakage of amniotic fluid. Lung compression and impaired lung growth also occur with congenital diaphragmatic hernia, eventration, ascites or pleural effusion, skeletal dysplasias with chest cage abnormalities as well as neuromuscular disorders, e.g. myotonic dystrophy.

Infants with pulmonary hypoplasia present immediately after birth with respiratory distress and severe, unremitting respiratory failure with early onset of hypercarbia, pneumothorax and persistent pulmonary hypertension. The clinical diagnosis of hypoplasia may be difficult to make without associated signs of Potter's or other syndromes or a history of chronic amniotic leak.

Radiologically there are small clear lungs with air leaks often complicating the picture. The determination of lung volume radiologically usually consists of an estimation of lung size compared to the overall size of the infant.

Pleural effusion

Fluid accumulates in the pleural space with an increase in either systemic or pulmonary venous pressure and with hypoproteinaemia. Pleural effusions should therefore be suspected in any infant with respiratory difficulty who is oedematous or has signs of congestive heart failure. Small pleural effusions may be seen with pneumonia or transient tachypnoea of the newborn, whereas infants with immune or non-immune hydrops fetalis may have large effusions that impair ventilation and require drainage of the pleural fluid in the delivery room. In this situation both intrapleural chest tubes and occasionally abdominal paracentesis may be necessary if diaphragmatic excursion is impeded. Central venous lines are occasionally complicated by superior vena caval obstruction, in which raised venous pressure contributes substantially to the large pleural effusions; perforation of a central venous catheter into the pleural space will also lead to accumulation of pleural fluid.

A unilateral pleural effusion may be suspected clinically by a decrease in breath sounds and shift of the mediastinum. The chest radiograph is usually diagnostic and shows diffuse opaque lung fields, wide intercostal spaces and horizontal ribs with a depressed diaphragm or obliterated diaphragmatic margins.

Thoracentesis may not only be therapeutic but also diagnostic in identifying effusions secondary to infection and to distinguishing chylothorax from other causes of pleural effusion.

Chylothorax

Chylothorax is the accumulation of chyle in the pleural space and may be congenital (spontaneous) or acquired. The aetiology of congenital chylothorax is unclear; it may result from intrauterine obstruction or a congenital malformation of the thoracic duct. Acquired chylothorax results from damage to the thoracic duct as a surgical complication following repair of diaphragmatic hernia, tracheo–oesophageal fistula or congenital heart disorders.

Chyle is clear and yellow and becomes milky after introduction of enteral feeding. It is distinguished by its high protein and lipid content and characteristic preponderance of lymphocytes (> 90 per cent, mainly T lymphocytes). Symptomatic treatment consists of drainage of chyle, supportive ventilation, supplementation of fluid losses and parenteral nutrition. Conservative management is usually successful and surgical intervention is rarely necessary even in cases with prolonged chyle production.[45]

Surgical causes of respiratory distress

Congenital diaphragmatic hernia (CDH)

This condition is discussed on p. 179.

Congenital cystic adenomatoid malformation (CCAM)

CCAM is a developmental lung bud anomaly with features of a hamartoma and dysplastic growth. Cystic malformation usually occupies one lobe or the lobes of one lung. Three presentations are described:

1. Stillbirth or early neonatal death in premature infants in which the pregnancy has been complicated by maternal polyhydramnios and fetal hydrops.

2. Respiratory distress in term infants at the time of birth.

3. Presentation with pulmonary infection in older infants.

Physical examination in the newborn reveals prominence of one side of the thorax, hyperresonance of the affected side, decreased breath sounds, distant or shifted heart sounds and possibly hepatomegaly secondary to hyperexpansion of the thorax.

Radiologically there is intrapulmonary opacification with the radiolucent curvilinear markings of cysts within the lung parenchyma. Mediastinal shift with depression of the hemidiaphragm is seen. The cystic nature of the condition may not be evident if the cysts are fluid–filled on initial films. In order to exclude CDH, it is essential that a chest radiograph be taken with a nasogastric tube in–situ, to demonstrate the normal situation of the stomach and intestine in CCAM. Ultrasound and/or CT scan may be required for confirmation of the diagnosis. Definitive therapy is surgical intervention and lobectomy.

Congenital lobar emphysema

This condition is discussed on p. 177.

Less common surgical congenital anomalies

Other developmental lung bud anomalies include bronchogenic cysts and pulmonary sequestration. Bronchogenic cysts are usually unilocular cysts adjacent to major bronchi. They occasionally present in the newborn period with respiratory signs, as they may compress the trachea or a major bronchus, giving rise to emphysema or atelectasis.

Pulmonary sequestration is an anomaly in which lung tissue is supplied by systemic vessels originating in the aorta or its branches. Intralobar and extralobar sequestrations are described, each associated with a pattern of other malformations. Sequestration is more common on the left (particularly in the lower lobe). Signs are occasionally produced in the newborn if the affected portion of the lung is sufficiently large.

Congenital pulmonary cysts and pulmonary lymphangiectasia must also be included in the differential diagnosis of congenital cystic diseases of the lung.

Congenital pulmonary cysts are uncommon; they may be single or multiple, although always confined to one lobe of the lung. As they communicate with peripheral airways, rapid expansion of a cyst may present with severe respiratory distress due to air trapping or a pneumothorax. The diagnosis of a congenital cyst is usually readily made on chest radiograph, although large cysts filled with air may be mistaken for a tension pneumothorax. Symptomatic infants will require immediate treatment and lobectomy.

Pulmonary lymphangiectasia due to congenital cystic dilatation of the pulmonary lymphatics has a wide spectrum of respiratory impairment. It may be associated with congenital heart disease particularly TAPVD, hypoplastic left heart syndrome and pulmonary stenosis. Those not associated with congenital heart disease may present with severe respiratory failure in the first hours after birth or may be seen later in infancy. The condition is usually bilateral and the diagnosis suspected by chest radiograph which shows dilated lymphatic vessels with small pleural effusions. Lung biopsy may be required to confirm the diagnosis of pulmonary lymphangiectasia prior to undergoing lobectomy or in unilateral cases total pneumonectomy. Diffuse bilateral lymphangiectasia is usually not amenable to treatment and most infants with this condition die early in the neonatal period.

Retinopathy of prematurity

The retina becomes vascularized from the nasal to the temporal side, the process being completed by the 44th week of gestation. If, during this process, the less mature side is exposed to high arterial PO_2, vascular spasm occurs, causing sensitive retinal tissue to become necrotic and heal with fibrosis. New vessels are formed in the fibrotic areas and these proliferate throughout the vitreous eventually causing retinal detachment and blindness. This pathological state is known as retinopathy of prematurity (ROP) or retrolental fibroplasia (RLF)

and is classified into four grades of severity. Fortunately only a small number of babies develop grade IV scarring (up to 10 per cent), but many have lesser problems such as nystagmus, squint or myopia. Babies with the lowest postconceptual age are the most likely to develop ROP and oxygen therapy is often involved.[46] Hyperoxia causes vasoconstriction and interrupts the cell cords that eventually form vessels. It may allow the release of angiogenic substances and oxygen free radicals which may be toxic, though trials with the antioxidant vitamin E have not proved successful. It is now recognized that the disease is multifactorial; an exchange transfusion with adult blood may also increase the risk and animal work suggests that the severe cicatricial form may occur when $PaCO_2$ is raised and also in the presence of drugs such as salicylates. Bright lights in the intensive care unit shining through very thin eyelids may also be a factor.[47]

It is recommended that the arterial PaO_2 be maintained between 6.7 and 9.1 kPa (50–70 mmHg) by very careful monitoring of inspired oxygen and arterial PO_2. The continuous use of a transcutaneous PaO_2 monitor may be better because PaO_2 is not easy to predict for a given FiO_2 as changes in cardiac output and pulmonary shunting may vary, especially during anaesthesia. It is not known whether a short period of high PaO_2 or a longer period of lower PaO_2 carry the same risk, although there is a report of a baby developing ROP whose only exposure to increased FiO_2 was during anaesthesia.[48] A type of ROP has been reported in babies who have never had an increased FiO_2 and also in babies with acyanotic congenital heart disease. However, during anaesthesia FiO_2 should not be taken to the absolute minimum, but rather an allowance made for reduction of FRC and other pulmonary and cardiac changes that may occur. Modern pulse oximetry allows a reasonably accurate monitoring of oxygen saturation to between 90 and 92 per cent.

A retinal examination should be undertaken by an ophthalmologist before discharge from hospital for all preterm patients who have received oxygen therapy.

Cardiovascular physiology

The changes in the circulation that take place at birth with the lungs taking over gas exchange from the placenta and the subsequent immaturity of the myocardium and the cardiovascular system as a whole have the greatest significance for the anaesthetist or intensivist.

Fetal circulation

In the fetus, the blood with the highest oxygen saturation flows to the developing brain whereas the less saturated blood goes to the lower body and placenta. Blood going to the latter has a PaO_2 19–22 mmHg (3–3.5 kPa) with a saturation of 38 per cent, but aortic blood has a saturation of 60 per cent (PaO_2 25–28 mmHg (3.5–4 kPa)).

Because the fetal ductus arteriosus is usually very large it allows equal pressures in the aorta

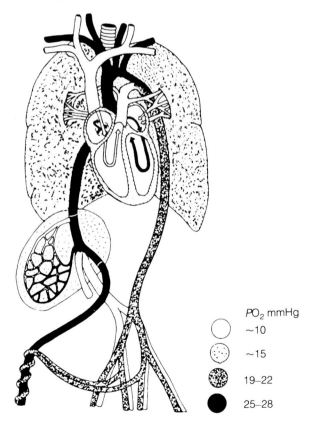

PO_2 mmHg

○ ~10

◌ ~15

◍ 19–22

● 25–28

Fig. 1.9 Diagram of fetal circulation. (Reproduced with permission from [49]).

and pulmonary artery, so that the flow to the lungs depends solely on the relative resistances of the lungs and placenta. The fetal circulation has a very low pulmonary blood flow (10 per cent of the output of the right ventricle) because the pulmonary vascular resistance is high; the muscularity of the small pulmonary vessels allows intense vasoconstriction mediated by the low PaO_2. Placental blood flow is high because the vascular bed has a low resistance and carries at least 50 per cent of the combined output of the two ventricles and fetal blood is oxygenated from the maternal blood. As gestation proceeds fetal cardiac output increases with fetal weight in a fixed relationship, but placental flow gradually falls towards term. Higher regional demands for oxygen and nutrients are met by redistribution of flow and not by increased cardiac output. The increase in pulmonary blood flow towards term which is seen with the production of surfactant is probably caused by the local vasodilating action of metabolites.

The ductus venosus takes umbilical oxygenated blood through the liver into the very short inferior vena cava with only minimal mixing of desaturated blood from the gut. The crista terminalis (the superior margin of the foramen ovale) divides the blood into two streams. Sixty per cent passes directly through the foramen ovale into the left atrium and thence to the aorta via the left ventricle. The rest passes into the right atrium where it mixes with less saturated blood draining from the head and neck via the superior vena cava together with coronary sinus blood. A small percentage of this blood crosses the foramen ovale, but the majority is ejected by the right ventricle into the main pulmonary artery. Less than 10 per cent reaches the lungs by right to left shunting through the patent ductus arteriosus (PDA) because the pulmonary vascular resistance is so much higher than the systemic. This also explains why 70 per cent of the cardiac output returns via the inferior vena cava and 20 per cent via the superior vena cava; the remaining 10 per cent comes from the lungs and coronary sinus.[50]

Adaptation to extrauterine life

The transition from intra- to extrauterine life requires the successful management of a series of well-synchronized cardiopulmonary manoeuvres.

For example, ventilation improves both pulmonary perfusion and releases surfactant which in turn further improves ventilation allowing the pulmonary vascular resistance to fall gradually and cardiovascular changes to take place.

With the very first breath and clamping of the umbilical cord, cessation of umbilical blood flow causes a reduction in right atrial pressure. At the same time, increasing pulmonary blood flow causes the left atrial pressure to rise and this rise is sustained with the onset of regular respiration. This reversal of the pressure difference between right and left atria results in the closure of the foramen ovale. Although potentially patent in up to 30 per cent of normal adults, it is held closed by the pressure difference between the atria and eventually seals in most cases, though it may reopen in some babies during prolonged crying episodes. Pulmonary vascular resistance (PVR) falls gradually, partly with gaseous expansion independent of changes in arterial blood gases, and partly under the influence of increasing arterial oxygen tension (PaO_2), decreasing carbon dioxide tension ($PaCO_2$ and a rising pH.[51] This leads to a further reduction in right atrial pressure, making closure of the foramen ovale even more secure. Bradykinin release from inactive precursors into the pulmonary

circulation also contributes to the fall in PVR. This release may be triggered by the fall in temperature and pH of umbilical venous blood at birth.[52] In the normal infant, pulmonary artery pressure falls to adult levels in about two weeks, with most of the changes occurring in the first three days.

This circulation represents a transitional phase of circulation between the true fetal circulation with the placenta and that of the adult where the left and right sides are completely separated.

The media of the ductus arteriosus differs markedly from the other vascular structures and has spirally arranged, dense, smooth muscle with very few elastic fibres. The wall contains a large amount of mucoid substance not seen in other arterial tissue. Closure of the PDA by contraction of the smooth muscle begins at the pulmonary artery end and is dependent on two processes: firstly the prenatal development of internal cushions formed by coalescence of the mucoid substance which protrude into the lumen[54,55] and secondly a humoral mechanism under the stimulation of increasing PaO_2 after the first breath and closure of the foramen ovale. This physiological closure is completed in 10–15 hours, but permanent closure requires 2–3 weeks during which fibrosis occurs caused by the now ischaemic layers of the ductal walls. The identity of the constrictor agent is still unknown, though its formation from a cytochrome P-450 dependent monooxygenase pathway is likely.[56]

During fetal life, patency of the ductus is maintained by a combined relaxant effect of low oxygen tension together with a combination of endogenous and bloodborne prostaglandin E_2 (PGE_2). Ductal tissue in tissue culture produces prostaglandin E_1 and E_2 and the assumption is that it is these which ensure patency of this vital channel during fetal life. At this time increases in PaO_2 cause the ductus to narrow and as gestational age increases towards term more constriction is seen for a smaller rise in PaO_2. Failure of the ductus to close normally may be due to immaturity of the ductus, hypoxia or a primary structural abnormality of the wall resulting in unresponsiveness to a rise in PaO_2. This latter is the most likely cause of PDA in the mature infant but the premature ductus is much less sensitive to the factors which cause closure and many more remain open in these babies. Continued patency is caused not only by exposure to a low PaO_2 but also because of other factors such as fluid overload at a time when the oxygen mechanism for closure of the duct may not be fully developed.

After closure of the ductus arteriosus, normal

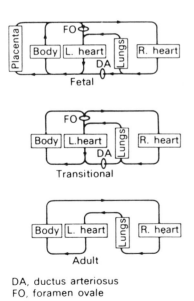

DA, ductus arteriosus
FO, foramen ovale

Fig. 1.10 Changes in the circulation after birth. (Reproduced with permission from [53])

'adult' separation of the pulmonary and systemic circulations is complete.

The cardiovascular system at birth

Modern pulsed Doppler echocardiographic techniques show that left ventricular (LV) output increases by 2–3 times immediately after birth. This results mainly from increased stroke volume associated with increased LV end diastolic diameter (LVEDD) and percentage shortening fraction (per centFS).[57] This increase in cardiac output occurs without any great changes in heart rate. Although detection of per centFS has some limitations in the newborn because of the high right ventricular pressure, it is very likely that the neonatal heart is working at a high level of the Frank–Starling curve. The high LV output in the first few hours of life is related to the widely open ductus arteriosus. The surge of endogenous catecholamines seen during and just after birth presumably also has a great effect on cardiac performance and is certainly a possible cause for the greatly increased performance of the LV at this stage. As stroke volume increases at this stage, it can do so because systemic vascular resistance is at its lowest level. Subsequently, the cardiac output falls from the average initial value of 400–500 ml.kg^{-1}.min for the output of both ventricles. By the end of the first week of life the output of the two ventricles becomes the same, as the fetal channels close, and reaches 150–200ml.kg^{-1}.min. The heart rate decreases significantly in this time which accounts for at least half the total fall in LV output. Shaddy et al.[58] have suggested that the relative inability of the neonatal heart to increase stroke volume, for example as a response to bradycardia, is because the heart is working at a relatively high level of the Starling curve and all evidence points to this. Bradycardia will cause a fall in cardiac output, an effect which lasts well into the neonatal period. Similarly increases in cardiac output come mainly by increasing the heart rate and increases in the rate of up to 200/min can increase the output. In the newborn, hypoxia causes bradycardia followed by heart block and asystole. Ventricular fibrillation is very uncommon in the newborn with a normal heart.

Premature infants have a relatively higher cardiac output than term babies with an average cardiac index for a 'normal' preterm baby of 5.5l.min^{-1}.m^2 (term baby 3.3l.min^{-1}.m^2).

Animal work shows that strips of fetal myocar-dium develop much less active tension during isometric contraction than do those from an adult. Also in the adult 60 per cent of cardiac muscle is contractile mass, whereas in the fetus and newborn, the myocardium is much less compliant and the figure may be as low as 30 per cent, resulting in less myocardial contractile ability. Myofibrils are sparse and randomly organized in the fetal heart so it is likely that newborns require a higher filling pressure than adults to optimize myofilament alignment. Van Hare et al.[59] have shown that even at these higher filling pressures, the Starling mechanism can still operate as long as afterload does not rise. However, with increases in end-diastolic pressure newborn hearts greatly increase their force/oxygen consumption ratios as compared to adults (300 per cent over base line compared to 160 per cent)[60] and if afterload increases, stroke volume falls.

At birth the morphology of the two ventricles is quite similar, but as the pulmonary vascular resistance falls, the right ventricle rapidly loses power as it pumps to a low resistance system without requiring as much muscular effort.

Neonatal cardiac muscle is much less susceptible to hypoxia than is mature muscle if the pH is normal, reflecting a greater ability for anaerobic metabolism. There is also a greater resistance to acidosis, partly attributable to a greater buffering capacity of the immature cells which allows smaller changes in intracellular pH as well as the presence of different troponin I isoforms in the newborn myocardium. Falls in cardiac output of only 20–25 per cent occur in hypoxia (PaO$_2$ <2.7 kPa) (20 mmHg) in association with severe metabolic acidosis (pH < 7.15).

Because there is less sarcoplasmic reticulum in the newborn myocardium, it is more dependent on trans-sarcolemmal calcium influx than in the adult which has calcium stored in the sarcoplasmic reticulum. This explains the significant, though short lived increase in ventricular performance with bolus doses of calcium as well as the marked depressant effect of calcium channel blocks.[61]

Stimulation of the sympathetic nerves to the heart in newborn experimental animals produces a myocardial contractile response comparable to that of the adult, although in the human there is some evidence that innervation of the fetal and neonatal myocardium may be incomplete. Responses elicited, although similar in sensitivity to the adult may be of shorter duration and there is considerable postnatal development. From histological findings it seems that reflex control of the heart is dominated by the parasympathetic nervous system up to and for some time after birth.

The response of immature myocardium of human and other animal species to catecholamines increases with increasing gestational age, but at all times is more sensitive to both α and β-adrenergic stimulation than adult myocardium.[62] These researchers found that the response of infant myocardium to phenylephrine was five times greater and the effect of isoprenaline was three times greater than for the adult. However, in the clinical situation higher doses of inotropic agents may be necessary to improve ventricular performance in a newborn than an adult, in situations where the receptors may have been 'downgraded' by previous stress such as hypoxia or acidosis. For babies of gestational age below 31 weeks it may be difficult to elicit any positive inotropic effects at all with drugs such as dopamine or dobutamine, presumably because of the structural and functional immaturity of the myocardium at this age.

At birth, the heart rate is rapid – averaging between 130 and 160 per minute – and this gradually falls to around 100 by five years of age.

Neonates have a lower blood pressure than older children or adults mainly because the systemic vascular resistance is so low, because the cardiac output is actually high. The mean systolic blood pressure is $10.7 + 2.1$ kPa (80 ± 16 mmHg) and the mean diastolic blood pressure is 6.1 ± 2.1 kPa (46 ± 16 mmHg). In the two hours after delivery, there is a fall in blood pressure from an initial higher level, which has been partly caused by compensation for the placental transfusion and partly because of mechanisms operating during birth which tend to cause hypertension such as a surge of catecholamine release and hypoxia induced angiotensin.[63]

Arterial baroreceptors in the carotid sinus and aortic arch maintain homoeostasis in the cardiovascular system by adjusting cardiac output and peripheral vascular resistance to acute changes in blood pressure that may occur with posture, exercise or blood loss. Afferent impulses pass through the vagus to nuclei in the brainstem. The efferent pathway passes through the sympathetic adrenergic nerves and the cardiac vagus nerve. Although these reflexes function even in the premature infant there is no agreement on whether these reflexes have decreased function and immaturity. Palmisaro *et al.*[64] have shown that there is increased baroreceptor sensitivity at birth which decreases with increasing age together with a resetting to a lower heart rate and higher blood pressure. However, the neonatal response to posture is less efficient and marked hypotension is seen with the baby lifted into a head-up position. If 25 per cent of the blood volume is removed at exchange transfusion there is a marked tachycardia mediated by carotid sinus baroreceptors which does not compensate for a fall in blood pressure and which takes up to 15 minutes to recover. Peripheral vasoconstriction occurs most severely in the skin, muscles, liver, intestines and kidney.

These inadequate responses do seem to suggest that the mechanisms associated with circulating catecholamines are immature at birth and the renin-angiotensin system may be more important in the neonate for the maintenance of the circulation in stressful situations such as birth asphyxia. Renin activity is high in the fetus and fetal tissues respond to angiotensin II. In experimental animals nephrectomy abolishes the response to haemorrhage in the newborn. Although very high levels of angiotensin II, which is a very powerful vasoconstrictor, are found after severe birth asphyxia, it may not be as important in maintaining the resting levels of blood pressure and cardiac output as it is in the stressful situation. The aortic chemoreceptors are important in the fetus to respond to hypoxia by constriction in peripheral vascular beds and to maintain the placental blood flow at all costs and to divert flow to the brain and myocardium.

The pulmonary circulation

Normally pulmonary vascular resistance (PVR) is low and falls from systemic levels to adult levels within the first weeks of life. At birth the media of the peripheral pulmonary arterioles has abundant smooth muscle which is essential in fetal life to allow intense vasoconstriction and therefore to limit pulmonary blood flow in fetal life. This muscle normally regresses gradually but until it does so, the pulmonary vascular bed is very reactive and rises in PVR can easily occur, the vasculature reacting in particular to hypoxia, hypercarbia, acidosis and to a low FiO_2 via an adrenergic mechanism since it is abolished after sympathectomy.

If PVR rises to the level of systemic resistance, the fetal channels, ductus arteriosus (DA) and foramen ovale (FO) may reopen since in the early days of life they are only closed in a physiological way. Blood then flows from right to left and the physiological right-to-left shunt of 20 per cent (adult 7 per cent) immediately at birth may increase to 70–80 per cent, in which case the infant will be cyanosed even when breathing 100 per cent oxygen. This state is known as transitional circulation (persistent fetal circulation) or persistent pulmonary hypertension of the neonate (PPHN).

The rate of fall of PVR may be delayed by the presence of hypoxia and also in congenital cardiac disease with increased pulmonary blood flow such as VSD, PDA, etc. At post mortem examination all alveolar duct and wall arterioles, normally non-muscular, are found to be fully muscularized and where muscle is normally found in the intra-acinar arteries the width of muscle is doubled. It is possible that this abnormality is a failure of the normal postnatal regression of muscle followed by a rapid differentiation of pericytes and intermediate cells into mature smooth muscle cells. The overgrowth may be triggered by vasoactive substances released from endothelial cells in the presence of hypoxia.[65]

Pathophysiologically PPHN has been classified as occurring secondary to one or more of the following mechanisms:

1. *Postnatal maladaptation of the pulmonary vasculature*: functional, reversible pulmonary vasoconstriction associated with normal cardiopulmonary anatomy which is precipitated by hypoxia, hypercarbia, acidosis and/or sepsis.
2. *In utero excessive muscularization of the pulmonary arterioles*: this is associated with chronic *in utero* stress, premature closure of the ductus arteriosus and is also occasionally considered to be primary in origin.
3. *Underdevelopment of the pulmonary vascular bed*: decreased cross sectional area of the total pulmonary vascular bed is seen in hypoplastic lung syndromes, e.g. CDH, Potter's syndrome, and results in severe, unresponsive, fixed pulmonary artery hypertension.
4. *Obstruction to flow*: this may occur secondary to hyperviscosity associated with polycythaemia or to pulmonary venous hypertension associated with TAPVD, pulmonary vein stenosis or left outflow tract obstructive lesions.

One or more of the above mechanisms is therefore invoked in the following clinical disorders in which PPHN may occur:

1. lung disease, particularly meconium aspiration, RDS, pneumonia, TTNB;
2. birth asphyxia;
3. sepsis, particularly group B streptococcal pneumonia (GBS);
4. congenital diaphragmatic hernia/pulmonary hypoplasia;
5. polycythaemia;
6. congenital or acquired heart disease.

Infants with the above disorders have hypoxaemia and pulmonary hypertension for a number of reasons including ventilation-perfusion mismatching, intrapulmonary shunting, structural cardiac abnormality or pulmonary vasoconstriction secondary to alveolar hypoxaemia and hypercarbia. To be accurate in describing these conditions as complicated by PPHN, the distinguishing feature of extrapulmonary right-to-left shunting through the PDA and/or PFO must be demonstrable.

Signs of respiratory distress are usually present from birth. In a number of infants this is often initially only mild in degree; however, within 6–12 hours infants become increasingly distressed with cyanosis and tachypnoea. Lability of the systemic arterial saturation, particularly with any handling of the infant, is the key clinical feature; the severe hypoxaemia is not usually accompanied by hypercarbia. Hypoxaemia results in further pulmonary arteriolar vasoconstriction, intrapulmonary shunting and a vicious cycle of hypoxia and acidosis; this may lead to right heart failure, tricuspid or pulmonary regurgitation, low cardiac output and further tissue hypoxia.

To confirm the diagnosis of PPHN, right-to-left shunting through the ductus arteriosus can be demonstrated by comparison of the PO_2 in blood sampled simultaneously (or via transcutaneous electrodes) from arteries proximal to and distal to the ductus arteriosus. Echocardiography is also usually required to confirm the diagnosis, as well as to exclude underlying structural CHD. The chest radiograph may show the primary underlying disease process, may be relatively normal or may demonstrate oligaemic lung fields.

An element of adult respiratory distress syndrome (ARDS) may occasionally be seen in infants with PPHN.[66] Although difficult to define exactly, ARDS is characterized by severe refractory arterial hypoxaemia, decreased compliance, decreased lung volume and capacity and dense, bilateral alveolar infiltrates on chest X–ray. The pathogenetic mechanism is injury to the alveolar–capillary membrane leading to high permeability pulmonary oedema. The main triggering event is intrauterine/perinatal asphyxia, but it is also seen with severe septic shock (particularly GBS).[66,67]

If all the fetal channels have been closed surgically during cardiac surgery, a rise in PVR will provoke a 'pulmonary hypertensive crisis' and a vicious circle of falling cardiac output will be set up (see p. 242).

Control of the pulmonary circulation until recently has centred on the use of vasodilator substances infused into the circulation and manipulation of gas exchange by mechanical ventilation.[68] PVR may fall with ventilator-induced respiratory alkalosis and high FiO_2 if the lungs are compliant.

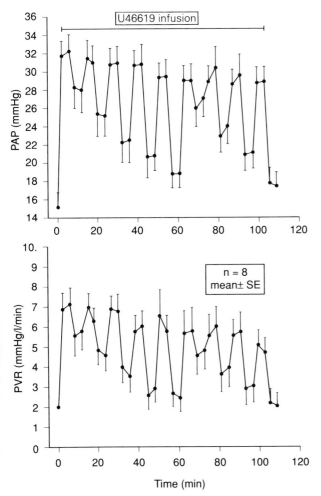

Fig. 1.11 Plots of mean pulmonary artery pressure (PAP) and pulmonary vascular resistance (PVR) during a continuous infusion of U46619. Lambs breathed various levels of nitric oxide (5–80 ppm) at FiO_2 0.6 for six minutes, then breathed a gas mixture of FiO_2 0.6 for six minutes without nitric oxide (n = 8, mean SEM). (Reproduced with permission from [71]).

Vasodilation by such agents as nitroglycerine and nitroprusside may take place via endothelium-derived relaxing factor (EDRF)[69] which is now known to be nitric oxide (NO)[70] (Fig. 1.13).

Nitric oxide itself, if given to lambs with increased PVR (induced by U46619, an analogue of thromboxane) in an inspired concentration of up to 80 ppm, reduces pulmonary artery pressure within seconds to resting levels without any change in systemic resistance[71] NO reacts with haemoglobin so that its effects only occur in the lungs. The toxicology and any deleterious effects of long-term exposure to nitric oxide are not yet known.

The inotropic agent dopamine may increase PVR in babies with a reactive pulmonary vasculature and it may be more logical to use dobutamine if inotropic support is needed in these babies.

Cardiac disease

History

The following points on history may suggest underlying heart disease in the newborn.

Maternal disease or drugs
Maternal illness during pregnancy may be associated with the occurrence of congenital heart disease. In mothers with systemic lupus erythematosus (often not clinically evident) the newborn may develop congenital heart block due to isoimmune damage to fetal cardiac conduction tissue. Maternal diabetes is associated with a spectrum of cardiac malformations as well as a specific form of hypertrophic cardiomyopathy. Maternal PKU is associated with congenital heart disease in the offspring. Rubella in the first trimester is teratogenic for congenital heart disease, particularly patent ductus arteriosus and peripheral pulmonary artery stenosis, and viral infection in the third trimester may lead to myocarditis in the newborn (particularly Coxsackie virus).

Maternal drug use is also associated with cardiac defects, e.g. alcohol (fetal alcohol syndrome), various anticonvulsants and retinoic acid.

Maternal polyhydramnios
A sudden increase in amniotic fluid over 1–2 weeks may be associated with non-immune hydrops fetalis, the most common cause of which is fetal supraventricular tachycardia.

In utero detection of a cardiac abnormality

The indications for fetal echocardiography include fetal factors (arrhythmias, hydrops), maternal factors (maternal congenital heart disease, Rh or other high risk conditions, polyhydramnios) and familial factors (previous sibling with congenital heart disease, unexplained stillborn or neonatal death).

Virtually all forms of structural abnormalities have been detected *in utero*. However, the following may be difficult to identify: small to moderate VSD; minor semilunar and AV valve abnormalities; anatomy of the distal aortic arch, specifically at the isthmus; and occasionally pulmonary venous drainage.[72]

Identification of an *in utero* fetal cardiac abnormality has not only changed the population for evaluation of structural heart disease in the newborn period, but has also resulted in maternal drug therapy where fetal congestive heart failure has been diagnosed. Sustained fetal tachycardia, >200 bpm, is most frequently due to supraventricular tachycardia (SVT). Treatment of fetal arrhythmias via administration of digoxin to the mother is generally instituted as SVT may be fatal or lead to persistent neonatal heart failure. However, the optimal therapeutic approach to fetal therapy, the choice of second-line antiarrhythmic agents and many other issues require very careful thought and are as yet not defined.[73]

Family history of CHD

A familial occurrence of virtually all forms of congenital heart disease has been noted; there is a higher recurrence rate for first degree relatives, particularly the offspring of mothers with CHD or siblings with CHD. The aetiology of most congenital heart disease remains, however, multifactorial in origin and most defects do not segregate as Mendelian traits. If a patient does have congenital heart disease in association with a Mendelian malformation syndrome, e.g. dysplastic pulmonic valve stenosis in Noonan's syndrome, relatives should be evaluated for evidence of that syndrome.[74]

Dysmorphic syndromes

Congenital heart defects are an integral part of many dysmorphic syndromes or chromosomal disorders such that even where clinical signs of heart disease are not evident in the first few days of life the probability of underlying CHD must be strongly suspected (e.g. atrioventricular septal defects in Down's syndrome).

Perinatal distress

A history of perinatal distress, difficult labour or low Apgar scores may be associated with poor myocardial function in the first few hours to days of life. This may manifest as congestive heart failure or cardiogenic shock with or without cyanosis.

Feeding difficulties

Difficulty with feeding, extreme tiredness or the inability to take more than a small amount of feed before becoming distressed, associated with diaphoresis, tachypnoea and tachycardia are suggestive of congestive heart failure. Infants will fail to thrive until the cardiac abnormality is recognized.

The age at which symptoms appear may aid in distinguishing the cause of congestive cardiac failure. Signs present at birth suggest an intrauterine arrhythmia, anaemia or over-transfusion (e.g. twin–twin transfusion); congestive heart failure at one to two days of life suggests left heart hypoplasia; signs of failure at the end of the first week are probably due to coarctation of the aorta.

Presentation of heart disease in the newborn

Cardiac disease in the newborn usually presents in one or more of the following ways.

Cyanosis

Cyanosis is defined as a blue discoloration of the mucous membranes resulting from the presence of more than 4–5 $g.dl^{-1}$ of circulating reduced haemoglobin. Its clinical detection depends on the arterial oxygen saturation, the haemoglobin concentration and the rapidity of the peripheral circulation. It is often difficult to detect visually, since oxygen saturation must decrease to approximately 80–85 per cent before it can be clinically recognized with certainty.

Acrocyanosis due to marked peripheral arteriolar constriction is transient and is seen in normal infants in the first 1–2 days of life. Peripheral cyanosis may be seen in many conditions in which there is a prolongation of the circulation time and an increase in tissue oxygen extraction (with normal arterial

Table 1.3 Clinical approach to congenital heart disease

History

Maternal illness: diabetes, collagen vascular disease

Factors associated with congenital anomalies

Family history of CHD

Delivery, Apgar scores, etc.

Infant's feeding history, other symptoms

Examination

General
Signs of distress, tachycardia, respiratory rate >60 after the first day

> Colour: central and peripheral cyanosis
> Temperature, perfusion of extremities
> Nature of pulses, brachial, axillary, femoral
> Blood pressure, all four limbs
> Oedema, generalized or localized
> Bruits, cerebral, hepatic

Specific
Cardiovascular system:

> Active precordium, LV and RV impulses, maximal cardiac impulse, palpable thrill (uncommon)
> Heart sounds, first, second (single at birth, split normally by 48 hours, 80 per cent of newborns)
> Presence of gallop
> Extra sounds, ejection clicks
> Murmurs, location, radiation, quality, intensity

Liver >2–3 cm, size, location (e.g. central or left sided), pulsatile, splenomegaly

---

saturation), e.g. in infants with poor cardiac output, sepsis, polycythaemia or metabolic acidosis.

Central cyanosis is either cardiac in origin (systemic venous blood bypassing the lungs) or caused by pulmonary venous desaturation due to ventilation/perfusion imbalance in the lungs or airway obstruction preventing normal gas exchange. Central cyanosis during crying in the first day of life may not be indicative of heart disease, but must be evaluated if it persists or is associated with any other cardiac signs. (Crying will increase the degree of cyanosis if a right-to-left shunt is present due to increased intrathoracic pressure.)

Some forms of congenital heart disease with right-to-left shunts have increased pulmonary blood flow and may achieve oxygen saturations sufficiently near normal, making the clinical appreciation of cyanosis very difficult.

Differential cyanosis of the skin may occasionally be seen with the upper body pink and the lower body cyanosed; this occurs in PPHN or left heart outflow tract obstruction with right-to-left shunting through the ductus arteriosus.

Although the early onset of severe generalized cyanosis is usually indicative of heart disease, the following extracardiac causes of cyanosis must first be excluded.

Pulmonary disease

In respiratory disorders other signs of respiratory distress are evident, including tachypnoea, tachycardia, flaring of the alae nasi, retractions and grunting. The distinction between respiratory and cardiac causes of cyanosis is usually readily made with the aid of a chest radiograph, arterial blood gases and, where necessary, response to 100 per cent oxygen (hyperoxia test). The hyperoxia test is the response to 10–15 minutes of 100 per cent O_2; arterial oxygen tension should be measured from the right radial artery or via $TcPO_2$ electrodes placed on the right upper chest and lower abdomen reflecting pre- and postductal sites. In lung disease there is evidence of parenchymal disease on chest films, CO_2 retention is usual and arterial $PO_2 > 150$ mmHg can usually be achieved when the environmental oxygen is increased to 100 per cent. In cyanotic CHD the arterial O_2 tension will not increase by more than a few mmHg. Occasionally, however, in an infant with cyanotic CHD and pulmonary hypertension, 100 per cent O_2 may increase the dissolved oxygen as well as lower pulmonary vascular resistance such that the value may rise, but rarely beyond 150 (e.g. TAPVD, partial APVD).

An infant with an arterial $PaO_2 < 150$ in 100 per cent oxygen with or without respiratory distress must be suspected of having either cyanotic congenital heart disease or PPHN. The distinction between PPHN and cyanotic CHD is aided by the rapid evolution of the PPHN clinical picture and its associated or precipitating conditions, e.g. meconium aspiration, perinatal asphyxia or sepsis. The degree of hypoxaemia may occasionally aid in the differentiation in that the PO_2 in PPHN is usually > 40 mmHg; in cyanotic CHD, e.g. TGA with intact ventricular system, the PO_2 is often < 30 mmHg. The distinction between

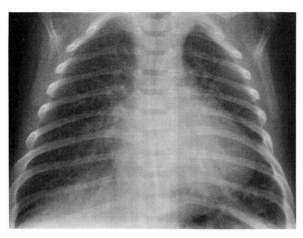

Fig. 1.12 Atrioventricular septal defect. There is marked cardiomegaly. The pulmonary arteries are very prominent and are somewhat indistinct in outline with a linear pattern in the lungs consistent with pulmonary oedema.

PPHN and cyanotic CHD may be further aided by the response to hyperventilation whereby the induction of hypocapnia and respiratory alkalosis results in an increase in the postductal PO_2 tension in PPHN and not in structural CHD. Finally, two-dimensional echocardiography may be required to confirm definitively right to left ductal and atrial shunting in PPHN or the presence of structural CHD.

Hyperviscosity syndrome/polycythaemia
Hyperviscosity and polycythaemia may mimic cyanotic heart disease despite normal oxygen saturation, owing to increased viscosity and capillary stasis.

Sepsis and other neonatal conditions
Sepsis, hypothermia, hypoglycaemia and acidosis may also produce cyanosis by altering peripheral tissue perfusion.

Depression of the central nervous system or neuromuscular disease
CNS depression or neuromuscular disease may result in hypoventilation and cyanosis; other signs of nervous system involvement are usually clearly evident.

Methaemoglobinaemia or other haemoglobin abnormalities
These should be suspected when the infant is cyanosed without cardiac or respiratory signs, there is little or no improvement in colour following oxygen administration, the PaO_2 is normal despite low arterial saturation and the blood remains dark when mixed with air.

Cyanotic congenital heart disease
The presence of cyanosis may be the sole evidence of CHD; in a third of lethal CHD, cyanosis is the major presenting symptom.

Cyanotic congenital heart disease can be divided into:

- conditions in which there is normal or increased pulmonary blood flow, and
- conditions with definitively decreased pulmonary blood flow.

Conditions with normal or increased pulmonary blood flow include:

1. *Transposition of the great arteries (TGA)*: TGA is the most common form of cyanotic congenital heart disease in the immediate newborn period and is more common in males. It usually presents in the first two days of life dependent upon the degree of mixing between the pulmonary and systemic circulations. Those with an intact ventricular septum present with early profound hypoxaemia as the ductus closes; the presence of a VSD will ameliorate the hypoxaemia to a degree.
2. *Total anomalous pulmonary venous drainage (TAPVD)*: Marked tachypnoea in the obstructed form of this disorder often leads to an initial diagnosis of pulmonary disease.
3. *Truncus arteriosus*: Bounding peripheral pulses and a loud single second heart sound with an ejection click are very suggestive of this lesion.

   Lesions with increased pulmonary blood flow tend to produce both cyanosis and heart failure; the newborn is usually in distress; there is an active precordium, usually a single second heart sound (with the exception of TAPVD) as well as systolic murmurs.
4. *Atrioventricular septal defect: see Fig. 1.12.*

Conditions with decreased pulmonary blood flow include:

1. Tetralogy of Fallot with severe pulmonary stenosis or atresia.

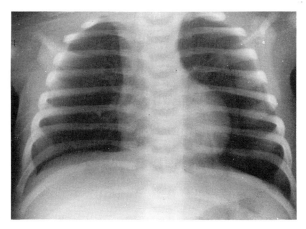

Fig. 1.13 Tricuspid atresia. The left margin of the heart is prominent. The pulmonary vascularity is diminished.

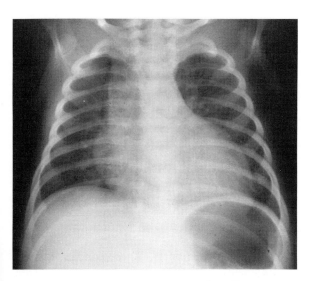

Fig. 1.14 Cardiomegaly (with normal cardiac structure) due to intracranial arteriovenous malformation. Pulmonary vasculature is normal and lungs are clear.

2. Hypoplastic right heart syndromes, tricuspid and pulmonary atresia/stenosis (Fig. 1.13).
3. Ebstein's disease of the tricuspid valve with tricuspid regurgitation, massive cardiomegaly and congestion on chest X-ray.

Cyanosis without failure is the usual clinical presentation in this group of infants. The precordium is quiet, the infant is not distressed and pulmonary outflow obstruction leads to inaudible pulmonary valve closure and a single second heart sound. Some of the conditions characterized by a decrease in pulmonary vascularity produce right ventricular hypertrophy on ECG with a QRS axis $> 90°$, others produce LVH. If the QRS axis is superior, i.e. 0 to $-90°$, tricuspid atresia is more likely; an inferior axis of 0 to $+90°$ suggests pulmonary atresia with intact ventricular septum.

The initial differentiation of cyanotic congenital heart disease based on clinical findings, chest X-ray and ECG may not identify the more complex forms of cyanotic heart disease, i.e. single ventricle, atrioventricular canal defects with pulmonary stenosis or atresia, etc. These will require echocardiography and/or cardiac catheterization for definitive diagnosis.

Table 1.4 Cyanotic congenital heart disease

Distress/CHF		Not distressed/no CHF		
CXR				
Increased PBF		Decreased PBF		
ECG		ECG		
RVH	LVH or CVH	RVH	LVH	CVH
TGA/IVS	TGA/VSD	T of F	TA	TGA/PS
TAPVD	Truncus	Ebstein's	PA	Truncus/PA
	Single ventricle			Single vent./PS

Congestive heart failure (CHF)

The signs of cardiac failure in the newborn include tachypnoea, tachycardia, gallop rhythm, abnormal pulses, cardiomegaly, hepatomegaly, cyanosis, diaphoresis, feeding difficulty and occasionally periorbital or peripheral oedema.

Congestive cardiac failure in the newborn may be due to:

Non-cardiac causes

An element of CHF may complicate many neonatal disorders including perinatal asphyxia, septicaemia (group B streptococci, viral infections), anaemia, polycythaemia, hydrops, fluid overload, hypoglycaemia, arteriovenous fistulae (Fig. 1.14) and conditions associated with infants of diabetic mothers with or without hypoglycaemia.

Infants with arteriovenous fistulae (usually an aneurysm of the vein of Galen or occasionally within the liver) present with congestive failure, bounding pulses, a structurally normal heart and cerebral or hepatic bruits.

Infants of diabetic mothers are large for their gestational age and demonstrate macrosomia, cardiomegaly and mild CHF. This may be the result of hypoglycaemia, associated respiratory distress or hyperviscosity. Infants of diabetic mothers may also have structural congenital heart disease: most commonly transposition of the great vessels, septal defects, coarctation or hypertrophic cardiomyopathy.

Cardiac causes

Causes of non-structural heart disease include:

1. *Transient myocardial ischaemia (TMI)*: The signs of TMI may be seen following intrapartum hypoxia. Frequently these infants, born at term via a complicated delivery, have low Apgar scores, early onset of respiratory distress and congestive heart failure with or without cyanosis. A spectrum of cardiac dysfunction may be seen clinically: CHF with a gallop rhythm and systolic murmurs of tricuspid or mitral regurgitation; a persistent pulmonary hypertension picture with right-to-left atrial shunting, cyanosis and marked hypoxaemia; or a low output state with cardiovascular collapse and shock.

   The chest X-ray shows cardiomegaly; decreased pulmonary blood flow is seen in those infants with right-to-left shunting at atrial level; those with dominant left-sided failure show pulmonary venous congestion. The ECG shows right atrial enlargement, diffuse ST and T wave changes with ST depression and T wave inversion over the left precordium and possibly pathologic Q waves.

   Echocardiography in TMI will not only rule out structural congenital heart disease but will also provide an assessment of ventricular function, pulmonary artery pressures, right-to-left shunting and the degree of tricuspid or mitral regurgitation. Serum CK-MB fraction may be elevated, particularly in the presence of significant tricuspid incompetence.[75] Although the cardiovascular sequelae of myocardial ischaemia are usually transient, atrioventricular valve regurgitation and ECG abnormalities may persist for months.[76]

2. *Arrhythmias*: In the newborn or *in utero*, arrhythmias may lead to fetal death or varying degrees of cardiac failure either before or immediately after birth. Supraventricular tachycardia, if prolonged, has a high incidence of congestive heart failure. Congenital heart block is associated with an increase in heart size in more than 50 per cent of cases.

3. *Myocardial dysfunction*: This occurs for example in infants with myocarditis (Coxsackie or rubella virus), glycogen storage disease type II or endocardial fibroelastosis. The ECG is virtually diagnostic in myocarditis and reveals reduced QRS voltages, ST segment abnormalities and arrhythmias.

Causes of structural heart disease include:

1. *Cyanotic congenital heart disease*: The most common causes of failure in this group are those lesions with increased pulmonary vasculature and include TGA, TAPVD and truncus arteriosus.

2. *Acyanotic congenital heart disease*: Congestive heart failure in this group of disorders is due to either:

   • volume overload with left to right shunt lesions, or
   • pressure overload secondary to varying degrees of left ventricular outflow tract obstruction.

Left-to-right shunt lesions are generally not evident until the pulmonary vascular resistance has dropped sufficiently over the first few days to weeks of life; conditions in the newborn include patent ductus arteriosus, aortopulmonary window (rare), VSD or a VSD with PDA, and atrio-ventricular septal defects. These conditions show cardiomegaly, a dilated main pulmonary artery and increased pulmonary vasculature on X-ray.

Left ventricular outflow tract obstructions include coarctation of the aorta, interrupted aortic arch, aortic valvular or supravalvular stenosis and hypoplastic left heart syndrome. In outflow tract obstructions due to arch anomalies the pulses are usually asymmetric with an increase in the right arm proximal to the obstruction and decrease of pulses in the lower limbs. The left arm pulses are variable dependent upon whether the coarctation or interruption is proximal or distal to the left subclavian artery. Most coarctations are juxtaductal or preductal; thus the pulses in the left arm are usually decreased. These lesions show varying degrees of congestive failure, cardiomegaly and pulmonary oedema and often present in acute cardiogenic shock at the time of closure of the ductus arteriosus (see below).

Cardiogenic shock

The first presentation of congenital heart disease in its most severe form may be cardiovascular collapse and cardiogenic shock. Heart failure develops rapidly in the newborn because of limited intrinsic myocardial reserve, little compensatory hypertrophy and often less response to the effect of catecholamines on heart rate and velocity of ejection than in older children (only partial innervation of adrenergic receptors at birth).[77] In addition, the newborn is limited in its ability to unload oxygen at tissue level because of the presence of fetal haemoglobin.

Non–structural heart disease may present in this acute shock-like manner, particularly secondary to transient myocardial ischaemia, supraventricular tachycardias, myocarditis or other metabolic conditions (as described in CHF).

Obstructive lesions of the left ventricular outflow tract

Infants with this condition are usually normal at birth but develop tachypnoea, poor feeding and congestive heart failure when the ductus constricts and obstructs systemic blood flow. They may present with acute cardiovascular collapse, gasping respiration, poor pulses, a grey and mottled colour, indistinct heart sounds, large liver and heart and an acute metabolic acidosis.

Valvular aortic stenosis does not usually present as acutely as hypoplastic left heart syndrome; the signs of failure tend to occur later but once present, progress rapidly. A systolic ejection murmur with a click may be heard on the right or left upper sternal border. The chest X-ray shows cardiomegaly with both pulmonary venous hypertension and increased pulmonary blood flow. The ECG shows left ventricular hypertrophy with a strain pattern.

While all pulses are low volume or poorly felt in HLHS or aortic stenosis, asymmetric pulses are seen in coarctation or interrupted aortic arch. The femoral pulses may come and go with the closure of the duct and repeated four limb blood pressure measurement may be required if any difficulty exists in palpation of the femoral arteries. The murmur of coarctation is loudest at the lower left sternal border or into the axilla, but generally murmurs are not impressive or helpful. The chest X-ray shows cardiomegaly with increased pulmonary vascular markings but there is no specific abnormality on CXR or ECG to aid in the distinction between an interrupted arch or coarctation of the aorta. In HLHS the CXR shows pulmonary venous congestion and cardiomegaly; the ECG shows right axis deviation with right ventricular dominance and decreased left sided forces.

Heart murmurs

Murmurs in the immediate newborn period are subject to marked fluctuation due to the postnatal cardiopulmonary adaptation, i.e. the decrease in pulmonary vascular resistance, right ventricular and pulmonary artery pressures and increase in pulmonary blood flow. Careful auscultation of the heart in the first few days of life will often detect short systolic murmurs due to increased flow in the pulmonary arteries causing a degree of physiologic pulmonary stenosis; these infants do not subsequently show evidence of structural heart disease.

A murmur may not be audible because of the small pressure gradient at the site of the defect. Furthermore, a number of serious cardiac anomalies do not cause sufficient turbulence of blood flow to produce murmurs, e.g. hypoplasia of the left or right heart. Pure right-to-left shunting at atrial, ventricular or great vessel level does not usually produce loud murmurs.

Conversely, a systolic murmur that is loud and occupies most or all of systole, or one that radiates widely and is persistent on repeated examination in the first few days of life, or is accompanied by abnormality of the second heart sound or signs of failure, is likely to be haemodynamically significant and requires further investigation.

The nature of the cardiovascular defect determines when a significant murmur is first heard. Obstructive lesions, e.g. stenosis of the pulmonary valve, pulmonary artery or aorta, are more likely to produce murmurs soon after birth, whereas murmurs due to left-to-right shunts may not be noted until the pulmonary vascular resistance has decreased sufficiently postnatally. The systolic murmur of a PDA may be audible after a few days, while the classic continuous murmur may not be heard until further reduction in PVR has occurred. Similarly, the murmur of a ventricular septal defect is unusual after birth and tends to become audible only after several days or, in the case of large VSDs, only during the first 2–4 weeks of life.

The presence of a murmur in the newborn should alert the examiner to the possibility of serious disease and the necessity of distinguishing it from a functional haemodynamically benign murmur. Repeated clinical examination, electrocardiography and a chest radiograph are initially indicated; further investigation with two-dimensional echcardiography may subsequently become necessary.

Heart rate abnormalities

Bradycardia

1. *Sinus bradycardia*: Although the neonatal heart rate is normally between 120 and 140 bpm, considerable variation is found in otherwise healthy infants. Sinus bradycardia, < 100 bpm, with a normal P wave preceding each QRS complex occurs in about a third of term infants and a larger proportion of preterm infants.

   Bradycardia may be transient or persistent; transient episodes are associated with feeding, sleeping, yawning, defaecating, hiccuping or nasopharyngeal suctioning (secondary to increased vagal tone).

   Persistent or prolonged sinus bradycardia is associated with generalized abnormalities including raised intracranial pressure, hyperkalaemia, acidosis, hypothermia, hypoxia, obstructive jaundice and hypothyroidism. Occasionally a 24 hour Holter ECG recording will be required to ensure that more serious dysrhythmias do not coexist with a sinus bradycardia.

2. *Second degree heart block*: In second degree heart block there is intermittent failure of atrioventricular node conduction of the atrial impulse to the ventricles, either as a progressive prolongation of the PR interval followed by an unconducted atrial impulse (Wenkebach or Mobitz type I) or intermittent non–conducted P waves manifested as dropped ventricular beats and no progressive PR interval (Mobitz type II). Second degree heart block may be seen with anoxia, metabolic abnormalities, hyperkalaemia, hypocalcaemia, sepsis, supraventricular tachyarrhythymias and digitalis toxicity. Second degree heart block should be observed closely as it may lead to symptomatic bradycardia.

3. *Congenital third degree or complete heart block*: This is a rare disorder (1 in 20 000 live births) in which the ventricular rate is slow and regular (< 60 bpm) and is independent of the atrial rate with no fixed relationship between the P wave and the QRS complex. It may be associated with congenital heart disease in about 25–30 per cent of cases (congenitally corrected transposition, left atrial isomerism and AVSD). The mother of an infant with complete heart block may show clinical evidence of a connective tissue disorder at the time of delivery or subsequently develop evidence of such disease, particularly systemic lupus erythematosus. Complete heart block is often suspected *in utero*; occasionally the persistent slow fetal heart rate may be interpreted as fetal distress with inadvertent delivery by emergency caesarean section.

   Infants with congenital heart block are normally asymptomatic, particularly if the QRS complex is normal, the heart rate is > 50 bpm and there is no evidence of structural heart disease. However, the prognosis is not as favourable in those infants who demonstrate very slow heart rates (< 50 bpm), QT prolongation or those with associated structural cardiac malformations.

Tachycardia

The mean heart rate in term and premature infants is 130 to 145 bpm. Tachycardia greater than 160 bpm is a frequent finding in the normal newborn and many stimuli can increase the heart rate to approximately 200 bpm.

1. In a sinus arrhythymia there is a phasic variation of the heart rate with respiration. Sinus tachycardia is commonly seen with infectious illness, dehydration, anaemia, congestive heart failure, fever and shock. It is also produced by many medications used in the newborn (e.g. caffeine and inotropic agents). The ECG in sinus tachycardia shows visible P waves with a normal P wave axis. The heart rate seldom exceeds 200 bpm.

2. The main entity in the differential diagnosis of sinus tachycardia in healthy infants, or in those with sepsis or congestive heart failure, is supraventricular tachycardia (SVT). This is the most common type of supraventricular tachycardia seen in the newborn and may be life-threatening if not recognized and promptly

corrected. The heart rate (180–360 bpm) is often paroxysmal in nature, with episodes of tachycardia beginning and ending abruptly. It may precipitate congestive heart failure if the SVT is continuous for more than 24 hours; the infant may develop pallor, irritability, poor feeding and respiratory distress. No structural heart disease is found in the majority of infants with SVT, although re-entry tachycardia due to a bypass tract is associated with Ebstein anomaly, corrected transposition, tricuspid atresia and cardiac rhabdomyomas. The Wolff–Parkinson–White syndrome should be suspected in the presence of a delta wave, a shortened PR interval and a wide QRS complex, changing to narrow complexes and retrograde (inverted) P waves during tachycardia.

Associated Malformations

Extracardiac malformations occur in approximately 25 per cent of infants with structural congenital heart disease, many of whom have identifiable malformation syndromes[78]; 12 per cent of all infants with CHD have chromosomal abnormalities[79] and formal genetic evaluation including karyotype is usually warranted.

Table 1.5 Congenital heart defects in selected chromosomal aberrations. (Reproduced with permission from[80])

Conditions	Incidence of CHD, %	Common defects in decreasing order of frequency
5p – (cri-du-chat syndrome)	25	VSD, PDA, ASD
Trisomy 13	90	VSD, PDA, dextrocardia
Trisomy 18	99	VSD, PDA, PS
Trisomy 21 (Down's syndrome)	50	AVSD, VSD
Turner syndrome (XO)	35	COA, AS, ASD

AS = aortic stenosis; ASD = atrial septal defect; COA = coarctation of the aorta; PDA = patent ductus arteriosus; PS = pulmonary stenosis; VSD = ventricular septal defect; AVSD = atrioventricular septal defect

Special investigations

Chest radiography

This is used to determine:

1. *Cardiac size, shape and contour*: A cardiac to thoracic ratio > 60 per cent is usually indicative of enlargement. The shape of the heart, the prominence or absence of the pulmonary artery segment, right atrium and other chambers should be observed. Particular contours and shapes are described in many conditions, e.g. the "egg on side" appearance of the heart in TGA, massive cardiomegaly of Ebstein's malformation of the tricuspid valve, and the boot–shaped heart with upturned apex and concave pulmonary artery segment in patients with tetralogy of Fallot.
2. *Nature of the pulmonary blood flow*: An increase or decrease in pulmonary blood flow is made by assessment of the peripheral and hilar pulmonary vascular markings; the former is generally more reliable as a reflection of pulmonary plethora or oligaemia.
3. *Laterality of the aortic arch*: This is often difficult to determine, but abnormality is suggested by deviation of the trachea. A right-sided arch may be seen in truncus arteriosus or tetralogy of Fallot.
4. *Evidence of respiratory disease or respiratory complications of CHD*: For example, compression of left main bronchus by a dilated left atrium.
5. *Location of abdominal and thoracic viscera*: to determine situs inversus and situs ambiguous.
6. *Associated skeletal abnormalities of the spine and ribs*.

A number of caveats must be made in the interpretation of the chest radiograph:

(a) Maximal inspiration is often difficult and may lead to a spurious diagnosis of cardiomegaly;
(b) A prominent thymus is often misinterpreted as enlargement of the heart. Absence of the thymus should also be noted because of its association with DiGeorge syndrome;
(c) Associated respiratory disorders, e.g. TTNB, may make interpretation of the pulmonary vasculature difficult;
(d) Typical radiographic patterns may not be seen in the first few days of life owing to variation in the rate of the postnatal decrease in the

pulmonary vascular resistance and increase in pulmonary blood flow.

Electrocardiography (see Tables 1.6 and 1.7)

Two-dimensional echocardiography

Echocardiography has led to major advances in the diagnosis and management of CHD in the newborn. The diagnostic capability of two-dimensional echocardiography has been facilitated by the application of Doppler ultrasound and colour flow mapping, such that not only can accurate and rapid diagnoses be made at the bedside but quantitation of transvalvular gradients, cardiac output and shunt size can also be accomplished. Advances in equipment and image processing allow excellent visualization even in the small preterm infant.

Most neonatal cardiac lesions can be diagnosed with certainty so that cardiac catheterization is seldom required for diagnostic purposes. Leung[83] found a 96 per cent sensitivity and 98 per cent specificity using two-dimensional and pulsed–Doppler echocardiography in the diagnosis of anomalies in the newborn. Two-dimensional echocardiography is also extremely useful in differentiating CHD from non-structural cardiac disease, particularly PPHN and TMI, and qualitatively assessing myocardial function in any sick newborn.

Cardiac catheterization

Cardiac catheterization is still necessary for balloon atrial septostomy in TGA in most centres, as it is for definition of pulmonary arteries in neonates with pulmonary atresia/VSD and for definition of coronary arterial abnormalities. A list of neonatal cardiac conditions requiring cardiac catheterization is given in Table 1.8. The cardiac surgeon has developed sufficient confidence in the accuracy of echocardiography to operate without cardiac catheterization in most forms of neonatal heart disease.[84]

Patent ductus arteriosus

Persistent patency of the ductus arteriosus, a communication between the main pulmonary artery and the descending aorta, is one of the most common cardiac disorders in the newborn, particularly in premature infants. In the term infant the ductus starts to constrict soon after delivery, and functional closure in 90 per cent of infants is achieved by 48 hours of life.[85] Closure is in response to the postnatal rise in oxygen tension and developmental alterations in the sensitivity of the vessel to locally produced prostaglandins. Initially contraction of smooth muscle takes place, followed by breakdown of the endothelium and proliferation of connective tissue. In the premature infant the ductus fails to develop this anatomic obliteration of its lumen.

Incidence

The incidence of patency of the ductus is inversely related to gestational age. In premature infants the incidence is increased with RDS, asphyxia,[86] high fluid volumes and in infants with RDS given frusemide.[87,88] Some studies have suggested that the symptoms of PDA are more frequent with surfactant therapy of RDS[89,90] as surfactant exacerbates left-to-right shunting following reduction of pulmonary vascular resistance; this has not been borne out in other studies.[86,91]

Haemodynamic effects

The effects of prolonged ductal patency depend upon the size of the shunt and the cardiac and pulmonary vascular responses. Alterations in blood flow allowing a 'steal' away from the splanchnic or cerebral circulation have implicated PDA in the pathogenesis of NEC and IVH respectively. The increased flow in the ascending aorta and pulmonary circulation leads to an increase in pulmonary venous return and consequently increased LA and LV end diastolic pressures. Over time the increase in LV end diastolic pressure and pulmonary venous pressure causes pulmonary venous congestion, increased pulmonary capillary permeability and interstitial and alveolar lung fluid and a decrease in lung compliance. Decreased pulmonary compliance will delay weaning from the ventilator, prolong oxygen and mechanical ventilation requirements and further predispose the infant to the development of bronchopulmonary dysplasia. However, the changes in pulmonary mechanics occur only after some period of exposure to a PDA.[92] Little effect on pulmonary function in the first week of life was seen by Krauss[93] in infants with hyaline

Table 1.6 Summary of normal ECG values. (Reproduced with permission from[81])

Age Group	*Heart rate (BPM)	Frontal plane QRS ventor (degrees)	PR interval (sec)	**Q III (mm)§	**Q V6 (mm)	RV1 (mm)	SV1 (mm)	R/S V1	RV6 (mm)	SV6 (mm)	R/S V6	**SV1 + RV6 (mm)	**R + S V4 (mm)
Less than 1 day	93–154 (123)	+59 to −163 (137)	.08–.16 (.11)	4.5	2	5–26 (14)	0–23 (8)	.1–U (2.2)	0–11 (4)	0–9.5 (3)	.1–U (2.0)	28	52.5
1–2 days	91–159 (123)	+64 to −161 (134)	.08–.14 (.11)	6.5	2.5	5–27 (14)	0–21 (9)	.1–U (2.0)	0–12 (4.5)	0–9.5 (3)	.1–U (2.5)	29	52
3–6 days	91–166 (129)	+77 to −163 (132)	.07–.14 (.10)	5.5	3	3–24 (13)	0–17 (7)	.2–U (2.7)	.5–12 (5)	0–10 (3.5)	.1–U (2.2)	24.5	49
1–3 weeks	107–182 (148)	+65 to +161 (110)	.07–.14 (.10)	6	3	3–21 (11)	0–11 (4)	1.0–U (2.9)	2.5–16.5 (7.5)	0–10 (3.5)	.1–U (3.3)	21	49
1–2 months	121–179 (149)	+31 to +113 (74)	.07–.13 (.10)	7.7	3	3–18 (10)	0–12 (5)	.3–U (2.3)	5–21.5 (11.5)	0–6.5 (3)	.2–U (4.8)	29	53.5

*2%–98% (mean) § mm at normal standardization
**98th percentile U undefined (S wave may equal zero)

Table 1.7　Common ECG manifestations of some congenital heart defects. (Reproduced with permission from [82])

Congenital defects	ECG findings
Anomalous origin of the left coronary artery from the pulmonary artery	Myocardial infarction, anterlateral
Anomalous pulmonary venous return	
Total	RAD, RVH and RAH
Partial	Mild RVH or RBBB
Aortic stenosis	
Mild to moderate	Normal or LVH
Severe	LVH with or without 'strain'
Atrial septal defect	
Primum type	Left anterior hemiblock (superior QRS axis)
	rsR' pattern in V1 and aVR (RBBB or RVH)
	First-degree AV block (>50 per cent)
	Counterclockwise QRS loop in the frontal plane of vectorcardiogram
Secundum type	RAD, RVH or RBBB (rsR' in V1 and aVR)
	First-degree AV block (10 per cent)
Coarctation of the aorta	
Infants younger than 6 months	RBBB or RVH
Older children	LVH, normal or RBBB
Common ventricle or single ventricle	Abnormal Q waves
	Q in V1 and no Q in V6
	No Q in any precordial leads
	Q in all precordial leads
	Stereotype RS complex in most or all precordial leads
	WPW syndrome or PAT
	First- or second-degree AV block
Cor triatriatum	Same as for mitral strenosis
Ebstein's anomaly	RAH, RBBB
	First-degree AV block
	WPW syndrome
	No RVH
Endocardial cushion defect	
Complete	Left anterior hemiblock (superior QRS axis)
	RVH or CVH, RAH
	First-degree AV block, RBBB
Partial	See ASD, primum type
Endocardial fibroelastosis	LVH
	Abnormal T waves
	Myocardial infarction patterns
Hypoplastic left heart syndrome (aortic and/or mitral atresia)	RVH
Mitral stenosis, congenital or acquired	RAD, RVH, RAH, LAH ($\pm$)
Patent ductus arteriosus	
Small shunt	Normal
Moderate shunt	LVH, LAH ($\pm$)
Large shunt	CVH, LAH
Eisenmenger's syndrome (pulmonary vascular obstructive disease)	RVH or CVH

Congenital defects	ECG findings
Persistent truncus arteriosus	LVH or CVH
Pulmonary atresia (with hypoplastic RV)	LVH
Pulmonary stenosis	
Mild	Normal or mild RVH
Moderate	RVH
Severe	RVH with 'strain', RAH
Pulmonary vascular obstructive disease (Eisenmenger's syndrome)	RVH or CVH
Tetralogy of Fallot	RAD RVH, moderate or severe RAH ($\pm$)
D-Transposition of the great arteries (complete transposition)	
Intact ventricular septum	RVH, RAH
VSD and/or PS	CVH, RAH or CAH
L-Transposition of the great arteries (congenitally 'corrected' transposition)	AV block, first- to third-degree Atrial arrhythmias (PAT. atrial fibrillation) WPW syndrome Absent Q in V5 and V6 and qR pattern in V1 LAH or CAH
Tricuspid atresia	Left anterior hemiblock (superior QRS axis) LVH, RAH
Ventricular septal defect	
Small shunt	Normal
Moderate shunt	LVH, LAH ($\pm$)
Large shunt	CVH, LAH
Pulmonary vascular obstructive disease (Eisenmenger's syndrome)	RVH

membrane disease and PDA who did not have cardiac failure. Conversely, Stefano *et al.*[94] showed significant improvement in pulmonary compliance and ventilation parameters after successful closure of the ductus with indomethacin in infants being ventilated for RDS.

Diagnosis

Clinical
Signs of PDA usually appear between days 3–5 of life or may occur earlier with surfactant treated RDS. A generalized deterioration with poor peripheral perfusion, sudden increase in oxygen requirements or worsening of respiratory status may occur in the VLBW infant with associated RDS. Cardiac findings include bounding pulses, a hyperactive precordium, widened pulse pressure, tachycardia and a systolic murmur. The murmur is commonly intermittent, reflecting the fluctuating state of patency in relation to variation in the O_2 tension and the pressure gradient across the shunt as the pulmonary vascular resistance changes. Until the pulmonary vascular resistance has dropped sufficiently, the diastolic murmur may not be audible. The chest X-ray shows congested lung fields. Mild cardiomegaly may be seen over time but is usually not evident with short duration of ductal patency.

A PDA is considered haemodynamically significant if the pulse pressure is > 35 mmHg, if signs of failure are present with an increase in liver size, if there is an increase in oxygen requirements, and if pulmonary plethora or cardiomegaly are seen on chest X-ray.

Table 1.8 Reasons for cardiac catheterization before surgery in acyanotic and cyanotic congenital cardiac anomalies in neonates. (Reproduced with permission from [84])

Anomaly	Associated complicating lesions	Reasons
Acyanotic		
Coarctation (discrete or with arch hypoplasia)	VSD, mitral stenosis, aortic stenosis, aberrant right subclavian artery	Rarely needed preoperatively; Required postoperatively for residual coarctation
Critical aortic valve stenosis	Left ventricular hypoplasia, mitral stenosis, coarctation	Balloon dilatation is being considered
Aortic arch interruption	VSD, subaortic stenosis, aortopulmonary window, aberrant right subclavian artery	To clarify arch anatomy (rarely needed)
Hypoplastic left-heart syndrome	Coarctation, VSD, rarely anomalies of pulmonary venous return	Rarely needed
Isolated patent ductus arteriosus	Occasionally lesions masking coarctation	Imaging of aortic arch if coarctation is not clearly defined by echocardiography
Aortopulmonary septal defect (window)	Aortic arch obstruction (coarctation, interruption)	Diagnosis may be missed by echocardiography
Atrioventricular septal defects	Ventricular hypoplasia, subaortic stenosis, arch obstruction, parachute left atrioventricular valve, patent ductus arteriosus	Assessment of ventricular size and confirmation of arch abnormalities if unclear because of large ductus
Cyanotic		
Tetralogy of Fallot	Non-confluent pulmonary arteries, peripheral pulmonary artery stenosis, restrictive VSD, right ventricular or left ventricular hypoplasia, mitral stenosis	Definition of pulmonary artery anatomy prior to shunt
Pulmonary atresia with VSD	Non-confluent pulmonary arteries, aortopulmonary colaterals	Definition of pulmonary blood supply*
Truncus arteriosus	Aortic arch interruption, unusual origin of pulmonary arteries (ductal origin of left pulmonary artery), abnormal origin of coronary artery	Definition of pulmonary artery anatomy is the only usual indication
Tricuspid atresia	Pulmonary stenosis present or absent	Rarely needed prior to shunt or pulmonary artery band
Univentricular connections		
In situ solitus	Pulmonary stenosis present or absent	Rarely needed prior to shunt or pulmonary artery band
In situ ambiguous (left or right isomerism)	Anomalous pulmonary venous and systemic venous drainage, pulmonary atresia or stenosis	Complex mixed venous drainage when palliation is considered.
Total anomalous pulmonary venous drainage	Left ventricular hypoplasia, mixed sites of drainage, rarely other associated lesions	Complex mixed drainage present; no clear confluence identified by echocardiography
Transposition		
With intact ventricular septum	Very rarely coarctation	Coronary arterial anatomy**
With VSD (subaortic, subpulmonic, or remote)	Multiple muscular defects, pulmonary stenosis, mitral and tricuspid valve anormalities, hypoplasia of right and left ventricle, aortic arch abnormalities	Rarely needed prior to shunt or pulmonary artery band

*In some instances when aortopulmonary collaterals are obvious at echocardiography, cardiac catheterization may be deferred until two or three months of age
**In most centres not considered a reason for routine cardiac catheterization

Two-dimensional echocardiogram

The ductus can be readily visualized by two-dimensional echocardiography. The LA is larger than the RA or the aortic root, and the atrial septum may bulge towards the right. The left ventricle is dilated and hypercontractile. The shunt may be quantitated by Doppler ultrasound and colour flow has facilitated recognition of the characteristics of the flow patterns of PDA. Two-dimensional echocardiographic confirmation of PDA should always be attempted prior to the initiation of treatment as the shunt may be small and not require treatment, and more importantly, unsuspected associated congenital heart disease may be present for which ductal closure may be contraindicated.

Management of PDA

This usually involves:

Fluid restriction

In general fluid intake is maintained at a low normal level; fluid restriction is considered unlikely to lead to ductal closure and may not always be appropriate treatment, particularly if the nutritional consequences of fluid restriction are ignored.[92,95]

Supportive measures

Ventilatory management involves increasing the end expiratory pressure which decreases left-to-right shunting and improves systemic blood flow. Other supportive measures include maintaining adequate oxygenation, oxygen carrying capacity, neutral thermal environment and nutritional requirements.

There are no clear benefits from the use of diuretics; in fact it has been reported that frusemide increases the incidence of PDA via a prostaglandin mediated process.[88] Furthermore, if diuretics are used in conjunction with fluid restriction, electrolyte abnormalities are a likely complication.

Digoxin is not generally indicated as myocardial contractility is increased rather than decreased with PDA and true myocardial dysfunction is rarely a problem when prospective management of the PDA is initiated. Furthermore, digoxin is often associated with toxicity in the very low birthweight infant.

Indomethacin

Indomethacin is a powerful prostaglandin synthetase inhibitor and is widely used as the primary method to effect closure of a haemodynamically significant PDA.[96] The response to indomethacin varies according to many factors, but in particular gestational and postnatal age (less effective in extremely low birthweight infants and after the first week of life). The recurrence of a symptomatic PDA following a course of indomethacin is also significant, particularly in low birthweight infants. Although indomethacin is most effective in the first 48 hours after birth, this would require its use in a large number of infants in whom the ductus would close spontaneously; furthermore, early prophylactic closure of the PDA by surgical ligation in infants < 1000 gm did not affect the total duration of oxygen or ventilator requirements, nor the incidence of BPD.[97] Prophylactic use of indomethacin is therefore not recommended.[92]

The potential side effects of indomethacin must be considered prior to its use. It predictably decreases urine output and often leads to hyponatraemia and is therefore contraindicated in patients with significant renal impairment. Various methods of preventing oliguria have been tried, including low dose dopamine or the simultaneous administration of frusemide, but these are not of proven benefit.[98,99] In addition, indomethacin, via its effects of decreasing GFR, will prolong the half–lives of all renally excreted drugs.

Focal areas of necrosis and GI tract perforation have been described in several reports following the enteral or IV use of indomethacin.[100,101] Whether the findings of bowel necrosis are in fact distinct from those of NEC is uncertain, but the presence of any signs suggestive of NEC are generally considered a contraindication to the use of indomethacin. A number of studies have shown decreases in renal and superior mesenteric artery blood flow velocity and in cerebral blood flow velocity[102–4] particularly if a rapid infusion is given.[105] The clinical significance of these changes is uncertain.

Indomethacin impairs platelet function and is generally contraindicated if the platelet count is < 80 000. It is not used in infants with documented IVH of grade II or greater.

The standard dose of indomethacin is 0.2 mg.kg^{-1} IV, followed by 0.2 mg.kg^{-1} dose for two further doses, 12 and 24 hours after the first. This has been modified in a number of ways to offset side effects: delaying the third dose, using 0.1 mg in very low birthweight infants or administering prolonged maintenance therapy at lower dosages. These manoeuvres have led to lower PDA recurrence rates and lower requirements for surgical ligation without an increase in toxic side effects.[106,107]

Table 1.9 Contraindications to the use of indomethacin

Creatinine $> 100 \ \mu$mol.l^{-1}
Urea > 7 mmol.l^{-1}
Oliguria $< 0.5 - 1$ ml.kg^{-1}.hr
Necrotizing enterocolitis
Thombocytopaenia $< 80\ 000$
Bleeding diathesis
IVH
Hyperbilirubinaemia
Sepsis

Surgical ligation

Surgical ligation is usually reserved for infants with a haemodynamically significant PDA with contraindications to indomethacin such as NEC, sepsis or IVH. It is also used a priori in the ELBW infant because of the variable response to indomethacin, the high rate of recurrence and side effects and because of the low incidence of surgical complications in closure of the PDA. Despite this, it is important to note that closing the duct via surgical or medical means has not significantly improved the incidence of BPD in very low birth weight infants.[97,108]

Central nervous system

The nervous system at birth

The brain at birth is relatively large, being 10 per cent of the total body weight. By six months of age it has doubled in size and by one year has trebled. About 25 per cent of the adult number of brain cells is present at birth. The cells of the cortex and brainstem are complete in number after one year of life. The cerebellum has less of its total complement at birth but reaches its final number before other areas.

The rapid growth in the first year of life is the result of myelination and elaboration of the dendritic processes necessary for the full complex behaviour of the older child and adult.

Nutritional deprivation during the period of the postnatal growth 'spurt' of the infant brain may give rise to impairment of cerebral development and may explain the vulnerability of the brain in babies with inborn errors of metabolism. Certainly, infants who have suffered both prenatal and postnatal undernutrition have reduced quantities of brain cells, lipids and protein and decreased dendritic connections. There is now good evidence that newborn motor behaviour is not, as has previously been thought, entirely at subcortical levels. Cortical potentials are elicited during neonatal seizures which are manifest clinically, corresponding with the extent of dendritic growth in the motor cortex before birth. However, at birth, myelination of the nerve fibres is

incomplete and reflex responses not seen later (such as the Moro reflex) may be elicited. These reflexes depend on cutaneous stimulation and the resultant action is more widespread in immature babies. Such differences may be used to assess the gestational age of a baby.

Incomplete myelination in the CNS also explains the increased sensitivity to opioids and general anaesthesia.

In the very young, functional and anatomical immaturity give rise to low pain sensitivity and limited conscious behaviour, but even small preterm babies move away from noxious stimuli and the cardiovascular signs of autonomic stimulation and stress hormone release in response to pain are similar to the adult. Babies react to painful stimuli in a non specific way and do not appear to differentiate exactly the origins of the pain. Newborns have a higher circulating level of beta-endorphins than have adults and the immature blood–brain barrier may allow these easier access to the brain itself and may partly explain a reduced requirement for analgesics in this age group.

The sleep pattern depends on the degree of development of the CNS. Whether *in utero* or after premature delivery, the amount of slow wave sleep increases during the third trimester of gestation when about half of sleep is non-REM. Slow wave sleep is necessary for functional development of the respiratory control area of the brain. At the 36th week, the baby develops a biological rhythm with a definite pattern of slow wave, REM and transitional sleep.

The high incidence of convulsions in the first months of life is not fully understood but can be attributed to a number of factors, including poor myelination, immaturity of central inhibitory mechanisms, increased water content of the brain and a higher metabolic rate. Because dendritic connections are poorly developed at birth, fits do not spread throughout the cortex as they would in an older child and thus the clinical manifestation is often fragmentary.

By 12 weeks of gestational life, motor nerve fibres reach the extremities of the limbs, but by 28 weeks the neuromuscular junctions are more highly differentiated in the tongue and the diaphragm than in the hand. Gamma-efferent activity is less sustained than in the adult and this may contribute to the relative hypotonia of the newborn. At this stage the muscles are functionally a uniform group, having the characteristics of adult 'slow' fibres. Early in neonatal life the 'slow' and 'fast' groups develop at the same time that fibres lose their overall sensitivity to acetylcholine and the subneural apparatus of the neuromuscular junction appears. Together with this, an adult pattern of sensitivity develops restricted to the motor end–plate. Indirect tetanic stimulation is poorly sustained and there is some evidence of early tetanic fade. Because of the anatomical and physiological differences a different response to muscle relaxant drugs is elicited (see p. 130).

Cerebral circulation

In normal adults the process of autoregulation of cerebral blood flow tends to allow a constant flow with changes of mean systemic blood pressure between 60 and 130 mmHg. There is no reason to believe that this process is not present in the normal newborn, although in preterm babies the reflex is likely to be immature – slower in onset and less complete. Autoregulation is readily disturbed by hypercapnia and hypoxia and after severe hypotension, but in the newborn is regained by a period of mild hyperventilation of 30 minutes or so. Total cerebral blood flow may be lower in the preterm than the term baby, which in turn is less than in an older child on the basis of body weight. Animal work shows that the range of blood pressure

within which autoregulation takes place is narrower in the neonate, perhaps limited to 50–90 mmHg and beyond these limits cerebral blood flow varies directly with systemic blood pressure,[109] though the mechanisms determining the limits of CBF autoregulation are unknown. These researchers found a marked increase in cerebrovascular thromboxane, a potent vasoconstrictor, during hypotension and a large increase in vasodilator prostaglandins during hypertension. This explains why indomethacin used for treating PDA in preterm infants causes a reduction in CBF. The increase in cerebral vasodilators may limit the possibility of vasoconstriction in response to an elevated blood pressure and lead to the distension of cerebral vessels and the possibility of their rupture. An increase in thromboxane with hypotension may well contribute to ischaemic insults to the newborn brain as it does in the adult. Intraventricular cerebral haemorrhage is discussed in Chapter 5.

Surges of arterial pressure may occur if autoregulation has been disturbed by hypoxia followed by stressful manoeuvres such as tracheal intubation or venepuncture. Hypoxia also causes venous congestion and endothelial damage. Surges of venous pressure may come from high levels of airway distending pressure. In asphyxiated babies all attempts should be made to keep systemic blood pressure within the normal limits of 40–70 mmHg systolic. Low levels of blood pressure are associated with an increased incidence of subsequent IVH. Newer methods of measuring cerebral blood flow velocity using Xenon clearance or Doppler are being employed increasingly. Pryds *et al*[110] have shown increases in CBF which support cerebral metabolism during uncomplicated hypoglycaemia in preterm infants.

Neurological disease

History

It is important to elicit a full history in the evaluation of a newborn who presents with an abnormality of the central nervous system.

1. *The antenatal history* may reveal decreased fetal movements, an abnormal fetal position or polyhydramnios. Although these may be common non–specific indicators of underlying fetal abnormality, they may also suggest specific CNS disorders e.g. decreased fetal movement

may be the first manifestation of muscle weakness due to infantile spinal muscular atrophy, congenital myotonic dystrophy or congenital myopathy; a breech position may reflect lack of fetal tone or movement seen in these and other disorders; polyhydramnios may occur because of decreased fetal swallowing due to bulbar weakness.

2. A detailed history and review of the *labour and delivery* including fetal position, fetal heart rate, presence of meconium in the amniotic fluid, the method of delivery, duration of first and second stages of labour , intrapartum complications, Apgar scores, cord gases and the initial status of the infant in the delivery room may reveal evidence of intrapartum asphyxia. A history of a difficult delivery or one requiring forceps assistance or vacuum extraction may suggest birth trauma in addition.

   It is becoming increasingly evident that there may be an antenatal origin to the cerebral injury in infants who sustain intrapartum asphyxia, as the underlying disorder may lead to poor tolerance of the stress of delivery. In addition, neurologically abnormal fetuses may manifest abnormal fetal heart rate patterns because of neural mechanisms controlling heart rate, rather than because of intrapartum hypoxic events.[111] Therefore, although a positive history of difficulties in labour is often closely related to the neonatal neurological condition at birth this may not always be the case, and assumptions that an infant's neurological abnormality occurred because of intrapartum events may be erroneous.

3. *Maternal disease and drug history*: A number of maternal medical disorders have a direct effect on the central nervous system status of the newborn, e.g. myasthenia, thyrotoxicosis and myotonic dystrophy. A variety of agents taken by the mother during pregnancy may lead to malformations in the offspring, e.g. valproic acid and carbamazepine may interfere with neural tube closure resulting in spina bifida[112,113]

4. *Family history*: A history of siblings similarly affected in early infancy or in the neonatal period is suggestive of a familial inherited disorder. In particular, many of the causes of weakness and hypotonia due to peripheral nervous system disorders are genetic in origin and require detailed information from parents and relatives to determine patterns of inherit-

ance. The possibility of parental consanguinity should always be investigated in infants with congenital anomalies.

5. *In utero diagnosis*: A diagnosis of a CNS abnormality, particularly neural tube defects, will today usually have been made prior to delivery. Measurements of serum alpha–feto protein levels and/or the use of ultrasound allow the majority of these disorders to be detected. Ultrasound can be used to characterize the extent and location of spinal defects with great accuracy.[114] Furthermore, infants with myelomeningocele have identifiable cranial changes with indentations of the frontal regions of the skull, obliteration of the cisterna magna and distortion of the cerebellar hemispheres. The neural tube defect may not be an isolated finding and may be a component of a chromosomal disorder or multiple anomaly syndrome, necessitating a full and detailed fetal evaluation.

   In utero diagnosis should allow planning of the site and route of delivery (possibly, caesarean section)[115] as well as access to facilities where neonatal surgery can be performed.

Neonatal neurological examination

It is essential to assess the functional status of the newborn's nervous system in relation to gestational age; the interdependency of neurological signs, particularly tone and posture, with maturational change is underlined in a number of gestational age scoring systems[116]. In addition, the neurological assessment must take into account the behavioural state of the infant, as well as the level of systemic illness, as ill newborns tend to be relatively inactive, sleep more, cry infrequently and demonstrate a generalized depression of the nervous system.

CNS examination aims therefore, to determine: whether CNS findings are consistent with gestational age alone; whether CNS findings are consistent with systemic illness alone; or whether CNS findings are not accounted for and require repeat examination and/or further investigation.

While individual signs may appear minor, when grouped together they may be more indicative of an underlying diagnosis that has not been suspected or has been attributed to other causes, in particular to prematurity with associated respiratory distress.

Important components of the neurological examination include:

1. *General observation/level of consciousness.* Significant information can be gained from observing the infant's level of alertness, resting posture in prone and supine positions, degree of activity and spontaneous movement of limbs, as well as the nature of the infant's cry. It is important to appreciate the influence of external environmental factors (e.g. light, temperature, noise) on the state of the infant during the neurological examination.

2. *Accurate occipitofrontal head circumference measurement* and palpation of the skull, sutures and fontanelles should be performed. The status of the cranial sutures and anterior fontanelle are good indicators of intracranial pressure and should be evaluated with the infant quiet and in the sitting position.

3. *Evaluation of posture and muscle tone* involves examination of the resting posture and assessment of passive and active tone of each of the major muscle groups. This is best done with the infant awake, not crying and with the head in a neutral position. Normal term infants in the prone position assume a posture of partial flexion of the arms and legs, with the legs adducted such that the thighs are under the abdomen. In the supine position the normal term infant will assume a flexed posture of both upper and lower extremities and will show alternating flexion and extension in reciprocal fashion on the two sides. The supine posture of a hypotonic infant is one of abduction of the legs, flaccid extension of the arms or occasionally contractures with flexion deformities of the limbs.

   Muscle tone is evaluated by noting the amplitude of passive movements in a single joint. A certain degree of resistance is normally present at the elbows, knees and hips and tone is normally symmetrical when one side is compared with the other. Active tone can be evaluated by observing reflex head and trunk straightening reactions of the infant to ventral suspension (the examiner suspends the infant with the hand placed under the infant's chest and axilla) or to the traction response in which the infant is gently pulled up from the supine position while holding the infant's hands. With the latter manoeuvre, abnormality exists when the head lags passively and then drops forward (neck and trunk muscle hypotonia) or if the head is maintained extended and backward (neck extensor hypertonia).

   A decrease in muscle tone may reflect underlying dysfunction of either the central or peripheral nervous system. Hypotonia should not be equated with weakness (a reduction in muscle strength or power), despite the fact that the two may coexist in disorders of the peripheral nervous system. It is often difficult to differentiate decreased tone from decreased tone and weakness.

4. (a) *Evaluation of various primitive reflexes* is an essential part of the neurological examination of the newborn. The Moro reflex (sudden dropping of the head in relation to the trunk, resulting in opening of the hands, extension and abduction of the upper extremities and then drawing them together) is present, although incomplete, from 32 weeks gestation. The tonic neck response (rotation of the infant's head to the side, eliciting extension of the arm and leg on the side to which the face is rotated with flexion on the opposite side), and palmar and plantar grasp reflexes (elicited by pressure on the palm or soles of the feet), are all important components of the examination. The placing and stepping reflexes are less useful and these and other reflexes tend to add little further information to the examination.

   Absence of a reflex beyond the age at which it should appear, persistence of a reflex beyond the age of normal disappearance or asymmetry of any reflex clearly constitute abnormal findings.

   (b) *Deep tendon reflexes.* A variety of deep tendon reflexes can be elicited. They are often difficult to appreciate and the significance of an increase may be less significant than if the reflexes are asymmetric. Observation of the plantar response is of limited usefulness in the newborn. Loss of deep tendon reflexes is an important sign of neuromuscular disease in the newborn.

5. *Evaluation of the cranial nerves.* The cranial nerves are examined via the infant's reaction to light, and fixing and following of the examiner's head (II), ocular movements, pupil size, and doll's eye movements (III, IV, VI), facial muscle tone, particularly with crying (VII), startle response to loud noise (VIII), sucking reflex (V, VII, XII), swallowing (IX, X) and observation of the tongue (XII).

6. *Behavioural assessment.* The neurological exami-

nation is enhanced by evaluating the newborn's behavioural repertoire.[117] This encompasses aspects of the neurological examination (e.g. muscle tone and level of alertness), but goes further to include the level of vigilance or receptive state (enabling the infant to accept various stimuli), the ability to alter arousal states, the ability to suppress repetitive or intrusive stimuli (habituation), the level of irritability/consolability and other social interactions. It also includes assessment of physiological responses to stimuli (e.g. tremors, changes in skin colour, heart rate).

Behavioural studies in premature infants have shown that in the acute phase of their illness they are predominantly in a sleep state, they do not cry even when disturbed, they are generally not irritable and responsiveness is difficult to elicit. When stimulated to alertness, this is generally of short duration, poor orientation and often accompanied by signs of stress. This behavioural organization is felt to be a 'protective apathy', in that it conserves energy and attempts to maintain homoeostasis.[118] In time, with increasing physiological stability it evolves to more differentiated states of sleep, alertness and crying with an increase in activity and responsiveness.

Behavioural assessment not only enhances the appreciation of the CNS status of the infant, but also provides cues for caregivers to determine the appropriateness of particular interventions for the individual infant. The preterm infant may be particularly vulnerable to excessive or mistimed stimulation and generally should be protected from excessive interventions.

A single neurological examination may indicate that the infant is neurologically normal or overtly abnormal. However, in a large number of infants examination may only lead to suspicion of abnormality, implying that the infant requires repeated assessment to determine the persistence of such abnormalities.

Common signs of CNS dysfunction

Jitteriness

Jitteriness or tremulousness in the newborn is an extreme response to arousal or environmental stimuli in the first few hours to days of life. It is characterized by a rhythmic shaking of the limbs symmetrically and occasionally the jaw and is often elicited as an exaggerated or low threshold Moro reflex or increased muscle stretch reflexes. Jitteriness can be differentiated from seizures by the absence of extraocular movements, alteration in respiratory pattern or other autonomic changes (e.g. increase in heart rate, BP). Jitteriness is extremely stimulus–sensitive and the rhythmic movements can be obliterated with flexion of the affected limb or by gentle passive restraint or swaddling of the infant.

Mild jitteriness may be seen in otherwise normal newborns at the end of the startle reflex or as the infant shifts from sleep to awake states. Moderate jitteriness may be seen in several conditions, including:

1. birth asphyxia or haemorrhage;
2. SGA infants;
3. metabolic abnormalities, hypoglycaemia, hypocalcaemia and hypomagnesaemia;
4. hyperviscosity syndrome;
5. drug withdrawal states;
6. congenital CNS anomalies.

SGA infants are particularly prone to demonstrate jitteriness, with or without concomitant hypoglycaemia, hypocalcaemia or hyperviscosity.

Marked or persistent jitteriness in the presence of normoglycaemia and electrolyte homoeostasis may indicate CNS irritation and should be investigated as one would for seizure activity.

Seizures

Seizures are often the first sign of CNS dysfunction and represent the most distinctive signal of neurological disease in the newborn.[119] They are defined clinically as a paroxysmal alteration in neurologic function, i.e. behavioural, motor and/or autonomic function.

The clinical manifestations of seizures are variable in the newborn and other neurological signs may resemble seizure activity, e.g. jitteriness (as described above); clonus, a rhythmic alternating movement of the limbs of equal velocity (as opposed to clonic seizures in which the movement is alternating but of unequal velocity with rapid and slow components); tonic posturing movements which may be extremely difficult to differentiate from seizure activity; apnoea which may occasionally be a sign of seizure activity, but is generally rarely the sole manifestation (when apnoea is associated with eye deviation or other seizure movements it can be readily differentiated from non-convulsive causes of apnoea).

Difficulties in diagnosis and EEG correlation have led to recent attempts to characterize and classify neonatal seizures[119,120] (Table 1.10). The four seizure types described by Volpe are:

- subtle;
- clonic;
- tonic;
- myoclonic.

Table 1.10 Classification of neonatal seizures. (Reproduced with permission from[119])

	Common	Uncommon
Subtle		
Clonic*	+	
Focal		
Multifocal***	+	
Tonic		
Focal		
Generalized***	+	
Myoclonic		+
Focal,		
multifocal**		+
Generalized***	+	

*Indicates that the specific clinical seizure is commonly or uncommonly associated with simultaneous electrographic seizure. Only specific varieties of subtle seizures are commonly associated with simultaneous EEG seizure activity
**Multifocal refers to clinical activity that involves more than one site, is asynchronous and usually migratory
***Generalized refers to clinical activity that is diffusely bilateral, synchronous and non-migratory

1. *Subtle* seizures[119] or 'motor automatisms'[120] are common and repetitive. They include oral, facial, lingual or ocular activity (e.g. lip smacking, tongue thrusting, eye deviation and autonomic nervous system signs). They are related to many aetiologies and often occur with other seizure types especially in term asphyxia. The relative maturity of the temporal lobe compared with the cortex may explain the high frequency of temporal manifestations.[121]

Information from EEG studies suggests that subtle seizures are more common in premature than in term infants. In the latter, caution should be used in attributing an epileptic origin to subtle phenomena as they are often not consistent with EEG seizure activity, particularly if these phenomena are the only manifestation in the infant. Non-epileptic events may not require anticonvulsant drugs: this recommendation is related, first, to the fact that such events rarely interfere with ventilatory or circulatory function, second, to the lack of evidence that the phenomena per se are harmful to the brain, and third, to the fact that unusually high blood levels of depressant drugs such as phenobarbitone are needed to suppress the clinical activity.[119]

2. *Clonic* seizures may be focal or multifocal. Focal clonic seizures are rhythmic, repetitive jerking movements involving the face, upper and/or lower extremities on one side of the body, neck or trunk. They are often indicative of focal cortical pathology but may also be secondary to generalized disorders, including metabolic encephalopathies. Multifocal clonic seizures are movements in several different areas, often with migration from one part of the body to another. They are usually seen in full–term asphyxia and may be refractory to treatment.

3. *Tonic* seizures may involve one limb (focal) or the whole body (generalized) with a sudden increase in muscle tone, usually extension. They are often described as posturing of a limb or asymmetric posturing of the trunk and/or neck. They are associated with intraventricular haemorrhage in premature infants and with a poor response to anticonvulsant therapy.

4. *Myoclonic* seizures are distinguished from clonic movements by the more rapid speed of the myoclonic jerk and the particular predilection for flexor muscle groups. They are either focal, multifocal or generalized and are characterized by single flexion of an upper extremity or asynchronous twitching of several parts of the body or bilateral jerks of flexion of upper or lower limbs.

The time of onset of the seizures, associated physical abnormalities and the neurological status between seizures may aid in distinguishing the cause of seizures in the newborn. Common causes of seizures include the following:

1. *Perinatal asphyxia* accounts for the majority of seizures in term newborns (50–70 per

cent of acutely asphyxiated infants manifest seizures). Seizure types are often subtle, tonic or multifocal clonic in nature and usually occur within the first 6–24 hours. These seizures are often self–limiting even though they may be refractory to treatment for a period of time, requiring more than one anticonvulsant agent. In perinatal asphyxia the interictal state is usually abnormal.

2. *Intracranial haemorrhage* (ICH) may be due to birth trauma, hypoxic–ischaemic injury, thrombocytopaenia, coagulation disorders, vascular anomalies or tumours, or they may be secondary to invasive procedures, e.g. ECMO. Location of the haemorrhage may be intraparenchymal (usually secondary to HIE), cerebellar, subdural (either supra- or infratentorial and usually secondary to trauma) or extradural (also secondary to trauma and associated with skull fracture). Subarachnoid haemorrhage may occur as an isolated haemorrhage or in association with a subdural or epidural haemorrhage.

   Infants with ICH may present with seizures 24–48 hours after birth. Seizures are often focal, clonic or subtle in nature. The infant may appear well between seizures or the clinical picture may be one of systemic collapse with anaemia/shock, hypo/hypertonia, lethargy, vomiting, apnoea, bradycardia, localizing neurological signs and a bulging fontanelle. External evidence of birth trauma (forceps, vacuum marks) may be found.

   Intraventricular haemorrhage in the premature infant occurs within the first 12–72 hours of life, with sudden clinical deterioration and tonic or multifocal clonic seizures.

3. *Cerebral infarction/stroke* (focal necrosis in well–defined arterial territories) has a high association with seizures, particularly in full term infants.[122] Strokes occur in a number of diverse cerebrovascular disorders including asphyxia, polycythaemia, acute severe hypertension and embolization. Often no precipitating factor can be determined and the majority of neonatal infarctions follow apparently normal deliveries.[123,124] The infarct may go undetected if cranial imaging studies are not performed.

4. *Infection.* Seizures are commonly seen in infants with infection, particularly acquired bacterial meningitis. Congenital bacterial or viral infection may also lead to seizures at any time after birth up to several weeks of age.

5. *Metabolic causes of seizures* include hypoglycaemia (common within the first few hours of birth), hypocalcaemia either early (1–3 days) or late (end of the first week), hypomagnesaemia, hypo- and hypernatraemia and polycythaemia with hyperviscosity. Inborn errors of amino acid and organic acid metabolism, hyperammonaemia and pyridoxine dependency may also present with seizures.

6. *Cerebral dysgenetic disorders* may present with seizures. Malformations are suggested by dysmorphic features of the infant, abnormalities of head size and shape or other associated anomalies. Seizures occur at any stage in the neonatal period and tend to be of several types.

7. *Drug withdrawal* in the newborn secondary to maternal addiction is an uncommon cause of neonatal seizures. Occurrence is usually at 2–3 days of life.

Decreased Responsiveness/Level of Consciousness

As with the evaluation of all parameters of neurological integrity, decreased responsiveness must be assessed in relation to both the gestational age of the infant and the clinical and behavioural state in which the infant is examined. Brazelton[117] has described six states, ranging from deep or quiet sleep (I), light or REM sleep (II), drowsy (III), quiet wakefulness (IV), active wakefulness (V) and crying (VI). Repeated observation of an infant should determine that the infant does not remain in one state alone.

Alteration in level of consciousness may range from unarousable unconsciousness or coma to stupor or optundation in which only vigorous or repeated stimulation results in arousal, to lethargy, a milder degree of alteration in consciousness. The variable use of these terms requires that responses to specific stimuli, e.g. painful or caloric stimuli or loud noise, be accurately described.

The differential diagnosis of a decreased level of consciousness includes:

1. *Hypoxic–ischaemic encephalopathy (HIE).* This is the most common cause of an altered level of responsiveness in the immediate newborn period. The level of consciousness is the major clinical sign used in the staging of the severity of HIE in full–term infants.[125] In stage I (mild) the infant's level of consciousness is usually not impaired or is characterized by either

a brief period of lethargy immediately after birth or, more commonly, a hyperalert state with jitteriness and irritability. In this stage the infant's eyes are widely open and staring, with decreased frequency of blinking and prolonged periods of wakefulness. Stage II (moderate) is characterized by lethargy for the first few days and infants are often irritable when disturbed. Stage III (severe) is characterized by coma with little or no response to stimuli.

The clinical staging of the level of consciousness is useful and prognostic in the assessment of intrapartum asphyxia in term infants; it is not helpful in premature infants who do not demonstrate the same encephalopathic picture, and it is also obviously limited in those infants requiring anticonvulsants or paralyzing agents.

When neither the history of the labour and delivery nor the clinical picture reveal evidence of asphyxia, other possible causes of decreased responsiveness must always be considered. A decreased level of consciousness appearing after the first 24 hours should not be attributed to perinatal asphyxia.

2. *Intracranial haemorrhage (ICH)*. This is suggested by a history of a difficult delivery or abnormal fetal presentation. Trauma may give rise to focal or diffuse CNS signs, including a decreased level of consciousness. This may fluctuate over the first few hours to days. The signs of a subdural haemorrhage over the cerebral convexities may be non–specific lethargy and irritability; a subdural haemorrhage within the posterior fossa usually gives rise to symptoms after a few hours or days of birth with decreased responsiveness, apnoea, bradycardia, seizures and signs of raised intracranial pressure.

As trauma and HIE often coexist in term infants, when the degree of depression of the nervous system cannot be accounted for by the asphyxial episode alone, a CT scan to rule–out intracranial haemorrhage, particularly subdural haemorrhage, must always be considered.

3. *Metabolic abnormalities*. These commonly give rise to altered levels of consciousness. Hypoglycaemic infants may be stuporous, hypotonic or irritable or they may display jitteriness and seizures. Hypocalcaemia may also decrease responsiveness to stimuli with hypotonia and seizures in addition. Many inborn errors of amino acid metabolism present with altered levels of consciousness in the neonatal period; after the first protein feeding the infant may become lethargic, stuporous or comatose and develop seizures. Other signs including vomiting, an unusual odour to body or urine and a family history of affected siblings will direct attention to this possibility, requiring blood gases, ammonium, organic acid and amino acid determination.

4. *Electrolyte abnormalities*. Sodium and occasionally potassium abnormalities may give rise to altered levels of consciousness. Hyperbilirubinaemia may also result in lethargy and hypotonia.

5. *Infection*. Either congenital or acquired infection commonly leads to decreased responsiveness. Other associated CNS findings, e.g. full fontanelle, seizures or systemic findings, may be present. In any newborn with an abrupt change in neurologic status, sepsis and/or meningitis should always be considered and steps taken to exclude this possibility.

6. *Drug intoxication*. This is a fairly common cause of a decreased level of consciousness; maternal drug use (narcotics, alcohol), narcotics or magnesium sulphate used in labour, or the postnatal administration of anticonvulsants, lead to lethargy, hypotonia, decreased respiratory effort and diminished reflexes.

Hypotonia

Hypotonia implies a decrease in postural muscle tone resulting from an abnormality in the central nervous system, peripheral nervous system, skeletal muscle or combinations thereof. Classification of the hypotonic baby as either non–paralytic (hypotonia without significant muscle weakness) or paralytic (weakness with incidental hypotonia) generally depends on whether there is central or peripheral nervous system involvement respectively.

Nonparalytic Hypotonia

Non-paralytic or central hypotonia is the most common cause of hypotonia in the newborn. It is associated with a wide variety of conditions, the most common being an acute encephalopathy secondary to a major CNS insult, such as hypoxia–ischaemia, birth trauma, intracranial haemorrhage, infection or hypoglycaemia. Concomitant signs of decreased level of consciousness, convulsions or depressed primitive reflexes with variable deep tendon reflexes are usually present.

More chronic central causes of hypotonia include chromosomal and genetic disorders (e.g. Down's, Prader–Willi syndromes). Consciousness is usually not affected in these disorders. Hypotonia may also be a striking finding in the newborn with connective tissue disorders, metabolic, nutritional, endocrine or other miscellaneous conditions, such as familial dysautonomia.

Paralytic Hypotonia

The paralytic group of disorders is characterized by hypotonia, weakness, absence of reflexes and an alert level of consciousness. They result from trauma to the upper portion of the spinal cord, disease of the spinal anterior horn cells and abnormalities of the neuromuscular junction or muscle. These disorders include:

1. *Spinal cord trauma*. Infants present with respiratory depression, generalized hypotonia and flaccid weakness of extremities. There is absence of sensation below the level of injury and absent deep tendon reflexes (spinal shock). Infants with normal facial and cranial nerve function in the presence of either quadraplegia or paraplegia must be evaluated for spinal cord injury.
2. *Infantile spinal muscular atrophy (ISMA)*. In the acute fulminating form of ISMA, generalized and profound weakness is accompanied by absent deep tendon reflexes, an alert and expressive face, with atrophy and fasciculation of the tongue. The weakness leads to respiratory difficulty, and aspiration pneumonia frequently supervenes. There is no loss of sensory function or sphincter control.
3. *Transient myasthenia gravis*. This occurs exclusively in infants born to myasthenic mothers. It causes early feeding difficulty, generalized weakness, respiratory difficulty and hypotonia. Deep tendon reflexes are normal. Extraocular weakness and ptosis are uncommon in the transient form but are far more common in congenital myasthenia, which occasionally manifests as neonatal hypotonia. Reversibility of symptoms following injection of anticholinesterase drugs will confirm the diagnosis.
4. *Congenital Myopathies*. A number of congenital myopathies present with hypotonia in the neonatal period. They are clinically indistinguishable from each other and cerebral function and sensation are normally intact.
5. *Congenital Myotonic Dystrophy*. Infants with congenital myotonic dystrophy present with respiratory and feeding difficulties, facial diplegia, arthrogryposis, and hypotonia. A history of polyhydramnios in the mother, who may also show evidence of the facial features of myotonic dystrophy and elicitable myotonia, helps confirm the diagnosis.

Macrocephaly

Macrocephaly is defined as a head circumference of more than two standard deviations above the mean or above the 97th percentile for gestational age.

Macrocephaly may be indicative of subdural collections of fluid, hydrocephalus (either congenital or acquired), in which the cerebral ventricular system is dilated, or megalencephaly, in which the brain itself is abnormally large.

Congenital Hydrocephalus (see p. 176)

Congenital malformations which give rise to hydrocephalus include: aqueduct stenosis, the Dandy Walker syndrome (large cystic fourth ventricle with maldevelopment of the cerebellum) and the Arnold–Chiari malformation, characterized by downward displacement of the cerebellar tonsils through the foramen magnum, inferior displacement and elongation of the medulla oblongata and the fourth ventricle, with downward displacement of the cervical cord. Arnold–Chiari malformation is seen most commonly with neural tube defects. These range from craniospinal rachischisis to spina bifida occulta, in which the only clue to the underlying abnormality may be the presence of cutaneous signs: hypertrichosis, a port wine stain, palpable lipoma or dimpling in the lumbosacral area.

The most common neural tube abnormality is myelomeningocele. The neurological features related to the level of the myelomeningocele are given in Table 1.11. Congenital hydrocephalus is usually a feature of myelomeningocele, particularly if the level of the spinal defect is thoracolumbar, lumbar, or lumbosacral. If the head circumference is greater than the 90th percentile, there is approximately a 95 per cent chance of significant ventricular dilatation; if the head circumference is less than the 90th percentile, there is still an approximately 65 per cent incidence of hydrocephalus.[126] Clinical signs of increased ICP, bulging anterior fontanelle, and

Table 1.11 Myelomeningocele: Correlation between segmental innervation and motor, sensory, sphincter function and reflexes

Lesion	Major segmental innervation	Cutaneous sensation	Lower limb motor function	Sphincter function	Reflex
Cervical/thoracic	Variable	Variable	None	—	—
Thoracolumbar	T12	Lower abdomen	None	—	—
	L1	Groin	Weak hip flexion	—	—
	L2	Anterior upper thigh	Strong hip flexion	—	—
Lumbar	L3	Anterior distal thigh and knee	Knee extension	—	Knee jerk
	L4	Medial leg	Knee flexion	—	Knee jerk
Lumbrosacral	L5	Lateral leg and medial knee	Foot dorsiflexion and eversion	—	Ankle jerk
	S1	Sole of foot	Foot plantar flexion	—	Ankle jerk
Sacral	S2	Posterior leg and thigh	Toe flexion	Bladder and rectum	Anal wink
	S3	Middle of buttock	—	Bladder and rectum	Anal wink
	S4	Medial buttock	—	Bladder and rectum	Anal wink

diastasis of the cranial sutures should be sought. If the myelomeningocele is leaking CSF, the signs of increased ICP may not be evident.

Other congenital causes of hydrocephalus include the group of intrauterine TORCH infections (toxoplasmosis, rubella, CMV, herpes), vascular anomalies, other developmental anomalies of the CNS and rarely congenital tumours.

Acquired Hydrocephalus

Acquired hydrocephalus is usually secondary to intracranial haemorrhage, particularly intraventricular haemorrhage in the small premature infant or neonatal bacterial meningitis.

In the preterm infant the diagnosis of hydrocephalus requires ultrasonography or computed tomography (CT) scanning, since normal head circumference measurements can be associated with significantly enlarging cerebral ventricles (see IVH/PVH).

Subdural haemorrhages do not usually give rise to macrocephaly in the early newborn period; a chronic subdural effusion may result in an enlarging head circumference over the first few months of life.

Subdural effusions secondary to neonatal meningitis are usually not associated with increased ICP and tend to resolve spontaneously.

Megalencephaly

Familial forms of megalencephaly as well as generalized growth disorders such as cerebral gigantism, Beckwith–Wiedemann syndrome, achondroplasia and the neurocutaneous syndromes (phakomatoses, e.g., Sturge–Weber, tuberous sclerosis), may give rise to enlargement of the brain (macrencephaly). Macrencephaly is also caused by accumulation of metabolic products as in the lipidoses (e.g. Tay–Sachs disease) and the mucopolysaccharidoses (e.g. Hurler syndrome).

Microcephaly

Microcephaly (head circumference below the third percentile in an infant of normal length) occurs either as a result of craniosynostosis or micrencephaly, an undergrowth of the brain.

Craniosynostosis is a condition in which there is

premature closure of one or more cranial sutures, with limitation of skull growth in the affected area and compensatory growth from unaffected sutures. The infant's head may be small or normal in size at birth; the clinical appreciation of fused sutures will lead to the diagnosis of craniosynostosis. The skull ultimately assumes an abnormal configuration characteristic of the involved suture. For a craniosynostosis to produce microcephaly generally requires multiple suture involvement.

Micrencephaly may reflect either a primary defect of brain development (e.g. in the common autosomal chromosomal syndromes) or occurs secondary to a serious injury during pregnancy or in the perinatal period (particularly intrauterine infections, teratogenic agents (maternal alcoholism), meningitis, trauma or hypoxia–ischaemia).

Micrencephaly of even a moderate degree is associated with a poor prognosis for psychomotor development.

The sick premature infant may demonstrate a delay in normal head growth until recovery from systemic illness. In some infants this period may be prolonged. Though not true microcephaly, such a delay is cause for very careful serial neurological evaluation since it may indicate irreversible failure of brain development.

Feeding difficulty

The non-specific sign of feeding difficulty may appear as an isolated problem but is more commonly seen in infants with multiple, usually neurological disorders. It may be an acute feature of any systemic illness, particularly septicaemia, but is considered here more as a persistent problem in which it manifests predominantly as a slow or poor suck, prolonged time to complete a feeding, or regurgitation and choking associated with feeding. It thus requires evaluation of all phases of the suck–and–swallow mechanism. This common disorder occurs in infants who (1) are premature or ill, (2) have CNS or neuromuscular disorders, and (3) have anatomical or functional abnormalities of the GI tract.

1. Oral feeding is not usually feasible in the *premature infant* less than 32 weeks gestation; by 34 weeks sufficient coordination of the suck–and–swallow mechanism allows for concomitant respiration. Infants recovering from respiratory distress, a minor CNS insult, congenital heart disease, or renal failure may have difficulty in feeding, and show decreased interest or fatigue during a feeding.

2. *CNS or neuromuscular disorders*: Birth trauma, hypoxic–ischaemic encephalopathy, congenital infection or a CNS developmental abnormality are all likely to be associated with feeding difficulties.

   Specific conditions include infantile spinal muscular atrophy, Mobius syndrome, neonatal myasthenia gravis, congenital myotonic dystrophy, congenital myopathy and Prader–Willi syndrome.

3. *Anatomical or functional abnormalities of the GI tract* which lead to feeding difficulties include: tracheo–oesophageal fistula, cleft lip and palate, failure of relaxation of the upper oesophageal sphincter (cricopharyngeal achalasia) or a lack of coordination between the pharyngeal and oesophageal phases of swallowing (pharyngeal–cricopharyngeal incoordination). Incompetence of the lower oesophageal sphincter may cause gastro–oesophageal reflux; these infants are usually hungry and take feedings greedily, yet persistently vomit (non-bilious) with occasional choking or apnoeic spells. Gradual improvement is usually seen over a period of months.

   Feeding difficulties are extremely important to evaluate and ameliorate; they may lead to failure to thrive, apnoea, aspiration pneumonia and chronic lung disease and thereby compound any pre-existing condition.

Special investigations

Examination of the cerebrospinal fluid (CSF)

The single most important indication for CSF examination in the newborn is to determine the presence or absence of meningitis as it may coexist in up to a third of neonates with generalized sepsis.

The classic clinical signs of meningitis (e.g. neck stiffness) in the older child are usually absent in the newborn and the lumbar puncture therefore becomes an important consideration in the septic work–up of an infant, whether specific CNS signs are present or not. The decision to perform a lumbar puncture should be based on clinical judgement and the likelihood of a positive yield from a procedure which may compromise the status of a sick or unstable infant. The yield from an LP performed to rule out late onset or nosocomial infection after the first week of life is far greater than from an LP performed within the first 48 hours of life. In fact an early LP may not be appropriate in the routine work–up of early onset sepsis, particularly in asymptomatic infants or premature infants with respiratory distress.[128–31]

Examination of the CSF as a means of detecting the presence of intracranial haemorrhage is insufficient indication to perform a lumbar puncture; difficulties exist in differentiating a bleed from a traumatic tap and infants with clear spinal fluid may still have significant intracranial haemorrhage. More importantly, there are non–invasive means with greater accuracy to diagnose the various forms of ICH.

In the newborn who is too unstable to undergo an LP the procedure should be delayed and antibiotics administered empirically. The use of continuous non–invasive monitoring of pO_2, pCO_2, and saturation monitors should decrease any hypoxaemia associated with the procedure and prevent clinical deterioration. Other complications of LPs have been described, including seeding of organisms into the meninges in bacteraemic infants, spinal epidermoid tumours and brainstem herniation. These are all exceedingly rare.

Interpretation

The normal ranges of CSF values in newborn infants is given in the Table 1.12.[132]

In the normal infant the CSF is usually clear, although xanthochromia due to the presence of red blood cells or hyperbilirubinaemia may be seen, particularly in premature infants. A small number of WBCs per cubic millimetre may not be significant (see Table 1.12), particularly if all are mononuclear cells. Protein values up to 1.7 gm.l^{-1} have also

been considered normal. Glucose values range from 1.8–4.0 mmol.l^{-1} but should always be assessed in relation to the blood glucose value.

Although difficulty may exist in the interpretation of CSF findings in neonates, given the wide range of values considered normal, any one or a combination of the following CSF values should alert the clinician to the possibility of meningeal infection.[132]

1. WBC $> 30.mm^{-3}$ with > 60 per cent polymorphs
2. CSF protein > 1.7 gm.l^{-1}
3. CSF/blood glucose ratio < 0.5–0.6.

It is also possible for a relatively clear CSF with few cells to contain organisms. This necessitates that all CSF be gram–stained and cultured, irrespective of the cell count and other findings. The CSF findings interpreted together with a detailed clinical CNS examination will usually provide definitive clues for firmly establishing the diagnosis of a bacterial meningitis.[133]

Cranial sonography

Cranial sonography provides the definitive diagnosis of many neonatal brain disorders and may obviate the necessity for the use of other methods of investigation. It has emerged as the major tool for evaluating intraventricular/periventricular and intraparenchymal haemorrhage, ventricular dilatation and periventricular leukomalacia or echodensities in the premature infant. It is non–invasive, portable, free of ionizing radiation and provides excellent visualization of the ventricular system, basal ganglia, choroid plexus and corpus callosum.

Table 1.12 Normal ranges of CSF values in newborn infants. (Reproduced with permission from[132])

	Newborn infants		Infants and children
	Preterm	Term	
White blood cell count (cells/mm³)	0–29	0–32	0–6
Protein (gm.l⁻¹)	0.65–1.5	0.2–1.7	0.15–0.45
CSF/blood glucose (per cent)	55–105	44–248	60–90

Intraventricular haemorrhage/peri-ventricular haemorrhage(IVH/PVH) (Figs. 1.15–17)

Small haemorrhages remain confined to the subependymal germinal matrix areas (grade I) while larger haemorrhages rupture the ependyma and fill the ventricles and may lead to ventricular dilatation (grade II/III) (Table 1.13).

Large asymmetric intraparenchymal haemorrhages occur in the periventricular white matter mainly in the parietal region, but may extend from the frontal to occipital cortex. In more than 80 per cent of cases of intraparenchymal haemorrhage there is an associated intraventricular haemorrhage.

Ultrasound is not only extremely accurate in the documentation of IVH but is also essential in documenting progressive ventricular dilatation. Intraparenchymal haemorrhage with resultant tissue destruction and the development of

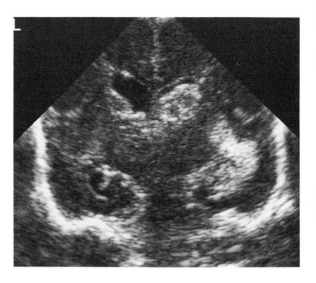

Fig. 1.16   Intraventricular haemorrhage. Coronal ultrasound of a premature infant shows a large left and a smaller right intraventricular haemorrhage with moderate dilatation of both ventricles. On the left there is haemorrhage extending into the parenchyma in the temporal lobe adjacent to the lateral ventricle.

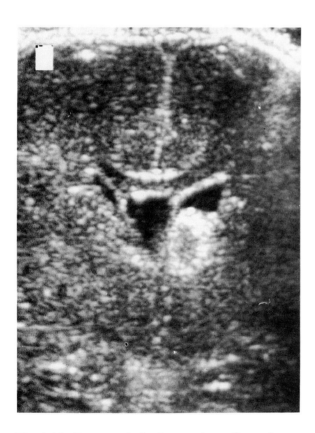

Fig. 1.15   Intraventricular haemorrhage. Coronal ultrasound of head in a premature infant shows a moderate sized left subependymal haemorrhage extending into the left lateral ventricle.

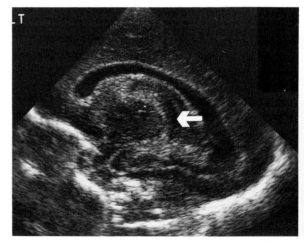

Fig. 1.17   Intraventricular haemorrhage. Left parasagittal ultrasound through the left lateral ventricle shows a resolving intraventricular haemorrhage (→). The resolving haemorrhage has a lower echogenicity than the more acute haemorrhages in Figures 1.15 and 1.16. A cast of the ventricle has formed at the time of the haemorrhage. Mild ventricular dilatation is evident.

porencephalic cysts is also well documented by serial scanning.

Periventricular leukomalacia (PVL) (Fig. 1.18)

Ultrasound is particularly useful in the detection of these watershed ischaemic injuries in periventricular white matter. PVL is seen as bilateral focal areas of increased echogenicity, either at the level of the frontal cerebral white matter adjacent to the superolateral angles of the ventricles or at the level of the optic radiation adjacent to the trigone of the lateral ventricle. Over two to three weeks after the appearance of echodensities, these areas may cavitate and form small cysts which do not communicate with the ventricles (cystic PVL). Small cysts may disappear ultrasonographically after 1–3 months; more extensive cystic necrosis of PVL may involve large areas of periventricular white matter.

Term asphyxia

In the term infant with hypoxic–ischaemic encephalopathy, ultrasound may show diffuse or focal areas of increased echogenicity. Florid echogenicity may involve the entire parenchyma with loss of normal anatomical landmarks. During the acute phase, diffuse increased echogenicity is usually associated with obliterated or slitlike ventricles due to cerebral oedema.

Follow–up sonography in HIE shows a variable degree of dilatation of the lateral ventricles and

Table 1.13 Classifying IVH and parenchymal echodensities. (Reproduced with permission from[135])

Class	Early scans	Late scans
Germinal matrix haemorrhage (GMH)	Grade 1 (1)	Germinal matrix cyst or complete resolution
Small intraventricular haemorrhage (IVH)	Grade 2a (2) GMH + IVH filling < 50 per cent of ventricle	Ventriculomegaly in 33 per cent; rarely posthaemorrhagic hydrocephalus
Large intraventricular haemorrhage	Grade 2b (3) GMH + IVH filling > 50 per cent of ventricle with ventricular dilation	Ventriculomegaly in 40 per cent; posthaemorrhagic hydrocephalus in 45 per cent
Intraparenchymal haemorrhage (IPH)	Grade 3 (4) bright triangular echodensity in white matter with its apex superolateral to the ventricle and its base toward the cortex merging with large IVH	Porencephalic cyst
Periventricular leukomalacia	Distinct triangular echodensity similar in appearance to IPH but less bright and separate from the ventricle	Cystic PVL
Flare	Diffuse echodensity parallel to the ventricle extending from the anterior horn to the atrium	Prolonged flare persists > 2 weeks to be significant
Intraparenchymal echodensity	Indistinct echodensity in the periventricular white matter	Resolves < 2 weeks = non-significant. May develop into cystic PVL or prolonged flare

Grades listed[135]; those in parentheses refer to the system of Papile sulci due to atrophy and the development of a degree of cystic encephalomalacia of the cerebral hemispheres. The cystic nature of these areas is better appreciated on sonography than on CT.

Focal areas of echogenicity are less frequently encountered in term asphyxia. The sites of focal lesions vary widely and include not only the cerebral hemispheres, but also the basal ganglia and thalami.

Although the vast majority of cranial sonographic studies are performed to determine the presence of haemorrhage and to follow the course of both haemorrhagic and hypoxic–ischaemic lesions of the brain, sonography is also able to define other

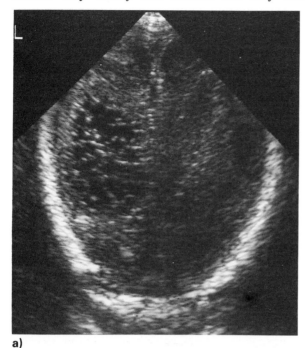

a)

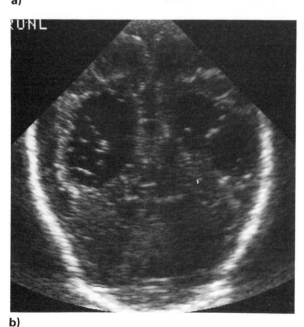

b)

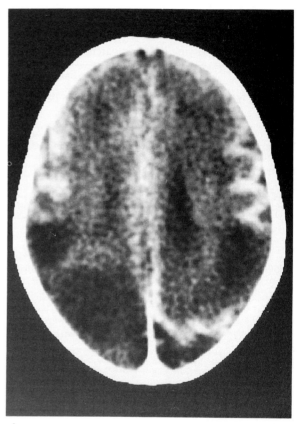

c)

Fig. 1.18 Periventricular leukomalacia. (a) Coronal ultrasound of the head through the occipital area shows leukomalacia on the right. Follow-up sonogram (b) shows an increase in the size of the cystic leukomalacia on the right and the development of similar changes on the left. Diffuse areas of low attenuation in the posterior parietal and occipital areas bilaterally (R > L) are seen on the CT scan (c).

pathological processes including congenital anomalies, tumours, infections (ventriculitis, abscess) and vascular and traumatic lesions.

Caveats to the usefulness of cranial sonography include difficulty in diagnosing posterior fossa haemorrhage, peripheral parenchymal haemorrhages and subarachnoid and subdural haemorrhages.

Duplex and colour Doppler ultrasound are being increasingly used because of their ability to visualize both the arterial and venous anatomy of the brain.

Computed tomography (CT) scanning

CT has a wide spectrum of application in the newborn with neurological disease, including intracranial haemorrhage, infarct (Fig. 1.19), hypoxic–ischaemic encephalopathy and congenital abnormalities of the central nervous system.

HIE in the term infant results in a diffuse change in the density of brain parenchyma, well detected on CT; in the preterm infant the decreased amount of myelin and relative increase in water make the detection of ischaemic lesions more difficult. Low attenuation or hypodense regions on CT do not, therefore, have the same prognostic significance as in the term infant.

Subdural, primary subarachnoid, intracerebellar and intraventricular haemorrhages are all readily identified on CT.

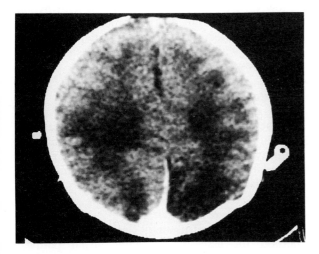

Fig. 1.19 Infarct. CT scan of the head shows areas of low attenuation mainly in the left posterior parietal and right mid parietal areas, consistent with infarcts in a term infant.

Focal cerebral infarction appears as a wedge-shaped, low attenuation area, usually best seen after the first three days of life if the insult occurred at the time of birth.

Magnetic resonance and ionic imaging

Magnetic resonance imaging (MRI) is a non–invasive procedure that provides information on both brain structure and function. To date, costs, availability, potential biological risks, the requirement for transport and the logistic difficulties in studying infants while being ventilated preclude

MRI scans are anatomical slices of the brain which provide great detail and enable subtle differences in grey and white matter density to be detected. The major indications for its use have been in the investigation of congenital CNS abnormalities, degenerative and demyelinating disorders, heterotopic grey matter, polymicrogyria and lissencephaly. Its role in acute brain injury has not been clearly defined, but it has been useful for evaluation of the sequelae of hypoxic–ischaemic lesions and in unusual seizure disorders.

MRI also provides a precise depiction of the location and extent of the white matter abnormalities of PVL beyond the neonatal period, and is useful in studying the progression and degree of myelination in the first months of life in very low birthweight infants.[137,.138]

Ionic imaging provides functional scans of brain chemistry and metabolism. Two methods of assessing brain oxygenation and haemodynamics have been utilized:[139,140]

1. MRS has been used to measure the concentration in brain tissue of phosphorus metabolites which are dependent for their synthesis on oxidative metabolism. Other metabolites such as lactate and neurotransmitters can also be measured.
2. Near infrared spectroscopy provides continuous information about cerebral oxygenation (both oxygen delivery and utilization) and haemodynamics, which is complementary to the information obtained by MRS.

    Measurement can also be made of cerebral blood flow, cerebral blood volume and other haemodynamic indices, providing a unique opportunity to observe cerebral cellular respiration on a minute–to–minute basis.

Electroencephalography (EEG)

It has often been difficult in the past to obtain EEG studies readily in the sick newborn because of limited access to the bedside, technical factors related to the application of multiple electrodes in small, sick and unstable infants, and electrical interference from surrounding electronic equipment. In addition the difficulties in interpretation of EEG findings tended to limit studies in newborn infants. However, the availability of portable monitoring equipment, greater reliability in interpretation and the increasing appreciation of the valuable information this investigation may yield has led to an increased demand for these studies in the NICU. Polygraphic recording of other variables including respiration, airflow, heart rate, muscle and eye movement, as well as transcutaneous oxygen and carbon dioxide changes at the time of the EEG recording, provide further physiological information. EEG and video recording of infants is a recent additional technique used in difficult diagnostic situations.

While the EEG has traditionally been used for the detection, characterization, localization and quantitation of seizures and the evaluation of the adequacy of anticonvulsant therapy, it may provide information in other clinical situations, e.g. infants with asphyxia who may not have demonstrated seizures, other high-risk infants without overt neurological signs or infants in whom CNS signs may be masked by their being paralyzed and ventilated. In addition, the ability of the EEG to detect the presence and character of maturational phenomena e.g., sleep–wake cycles has led to the increasing use of the EEG in premature infants.[141]

EEG findings

Periodic discharges confirm seizures in term infants or the presence of structural lesions in both term and preterm infants. Continuous EEG recordings have shown a high frequency of electrical seizures in infants without clinical manifestations.[120,143] The significance of these electrical seizures without clinically observable alterations in neonatal motor or behavioural function is uncertain.

As the EEG generally reflects functional impairment of the brain, EEG findings are generally non–specific from an aetiological perspective, although certain characteristic patterns have been described in premature infants with intraventricular haemorrhage in pyridoxine dependency , and in infants with periventricular leukomalacia.[144–6]

The significance of the background EEG activity with or without seizures has also been emphasized.[142,147] Normal background activity is usually associated with a normal clinical outcome whereas infants with excessively slow background activity rarely have a normal outcome.[142]

Despite difficulties in interpretation and the wide range of morphological characteristics of seizure activity, both the degree and duration of EEG abnormality are strongly predictive of outcome.[142,148] Early isoelectric, markedly low amplitude or burst suppression patterns are strong predictors of very poor outcome, whereas infants with acute neurological events and normal EEGs within one to two weeks usually have a more favourable outcome.

Evoked potentials

Evoked potentials represent cortical responses to external stimuli and can assess objectively and quantitatively the maturity and integrity of specific sensory pathways. The presence or absence of specific waves and their latencies are the main features used in these assessments.

Brain stem auditory evoked responses

These average and record electrical changes occurring along the auditory pathway and centres within the brainstem, in response to repeated auditory stimuli. They have been widely used in low birthweight infants and those with hypoxic–ischaemic encephalopathy, hyperbilirubinaemia, congenital infections and meningitis, as well as in infants with a family history of sensorineural hearing loss.

Somatosensory potentials

These are evoked by percutaneous stimulation of peripheral nerves and recorded in the contralateral parietal cortex, thereby assessing the afferent pathway passing through the periventricular region of the lateral ventricle and in close proximity to the pyramidal tract.

Visual evoked potentials

The response to diffuse light flashes is the simplest method for assessing neonatal visual pathway function and these have been used particularly in infants with hypoxic–ischaemic insults and in posthaemorrhagic hydrocephalus.

Evoked potentials have increasing clinical application as normative data at various gestational ages, postnatal maturational changes and the sensitivity and specificity in different neonatal conditions become established.[149,150] The variability of single recordings, however, implies that serial recordings should be performed to be of prognostic significance in the individual infant.

Renal function

Renal physiology in the newborn

The neonatal kidney has often been regarded as immature, but comparison with the adult kidney assumes that these neonatal and adult organs have similar tasks to perform. This is clearly not so, if only because of the effect of growth. Approximately 50 per cent of dietary nitrogen in the newborn is incorporated into new tissue, thus relieving the kidney of half of its excretory load. As will be seen below, the neonatal kidney appears to be well able to cope with the work it is normally required to perform, although it is less well equipped to counter the effects of severe dehydration, excessive water or solute load, trauma and acidosis.

During intrauterine life the human fetal kidney receives only between 3–7 per cent of the cardiac output, compared with approximately 20 per cent in the adult.[151] After an initial rapid rise in renal blood flow in the first few weeks of life, the rate of increased blood flow is more gradual and mature levels are not reached until about two years of age. This may account for the fact that neonates suffering from birth asphyxia or severe dehydration are particularly vulnerable to renal vascular insults such as venous thrombosis. The postnatal increase in renal blood flow (RBF) is due to a combination of decreased renal vascular resistance and increased cardiac output and mean arterial blood pressure. RBF is affected by changes in circulating levels of catecholamines and prostaglandins and the prostaglandin inhibitor indomethacin has been shown to cause a decrease in RBF.[152] Dopamine on the other hand increases RBF by vasodilatation of the renal vessels.

The kidneys produce dilute urine from as early as the third month of intrauterine life, although the excretory and regulatory requirements of the fetus are satisfactorily carried out by the placenta. The only known function of the fetal kidney is the maintenance of amniotic fluid volume; renal agenesis may lead to oligohydramnios and compres-

sion deformities. It is important to consider the possibility of absent kidneys in newborn babies with pneumothorax and pulmonary hypoplasia where amniotic fluid deficit may prevent proper maturation of the lungs. The contribution the kidneys make to fetal homoeostasis must, however, be small as infants born with absent kidneys may have normal plasma electrolytes, urea and creatinine. It is only at birth that the kidney must take up its role of excretion of the nitrogenous end-products of metabolism and play its part in stabilizing the volume, osmotic pressure and chemical composition of extracellular fluid.

Glomerular function

The low glomerular filtration rate (GFR) at birth increases in parallel with the changes in renal blood flow in the first weeks of life. While this applies to infants beyond 34 weeks gestational age in whom nephrogenesis has been completed, in younger infants structural immaturity limits the kidney's initial ability to increase function despite the postnatal increase in renal blood flow.[153,154] The increase in GFR continues until growth ceases, although on the basis of body surface area adult levels are reached between one and two years of age.

At birth, the glomeruli are smaller than in the adult, but their filtration surface in relation to body weight is similar. The tubules are not fully grown and may not extend into the medulla.

Tubular function

The ability of the neonatal kidney to modulate fluid and electrolyte balance depends largely, as in the adult, on tubular function.

Sodium balance

Renal tubular control of sodium is one of the

primary homoeostatic functions of the kidney. The term infant is able to conserve sodium under physiological conditions whereas the premature infant, particularly if less than 32 weeks, is considered a 'salt loser' and often demonstrates a negative sodium balance with high urinary sodium excretion rates after birth.[154]

Sodium conservation via tubular reabsorption is altered by hypoxia, hyperbilirubinaemia and intrinsic renal disease, with consequent increased sodium excretion and hyponatraemia. Urinary sodium losses are thus very common even in preterm infants with relatively uncomplicated neonatal courses and may be considerable during the diuretic phase following relief of urinary obstruction.[156] Beyond 34 weeks gestation the tubular reabsorptive capacity appears sufficient to maintain a positive sodium balance.

Sodium loading may exceed the kidneys' capacity to excrete sodium and result in hypernatraemia, fluid retention and oedema in the term infant. The premature infant has an even more blunted natriuretic response to sodium loading because of the inability to redirect renal blood flow toward the more mature salt losing nephrons in the cortex.[157] Adverse effects of sodium loading similar to those in the term infant will occur; in addition the opening up of a patent ductus arteriosus or the potentiation of an intracranial haemorrhage secondary to hypertonicity is of concern in these premature infants.

Potassium balance

The renal contribution to potassium homoeostasis is primarily a result of potassium secretion or reabsorption in distal nephrons. This is affected by many factors in the newborn including the low GFR with poor delivery of filtrate to the distal tubule, decreased tubular function with low aldosterone sensitivity, increased sodium losses and decreased potassium excretion, and leakage of potassium from cells due to the lower intracellular pH. This may lead to hyperkalaemia, particularly in extremely low birthweight infants.

Potassium levels are high at birth and well tolerated. Values greater than 6 mmol.l^{-1} can occur without changes in the ECG and without treatment necessarily being required. Such high levels would of course give rise to concern and levels above 5 mmol.l^{-1} demand investigation. Serum potassium levels fall gradually in the first 48 hours of life, but mainly because of a shift into the cells with correction of acidosis rather than by renal excretion.

Other solutes

The neonate has been shown to be similar to the older child in its tubular reabsorption relation to GFR. It has, however, poor reabsorption of filtered amino acids and the renal bicarbonate threshold is low. The restrained GFR probably prevents overperfusion of the poorly developed tubules and limits the loss of sodium and water, especially in response to water loading.

Water balance: concentration and dilution

The ability of the neonatal kidney to concentrate urine in response to water deprivation is less than in the adult. In the first week of life the neonate cannot concentrate urine much above 600 mmol.l^{-1}; even when no water has been given for three days following birth, concentrations above 500 mmol.l^{-1} are seldom reached. Diminished urinary concentrating ability in the neonatal kidney may be due in part to the low dietary protein intake which results in less urea availability for the medullary concentrating gradient. Alternatively, high levels of prostaglandins may be the cause. PGE$_2$ inhibits sodium transport into the medullary interstitium, and interferes with urea absorption also. Prostacyclin increases medullary blood flow and washes out the underlying medullary interstitial concentration gradient.

The limited capacity to concentrate urine in the term infant is further exaggerated in the premature. With maturation, concentrating ability improves, although high solute loads should be avoided and adequate free water always administered in the early neonatal period. The urine concentrating capacity reaches adult levels by two years of age.

The ability of the newborn kidney to excrete dilute urine in response to a water load is disputed. Some studies have shown that both term and preterm infants can produce urine with an osmolality of as low as 30 mosm.l^{-1},[158] whilst others have demonstrated water retention in low birthweight infants given high fluid intakes.[159]

Acid-base balance

The renal tubules' capacity to reabsorb filtered bicarbonate is reduced in the newborn with a consequent low bicarbonate threshold (i.e. the serum level at which bicarbonate appears in the urine). The tubule is also limited in its ability to excrete fixed acid. This may explain the relatively high urinary pH, ± 6, in the first few days of life. As tubular reabsorption of bicarbonate improves and the excretion of urea, ammonium and hydrogen ions increase, the urine pH is lowered to 5 or less. After the first few days of life the ability to acidify the urine is normal, but the excretion of titratable acid is low due to low phosphate excretion and ammonium excretion is reduced in proportion to GFR. During acidosis only a modest increase in acid excretion is possible, resulting in the rapid development of acidaemia in response to only a small increase in hydrogen ions. A persistently high urinary pH is seen in severe renal disease or renal tubular acidosis. (The urinary pH should always be evaluated in relation to plasma bicarbonate values. In term infants these are between 19–21 mmol.l^{-1} and only achieve a value of 24 by one year of age; in premature infants even lower values are considered normal.[160])

Extrarenal factors affecting neonatal metabolism

Growth
By the end of the first week of life, the normal term neonate on a diet of breast milk may be consuming 2 g protein kgBw^{-1}.day^{-1}. The growing infant, however, incorporates about 50 per cent of this protein into body tissues, together with water, phosphate, potassium and other substances. The phenomenon of growth thus relieves the kidney of some of its excretory load: growth has been described as 'the third kidney'.

Clinical Assessment of renal function

The functional reserve of the newborn kidney, and in particular that of the premature infant, is easily overcome by a number of neonatal disorders and assessment of renal function is therefore an essential part of the management of any sick or premature infant.

History

Abnormality of the renal system should be suspected when a history of any of the following is obtained:

Maternal oligohydramnios
From the time that fetal metanephric structures are identifiable (12th week of gestation), the fetal kidney produces urine into the amniotic fluid; therefore, a history of decreased amniotic fluid (if not due to chronic cervical leakage) should lead to the suspicion of renal agenesis, dysplasia or obstruction of the fetal urinary tract. In addition, the production of urine and its contribution to amniotic fluid is a critical factor in the growth and development of the lungs; thus, pulmonary insufficiency or hypoplasia in the newborn is commonly associated with renal agenesis or dysplasia. (The detection of oligohydramnios during pregnancy may have resulted in fetal ultrasound examination and identification of a renal malformation; in fact advances in fetal ultrasound have significantly altered the patient population: many infants are now referred with asymptomatic or non–clinically detectable renal abnormalities following fetal ultrasound diagnoses.)

Maternal drugs
Antihypertensive agents, indomethacin before delivery or cocaine use during pregnancy may have adverse effects on the newborn kidney.[161,162]

Family history of renal disease
The infantile or adult form of polycystic disease, the Finnish form of congenital nephrotic syndrome and nephrogenic diabetes insipidus may present at birth. In addition, a history of a previous sibling with a dysmorphic syndrome may suggest a renal abnormality.

Delay in voiding
More than 90 per cent of infants void within the first 24 hours of life; by 48 hours 99 per cent of newborns have voided at least once. Failure to pass urine within 24–48 hours of birth should suggest the inability to produce urine secondary to renal agenesis, an obstructive uropathy or severe acute tubular or cortical necrosis.

Abnormal urinary stream
The urinary stream of a newborn is usually continuous; a weak, intermittent or dribbling stream suggests urethral valves, congenital stricture of the urethra, a ureterocele or a neurogenic bladder. With lesser degrees of obstructive uropathy an infant may void normally.

Perinatal distress/oliguria
Although urine output is normally low on the first day of life (15–60 ml.kg^{-1}) and increases

thereafter (25–125 ml.kg^{-1}.day), a urine volume of < 1 ml.kg^{-1}.h in a sick or stressed newborn should be actively monitored. Perinatal asphyxia, hypotension or haemorrhage may lead to decreased perfusion to the kidneys with the redistribution of cardiac output; oliguria is a sensitive marker of the extent of neurological involvement in perinatal asphyxia and has been significantly correlated with neurological outcome.[163]

Physical examination

Many dysmorphic and chromosomal syndromes are associated with renal abnormalities; a complete general examination with particular attention to the facies, the ears and grouping of minor dysmorphic signs may lead to specific syndrome identification. In the fetal compression syndrome (Potter's) the infant characteristically has low set ears, a flattened nose, dimpled chin, marked epicanthal creases, contractures and malpositioning of the extremities. Renal abnormalities are also commonly associated with the Vater, Vacterl, Von Hippel–Lindau and many other syndromes.

Blood pressure
Measurement of the blood pressure, while routine in the sick newborn in the NICU, is often neglected in the standard physical examination of newborns. It should always, however, be part of the evaluation of an infant with suspected vascular or parenchymal renal disease. Blood pressure measurements are easily and accurately obtained by oscillometry devices or via direct intra–arterial indwelling catheters. BP values vary according to birthweight, postnatal age, the infant's state and the size of the blood pressure cuff. All these factors must be taken into account when evaluating the significance of an elevated measurement.

Systemic hypertension has been defined as a systolic and diastolic pressure > 90 and 60 mmHg respectively in the term infant, and > 80 and 50 mmHg in the preterm infant.[164] Many hypertensive infants are clinically asymptomatic and do not show evidence of renal insufficiency, congestive heart failure or neurological signs.

Oedema
The accumulation of excess extracellular fluid in subcutaneous tissues is abnormal in a term infant, but may be seen in premature infants without serious underlying disease due to excess body fluid (prior to physiological diuresis), increased capillary permeability and low colloid osmotic pressure.

Mild to moderate oedema due to either volume overload or fluid retention is often seen in sick infants whose renal or cardiac function has been compromised by asphyxia, hypotension, respiratory distress or congenital heart disease. It may also be seen less commonly in severe hypoproteinaemia due to poor nutrition, liver failure or protein–losing enteropathy.

Abdominal wall musculature
Abnormality of the musculature of the abdominal wall is seen in the prune belly (triad) syndrome: the skin appears wrinkled and hangs in folds. Renal abnormalities include megaloureter, cystic renal dysplasia and urethral obstruction.

Single Umbilical Artery
The umbilical cord (or placenta) should be examined for the presence of two umbilical arteries: infants with a single umbilical artery have an increased incidence of associated congenital malformations, most commonly affecting the genitourinary, musculoskeletal and cardiovascular systems. The relatively high yield of renal malformations and the ease of renal ultrasonography suggest that this examination is indicated in all such infants.[165]

Abdominal Examination
This should be specific for palpation of the kidneys, abdominal masses and the detection of ascitic fluid.

The kidneys are normally palpable in the newborn; the left is more easily felt than the right. Enlarged kidneys may be indicative of many renal disorders including renal vein thrombosis, acute cortical or medullary necrosis or cystic abnormalities. The distinction between an enlarged and a normal but easily felt kidney is often difficult and usually requires ultrasound examination for elucidation.

The majority of abdominal masses are of genitourinary origin. Hydronephrosis, the most common abdominal mass in the newborn, usually presents as a unilateral, soft and often cystic round mass. Bilateral masses in a male infant in the presence of a distended bladder suggest posterior urethral valves; in a female infant ureteroceles are more likely. Multicystic, dysplastic kidneys are usually unilateral and cystic or lobulated, whereas bilateral large symmetric firm masses, in the absence of a distended bladder, suggest infantile polycystic kidney disease. Renal venous thrombosis is suggested by the finding of an enlarged, firm, smooth kidney in association with haematuria, anaemia, thrombocytopaenia or renal failure. Adrenal haemorrhage is usually unilateral (right side more common) and presents as a flank mass with renal impairment. Other masses include mesoblastic nephroma, teratoma, neuroblastoma or a Wilm's tumour.

Newborn infants with obstructive urinary tract disorders (particularly posterior urethral valves) occasionally develop urinary ascites; this is thought to originate from a ruptured calyx or renal pelvis.

The External Genitalia

This requires careful examination of the urethral meatus, the presence of gonads and inguinal hernias, to detect hypospadias, epispadias, cryptorchidism, ambiguous genitalia or other associated anomalies. As the external genitalia are formed later in gestation than the upper urinary tract, the association between abnormalities of the external genitalia and renal abnormalities is infrequent.

Examination of the Placenta

Placental examination enables an immediate diagnosis of renal agenesis to be made by the detection of amnion nodosum; these small (1–5 mm) whitish specks on the fetal surface of the placenta are thought to be due to abrasion of keratinized fetal epithelium against the amnion, which adheres to the placental surface in the absence of fetal urine.

Laboratory assessment of renal function

Glomerular function

Serum creatinine

The serum creatinine is the simplest method for estimating glomerular function. At birth it reflects maternal levels; it then falls over the first few days of life with the increase in GFR and thereafter is stable at less than 45 mmol.l^{-1} in term infants. The number of factors affecting serum creatinine (maternal level, gestational age, fluid balance and muscle mass) make serial creatinine measurements imperative to estimate changes in renal function and glomerular filtration rate. In any newborn infant a significant increase in plasma creatinine concentration after the first day or two of life is abnormal (Table 1.14).

Blood urea

This depends on urinary flow rate, the level of hydration, protein intake and tissue catabolism and is not as reliable a measure of intrinsic renal function as the serum creatinine. Values in the newborn are higher than in older children and range between 2.9–10.00 mmol.l^{-1}.

Table 1.14 Median values of plasma creatinine: Normal ranges for infants form 28 to 40 weeks gestational age over first 28 days of life. (Reproduced with permission from[155])

Gestation (weeks)	Postnatal age (days)						
	2	2	2	7	14	21	28
	All babies	Breathing spontaneously	Ventilated	All babies			
28	116±40 (n=24)	108±20 (n=8)	121±45 (n=16)	84±32 (n=22)	72±32 (n=25)	60±33 n=25)	58±24 (n=24)
29–32	104±38 (n=50)	100±32 (n=36)	115±43 (n=16)	83±41 (n=56)	69±32 (n=42)	59±32 (n=29)	52±33 (n=30)
33–36	93±39 (n=36)	94±39 (n=32)	87±46 (n=4)	68±44 (n=31)	55±36 (n=27)	50±37 (n=20)	35±24 (n=12)
37–42	75±38 (n=27)	75±38 (n=27)		50±36 (n=39)	38±20 (n=19)	35±20 (n=19)	30±18 (n=15)

Mean plasma creatinine μmol.l^{-1}±2 SD.
Conversion SI to traditional units: 1 μmol.l^{-1} = 0.0113 mg/100 ml.

Tubular function

Estimation of the serum sodium and fractional excretion of sodium (FENa) are both extremely useful indicators of tubular function in the newborn.[160] FENa reflects the percentage of filtered sodium excreted in the urine and is calculated from the plasma and urine sodium and creatinine concentrations as follows:

$$FENa = \frac{urine\ sodium/serum\ sodium}{urine\ sodium/serum\ creatinine} \times 100$$

Term infants, after the first few days of life, are in positive Na balance, conserve Na efficiently and their FENa is < 0.5 per cent. Premature infants do not conserve sodium as efficiently and values of 5 per cent or higher may be seen in VLBW infants.

Serum potassium levels must be closely monitored and assessed in conjunction with urine flow rate and other indices of renal function.

Urine volume and osmolality

Urine output is low on day 1 due to the low GFR; from day 2–3 a diuresis and natriuresis occur with an increase in GFR and FENa. By day 4 GFR and FENa start to vary appropriately with intake and consequently urine output varies with fluid and electrolyte intake in a predictable manner.[166] Urine volume should be at least 1–2 ml.kg.$^{-1}$.hr after the first day. Although the rate of urine excretion cannot be used on its own to assess renal function (as renal failure can occur with a normal or even increased urine flow rate), it should be very accurately measured in all infants prone to the development of prerenal or renal azotaemia.

Urine osmolality is usually monitored by measuring urine specific gravity as there is a close correlation between these two measurements.[167] The range of urine concentration in the term newborn is 40–800 mmol.kg^{-1} H$_2$O corresponding to a urinary specific gravity of 1.001–1.020. The specific gravity in the premature is normally in the range of 1.002–1.010. In general the specific gravity provides an easy assessment of the functional concentrating reserve of the newborn kidney; serial measurements are particularly useful in the assessment of a response to a volume load. Molecules such as glucose and protein do affect the specific gravity and will substantially overestimate urine osmolality; therefore critical clinical decisions

regarding fluid management may occasionally require direct measurement of urine osmolality. This is particularly relevant in the evaluation of fluid requirements in infants with oliguria and oedema in the presence of prerenal azotaemia.

Urinalysis

Changes in urine composition occur with either primary genitourinary disease or systemic illness. Urinalysis should be routine for all infants in a neonatal ICU; it requires careful collection and interpretation of the following:

Colour

Urine in the newborn is normally pale, although the presence of uric acid crystals occasionally gives it a slightly pink tinge. A negative haematest will differentiate urates from red blood cells. Dark urine occurs in hyperbilirubinaemia and a smoky appearance may be indicative of haematuria.

Red blood cells

The dipstick readily detects free haemoglobin, myoglobin and intact red cells. Haemoglobinuria may occur with haematuria and therefore examination of fresh urine is required to distinguish haemolytic disease with free haemoglobin from intact red blood cells in the urine. Transient microscopic haematuria may be quite common in the premature infant, but the persistent finding of red cells in newborn urine is not normal and an underlying explanation should always be sought. Haematuria occurs in infants with shock, asphyxia, renal tubular or papillary necrosis, renal venous or arterial thrombi or as a manifestation of a generalized bleeding disorder.

White blood cells

A few white blood cells, up to 5 per high powered field, may be normal. Contamination of a urine specimen is very frequent and therefore the significance of bacterial colony counts is dependent upon the method of collection. In a regularly voided specimen less than 50 000 colonies per millimetre is not significant, whereas in a clean–catch specimen in a male infant in whom the urethral meatus has been thoroughly cleaned, these findings are suggestive of infection. Catheterization of the bladder is often traumatic and infection may be introduced by this means.

Suprapubic aspiration of the bladder is the

optimal means of obtaining uncontaminated urine for cell count, Gram stain, culture and bacterial antigen detection. A suprapubic specimen is not routinely indicated in the work–up of an infant with early onset infection since the yield is very low; in late onset or nosocomial infection it is an important component of the investigation as even small numbers of bacterial colony counts in a properly performed procedure may be indicative of infection.

Protein

Transient mild proteinuria may be seen in normal infants in the first few days of life. It is also seen in premature infants with asphyxia, congestive heart failure, dehydration and urinary tract infection. More significant proteinuria occurs in nephrotic syndrome or renal tubular disorders.

Glucose

The dipstick with glucose oxidase coating is specific for the detection of glucose; a small amount of glycosuria may be seen in normal newborn infants because of the low tubular maximum reabsorption threshold. However, glycosuria may be an indication of an osmotic diuresis and lead to dehydration, particularly in premature infants on a high intravenous glucose intake. Glycosuria may also be an early sign of neonatal sepsis.

Special Investigations

Diagnostic Imaging

Radiological studies play an extremely important role in the elucidation of renal disorders in the newborn.

Ultrasonography (Fig. 1.20)

This has become the primary method for imaging of the genitourinary system; it is non-invasive, does not have the potential hazards of intravenous contrast material or ionizing radiation and can be performed at the bedside. Images of the renal parenchyma, collecting system and blood flow can easily be obtained irrespective of kidney function. It is generally used as the first study; it may be definitive in itself or it may determine what studies are required for further investigation of specific conditions.

Ultrasound can readily determine kidney size

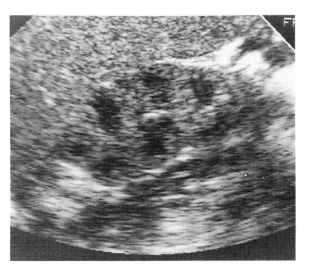

Fig. 1.20 Normal kidney. Longitudinal sonogram of the right kidney shows normal corticomedullary differentiation. The medullary pyramids appear echo poorer (blacker) than adjacent more echogenic cortex.

and position, the echogenicity of the medulla and cortex, the size of the collecting system and the nature and origin of other abdominal masses. Spectral and colour Doppler sonography facilitates evaluation of arterial and venous flow patterns.

Ultrasound should be considered in the following clinical situations:

1. The newborn with a prenatal diagnosis of urinary tract abnormality: significant changes noted antenatally need to be studied in the immediate postnatal period (Fig. 1.21). However, milder degrees of antenatal distension of the collecting system might be underestimated due to the low urine output in the first 1–2 days of life, and should therefore be studied after diuresis is established.
2. Dysmorphic infants, or those with anomalies identified in other systems, to identify associated renal malformations (Fig. 1.22).
3. Infants with a history of oligohydramnios, spontaneous pneumothorax or other clinical evidence of unexplained pulmonary insufficiency.
4. To demonstrate renal vascular accidents following hypovolaemia, polycythaemia or dehydration or in infants of diabetic mothers. Sonography may identify renal venous or IVC thrombosis, renal arterial thrombi or occasionally aortic thrombi following umbilical arterial

catheterization. Doppler ultrasound may aid in this regard. Serial examination may show the progression of renal venous thrombi in the renal parenchyma out into the major veins and IVC; it may also document progressive changes in the parenchyma with atrophy in severely affected infants.

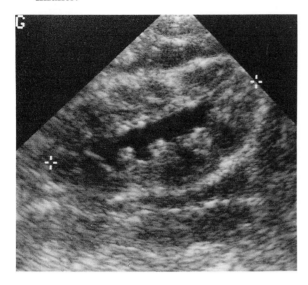

Fig. 1.21 Mild hydronephrosis. Longitudinal sonogram of the right kidney (between cursors) showing an echo-free (black) mildly dilated pelvicalyceal system in the central part of the kidney. The parenchymal volume remains normal. Similar pelvicalyceal changes can be seen with vesicoureteric reflux.

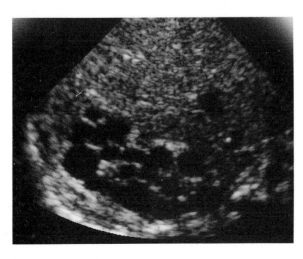

Fig. 1.22 Multicystic/dysplastic kidney. Transverse sonogram of the right kidney shows the parenchyma replaced by multiple cysts of varying sizes.

5. Following perinatal asphyxia or other precipitating events leading to renal failure: changes in the echogenicity of the renal cortex or medulla have been described in cortical necrosis and acute tubular necrosis respectively; sequential scanning may document a return to normal or progression with subsequent limited renal growth.
6. Infants with unexplained sepsis, prolonged jaundice or documented urinary tract infection to rule out underlying anatomic abnormalities of the renal tract.
7. To demonstrate nephrocalcinosis secondary to prolonged diuretic therapy.

Radionuclide imaging

Radionuclide imaging is an excellent method of assessing renal function and complements the information obtained by ultrasonography. Poorly functioning kidneys can be visualized with Technetium-99m-diethylenetriaminepenta acetic acid scans (DTPA). This study evaluates flow to the kidneys, provides a quantitative assessment of the GFR of each kidney, and determines drainage into the lower urinary tract.

Voiding Cystourethrogram

This is the preferred method for imaging the lower urinary tract to outline the bladder and urethra and in diagnosing the presence and degree of vesicoureteral reflux. Modification of the VCUG or genitography is used in infants with ambiguous genitalia and lower tract anomalies; this may involve selective catheterization of orifices and careful fluoroscopic injection of water soluble contrast material.

IVP (excretory urography)

IVP is not particularly useful to evaluate the renal parenchyma and the collecting system because of the low filtration rate and the poor concentrating ability of the newborn. It has a place in the evaluation of complex obstructive uropathy, but generally after ultrasound and renal scans have been performed. The high osmotic load of contrast media may produce dehydration.

Angiography

This is rarely used to evaluate the renal vasculature in newborn infants, but isotope blood flow studies and Doppler sonography demonstrate flow abnormalities without the hazards of angiography.

Normal water and electrolyte metabolism

Total body water

The total body water content of the newborn neonate is proportionately higher than the adult, due principally to a relative excess of extracellular fluid (Fig. 1.23). Normal babies receive little fluid for the first few days after birth until lactation becomes established, and during the first 72 hours after birth there is usually a weight loss of 5–10 per cent of body weight.

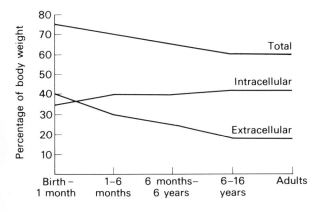

Fig. 1.23 Distribution of total, intracellular and extracellular water, expressed as a percentage of body weight related to age. (Reproduced with permission from [168]).

During this period of restricted food intake a negative balance develops for electrolytes (sodium, potassium, chloride), calories and nitrogen as well as water.[169]

As fluid intake gradually increases after the first 3–4 days of life there is a transition from negative to positive balance, though body weight usually continues to fall. By the end of the first week of extrauterine life with full feeding established there is a gradual increase in body weight.

These changes are summarized in Table 1.15 though the duration and severity of the changes, particularly during phase I, depend on the degree of stress which accompanies labour and delivery, and on the caloric intake; all three phases may be prolonged in premature infants.[170]

Insensible water loss (IWL)

Insensible water loss (IWL) refers to that water which is lost through the skin by passive evaporation and from the respiratory tract. IWL estimates are given in Table 1.16.

Very high insensible water losses from the skin occur in extremely premature infants with their decreased subcutaneous fat tissue, thin epidermal barrier to water diffusion and relative increase in surface area.[171–2] Newborn infants of less than 26 weeks gestation may have insensible water losses as great as 200 ml.kg^{-1}day.[173] These infants are significantly affected by the ambient humidity and airflow velocity; maintaining the ambient humidity high, for example, may reduce evaporative water loss and enable fluid intake to be kept low, particularly on the first to third day of life.[172]

Insensible water loss increases during exposure to radiant energy from overhead heaters and also during phototherapy. The increase with radiant heaters varies from 50 to 200 per cent, depending on the maturity of the infant and the type of heater used; water loss during phototherapy can be minimised by careful temperature control of the infant. Insensible water loss also increases during pyrexia, when environmental temperature is excessively high, as in the tropics, and will be affected by changes in the humidity of ambient air, although the magnitude of such changes in normal circumstances is relatively small. Water loss in the faeces is also usually small, except in the presence of diarrhoea.

Respiratory water losses do not appear to be as dependent on the maturity of the infant, but are more affected by the temperature and humidity of the inspired air, the infant's minute ventilation and the ability of the upper airway to dehumidify and cool the expiratory air.[174]

Response to surgery

In adults there is a well-defined metabolic response to surgery and trauma, including rapid utilization of glycogen stores, protein breakdown and the release of antidiuretic and adrenocortical hormones, causing water and salt retention. This is also seen in the newborn, particularly after fetal distress or birth trauma.

Recent work by Anand and others has shown that the metabolic response of neonates to the stress of cardiac and non-cardiac surgery is significantly greater than that of adults.[175–8] This metabolic

Table 1.15 Metabolic responses of a healthy newborn infant. (Reproduced with permission from[169])

Variable	Phase I	Phase II	Phase III
Age	0–3 days	3–7 days	7 days
Intake milk	None	Increasing breast milk	Full breast
Body weight	Decrease★	Further decrease★	Increase★
N metabolism balance	Negative balance	Transition to positive balance	Positive
K+ metabolism balance	Negative balance	Transition to positive balance	Positive
Na+ metabolism	Negative balance	Transition to positive balance	± Balance★
H₂O metabolism Balance★	Negative balance (oliguria)	Negative balance (diuresis)	±
Caloric metabolism	Negative balance	Transition to positive balance	Positive

★Balance may be slightly positive or slightly negative on any given day, but overall effect is slightly positive. In preterm infants all three phases can last longer and have more profound changes.[169]

Table 1.16 Insensible water loss (Modified from [169])

Birthweight (gm)	ml.kg⁻¹.day
<1000	60–70
1000–1500	30–65
1500–2500	15–30
>2500	10–15

response, which can be blunted either by the use of high dose opioids or by inhalational anaesthesia, has a variable effect on sodium and potassium balance, probably as a result of variation in renal responses, variable fluid and electrolyte regimens and concurrent drug therapy.

In acute renal damage the kidneys tend to retain salt and water because of the reduced GFR, although in chronic renal disease such as renal dysplasia, where salt and water retention is diminished, the antiduiretic response to surgery is not seen.

Thermoregulation

The ability of the neonate to regulate body temperature in a hostile environment is significantly limited compared with the older child and adult. As with many aspects of neonatal physiology, thermal regulation is less mature in preterm than term infants.

There are several reasons why heat balance in a new born infant can be seriously affected by environmental temperature. The surface area/weight ratio is approximately three times that of the adult, thermal conductance is increased and shivering thermogenesis is poorly developed.

Both the term and premature neonate are capable of vasoconstriction and vasodilatation[179] together with behavioural movements such as the adoption of nestling or huddling positions, but these processes can only compensate for a limited range of changes in environmental temperature. Term neonates can also increase evaporative heat losses by sweating in response to a warm environment, a response which gradually develops from 30 weeks gestational age onwards. Infants who are small for gestational age are capable of sweat production appropriate for this age though the onset of sweating is slower. The shivering mechanism, which in the adult is the main mechanism for heat production, is also less well developed in the neonate, even when term.

Heat Production

The main mechanism of heat production in the newborn is chemical non-shivering thermogenesis. This occurs principally through metabolism of brown fat, but can also occur in skeletal muscle and other tissue. Around 10 per cent of total body fat in the term neonate is located in the brown fat stores found at the base of the neck, in the axillae, between the scapulae, in the mediastinum and around the adrenal glands or kidneys. Morphologically, brown fat contains multinucleated cells with numerous mitochondria which appear densely packed with cristae and have increased respiratory chain components.[180] Brown fat has an abundant blood supply and rich innervation from the sympathetic nervous system.

Cold exposure releases noradrenaline at sympathetic nerve endings, depolarizes the cell membrane and, by activating adenylcyclases, increases the circulating level of 3'5'-cyclic AMP. This in turn activates protein kinases which enhance the action of hormone-sensitive lipase, causing hydrolysis of triglyceride stores to free fatty acid and glycerol. In addition to noradrenaline, glucocorticoids and thyroxine may also play a part in non-shivering thermogenesis.[181–3] Non-shivering thermogenesis can be inhibited pharmacologically by beta-blockade or surgically by sympathectomy. The extra calories produced by oxidation of triglycerides from brown fat stores have been shown to be capable of maintaining the cold-induced increase in heat production evoked by an environmental temperature of 25°C for about 3 days in the term baby.

Additional sites of heat production include the brain and liver where hepatic glucose production occurring by glycogenolysis provides the main source of energy.

Anaesthesia and hypoxia may interfere with thermal regulation in the newborn, though the mechanisms by which this interference occurs are unclear. Engleman and Lockhart[184] reported that halothane decreases rectal temperature more than pethidine, though Holdcroft and Hall[185] failed to demonstrate significant differences in heat loss between patients receiving either halothane or fentanyl in conjunction with nitrous oxide and oxygen. In studies on newborn rabbits by Nour *et al*.[186] the thermogenic response to a cold stress was similar regardless of whether the animals received general anaesthesia with pentobarbitone or local anaesthesia with lignocaine. Ryan[187] reported a twofold increase in oxygen consumption during anaesthesia and surgery in children during mild hypothermia, a clearly demonstrable metabolic response to cold stress even during anaesthesia.

Heat Loss

Newborn babies, like other homoeothermic organisms, lose heat in a cold environment by radiation, convection, evaporation and conduction. Hey[188] demonstrated that for newborn infants in incubators in a neutral thermal environment, these mechanisms accounted for 39 per cent, 34 per cent, 24 per cent and 3 per cent of heat loss respectively.

Radiation

Because the newborn infant has a large surface area to weight ratio, radiant heat losses are relatively large and form the major source of heat loss. Radiant heat loss decreases as environmental temperature rises (Fig. 1.24).

Convection

Convective heat loss depends on skin/air temperature gradients and air velocity. Even within an incubator the air circulation may be considerable and small neonates may only maintain their body temperature if they are covered or if other attempts are made to reduce air currents.

Evaporation

Evaporative heat loss occurs both from the respiratory tract and from the body surface. Evaporative heat loss from the skin surface is considerable at birth when the neonate is covered with liquor amnii, as in the labour ward, and loss from the lungs is increased with hyperventilation. Evaporative heat loss is practically unchanged over a wide range of ambient temperatures, so that losses by radiation and convection account for the greatest percentage of total heat loss in response to cold.

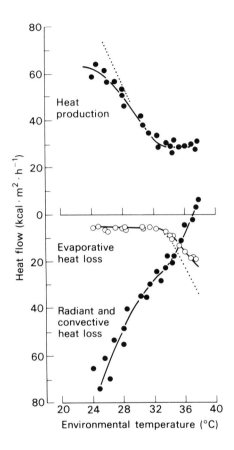

Fig. 1.24   The effect of environmental temperature on heat balance in a naked baby, weight 2.1 kg, gestation 36 weeks, when 3–7 days old, in surroundings of uniform temperature and moderate humidity. Conductive heat loss was small enough to be neglected. Heat loss by radiation and convection is large in a draught-free environment of 26°C, and falls to nothing when the environmental temperature equals body temperature (37°C). Heat production rises in a cold environment and evaporative water loss increases in a warm environment, but these changes are not enough to keep deep body temperature completely constant (the dotted lines indicate the changes that would be necessary for body temperature to remain consant). Neutral conditions are provided by an environment of 33°C. (Reproduced with permission from [188]).

Conduction

Conductive heat losses are generally small, since they depend on the temperature gradient between two contacting objects, and it is unusual for an infant to be laid in contact with a cold surface. Such losses will depend on the surface area of the contact, the conductivity of the material, cutaneous blood flow and subcutaneous thickness.

Neutral Thermal Environment

Although term newborns are capable of a threefold increase in metabolic rate over basal levels, the neonate is unable to maintain body temperature outside a narrow range of environmental temperatures because of the rapid rate of heat transfer. Even within that range body temperature may only be maintained at the cost of a significant increase in metabolic rate and oxygen consumption. The ideal thermal environment is therefore one in which oxygen consumption and metabolic rate are minimal – the neutral thermal environment or neutral temperature range. This temperature range is fairly high and narrow for the naked newborn baby and its mean on the first day of life increases from approximately 33°C in term neonates to almost 36°C in low birthweight babies (Fig. 1.25).

The neutral temperature range is widened and lowered by covering the baby with a layer of clothing (Fig. 1.26).

Limits of thermoneutrality are defined by upper and lower critical temperatures. Rise in environmental temperature above the upper critical temperature leads to recruitment of thermoregulating processes such as sweating and to an increase in body temperature, whilst an environment cooler than the lower critical temperature causes an increase in the thermogenic processes described above. Metabolism of brown fat increases metabolic rate and oxygen consumption, and any existing hypoxia is likely to be worsened. Silverman[190] and others have shown that mortality rates in premature infants are markedly reduced by increasing the environmental temperature.

Measurement of Temperature

Although Benzinger[191] suggested that tympanic membrane temperature probably gives the most reliable indication of core temperature, this is in

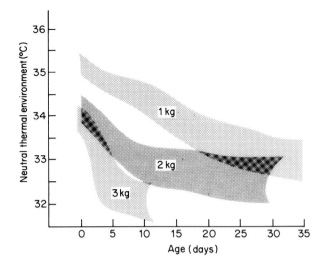

Fig. 1.25 Neutral thermal environment for babies of varying birthweight in the first few days of life. (Reproduced with permission from [189]).

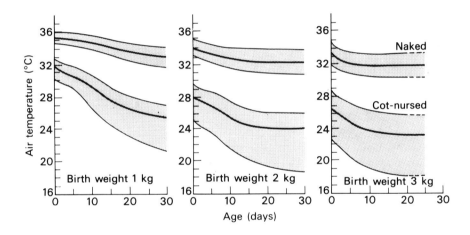

Fig. 1.26 Summary of the changes in optimum environmental temperature which occur with age in babies weighing 1, 2 or 3 kg at birth. The dark line indicates the 'optimum temperature (at the lower limit of the neutral environmental temperature range) and the shaded area the range of temperature within which a baby can be expected to maintain a normal body temperature without increasing either heat production or evaporative water loss more than 25 per cent. The higher temperatures are appropriate for a baby being nursed naked in a draught–free environment of moderate humidity (50 per cent saturation) and the lower temperatures are appropriate for a baby clothed and well wrapped up in a cot in a similar environment. It must be remembered that the environmental temperature inside a single-walled incubator is less than the internal air temperature recorded by the thermometer; the effective environmental temperature provided by the incubator can, however, be estimated by subtracting 1°C from the air temperature for each 7°C by which the incubator air temperature exceeds room temperature. (Reproduced with permission from[188]).

practice difficult to measure and may cause perforation of the tympanic membrane. Axillary temperature probes are unreliable and skin temperature is a poor reflection of core temperature. Rectal temperature is also unreliable. Core-peripheral temperature gradient may, however, be useful as an indication of volume status or cardiac output.

Both nasopharyngeal and oesophageal temperature probes give a reasonably accurate reflection of core temperature if properly placed, though both can be affected by the temperature of the inspired gas. The nasopharynx is probably the commonest and most satisfactory site for temperature measurement, though in cardiac surgery oesophageal temperature, which reflects aortic blood temperature, may be useful in addition.

Effects of Hypothermia

Increased oxygen consumption in response to hypothermia in a lightly anaesthetized infant may lead to a release of noradrenaline and consequent systemic and pulmonary vasoconstriction, acidosis and persistent pulmonary hypertension with right to left shunting. The immediate effect of cold stress in the neonate is an increase 'in metabolic rate and oxygen consumption, diverting oxygen supplies from the tissues, increasing tissue hypoxia and mortality, particularly in RDS. Hypothermia also decreases surfactant synthesis and is associated with coagulation abnormalities. In addition hypothermia lowers the minimum alveolar concentration (MAC) of inhalational anaesthetic agents and increases their tissue solubility. Unless inspired concentration is reduced anaesthetic depth will therefore increase. The pharmacokinetics of narcotic and analgesic drugs are also affected by hypothermia; non-depolarizing muscle relaxant requirements are decreased and their effects prolonged.

Effects of Hyperthermia

Although less common than reductions in temperature, raised environmental temperature can also be harmful to neonates. Increase in rectal temperature above 37°C can lead to a threefold increase in water loss by evaporation, although efficient sweating does not develop until 36–37 weeks of gestation. Neonates, including prematures, also vasodilate when their rectal temperature rises, enabling them to increase their heat losses fourfold. Oxygen consumption increases if the infant becomes restless or if his body temperature rises. Low birthweight infants exposed to raised environmental temperature or suffering from pyrexia may have an increased number of apnoeic attacks. It is known that a rise in temperature, as well as hypothermia, increases the mortality in premature infants but it is not known whether this is due to apnoeic attacks, to hypernatraemia from increased fluid loss or to cardiovascular strain from increased cardiac output. These harmful effects of a raised environmental temperature, however, occur below the temperature at which oxygen consumption increases and within the neutral temperature range.

Haematology

Fetal haematopoiesis

Haematopoietic activity can be detected in the human embryo by 14 days of gestation, starting in the yolk sac from aggregates of primitive mesenchymal cells (Fig. 1.27).

The peripheral cells become the first blood vessels and the central cells the primitive organ for formation of blood and although haematopoiesis begins in the bone marrow in the fifth month, the liver continues this role until the first week of postnatal life, but with decreasing importance. Neonatal red cells have a markedly shorter life span than the adult – between 45 and 70 days compared to the adult 120 days. Those of premature babies have an even shorter survival time.[192] Early erythrocytes are larger than at birth and contain large amounts of haemoglobin. Most are nucleated, though in the early fetus packed cell volume and red cell counts are very low. The reticulocytosis, which may be as high as 80 per cent (average 40 per cent) in early fetal life, falls to 5 per cent at birth and decreases rapidly to less than 1 per cent at five days of age. During the second trimester of pregnancy haematopoietic tissue is also found in the thymus, kidney and spleen, but by birth the contribution from these organs is negligible.

The three embryonic haemoglobins, Hb Gower 1 and 2 and Hb Portland, are restricted to the very primitive red cells in the yolk sac (Fig. 1.28).

Before birth, fetal haemoglobin (HbF $\alpha 2$, $\gamma 2$ globin chains) accounts for 90–95 per cent of all

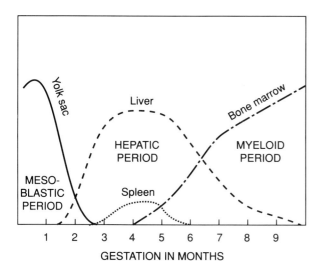

Fig. 1.27 Stages of haematopoiesis in the developing enbryo and foetus. (Reproduced with permission from [192])

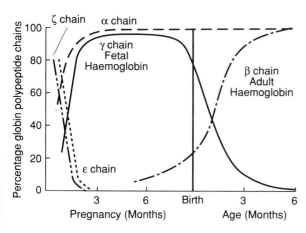

Fig. 1.28 Developmental changes in human haemoglobins. (Reproduced with permission from [193]).

Hb production and from 8–10 weeks becomes the major haemoglobin of fetal life. The maximum rate of synthesis declines after 35 weeks gestation and at term accounts for 50–60 per cent of haemoglobin production. The rate continues to decrease and at three months only 5 per cent of synthesis is HbF. Adult haemoglobin (HbA; $\alpha 2$, $\beta 2$) synthesis increases to 35–50 per cent of new Hb at birth so that at this stage the relative concentration of HbF is 80 per cent to HbA 20 per cent.[194]

Hb at birth

The mean cord haemoglobin of premature babies is 17.5 ± 1.6 gm.dl^{-1} and for term babies 17.1 ± 1.8 gm.dl^{-1}. One third of the fetal blood volume is in the placenta and one half of this volume goes to the baby held below the placenta within one minute. If cord clamping is delayed a greater transfusion takes place. Babies who are small for gestational age may be rendered relatively polycythaemic by placental insufficiency.

Table 1.17 shows the normal haematological values during the first week of life in the term infant. The concentration of Hb rises by up to 6 gm.dl^{-1} in the few hours after birth depending on the magnitude of the placental transfusion as the baby responds to this by reducing the plasma volume. A low fluid intake and the normal reduction in extracellular fluid volume also contribute to this rise. Hb values taken by heel or finger prick may be 1–2 gm.dl^{-1} higher than those taken from central venous or arterial access because of the sluggish peripheral circulation of the newborn. By one week the Hb level returns to the cord value but thereafter declines progressively and by 7–9 weeks of life the level has fallen to 9.5–11 gm.dl^{-1} irrespective of the size of the placental transfusion (Fig 1.29).

Table 1.17 Normal haematological values during the first week of life in the term infant[195]

Value	Cord Blood	Day 1	Day 3	Day 7
Hb (gm.dl^{-1})	16.8	18.4	17.8	17.0
Haematocrit (%)	53.0	58.0	55.0	54.0
Red cells (mm$^3 \times 10^6$)	5.25	5.8	5.6	5.2
MCV (μm^3)	107	108	99.0	98.0
MCH (pg)	34	35	33	32.5
MCHC (%)	31.7	32.5	33	33
Reticulocytes (%)	3–7	3–7	1–3	0–1
Nuc.RBC (mm^{-3})	500	200	0–5	0

MCV. mean corpuscular volume; MCH, mean corpuscular haemoglobin; MCHC, mean corpuscular haemoglobin concentration.

This phenomenon is known as the physiological anaemia of infancy and is caused by almost non-existent erythropoiesis, shortened red cell life span and the increasing blood volume of the developing infant. Premature babies have an even greater fall in Hb levels, the average being 8 gm.dl^{-1} at 48 weeks

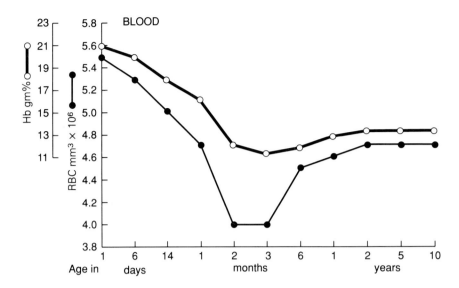

Fig. 1.29 The relation of haemoglobin and red blood cell count to age in infant and child. (Reproduced with permission from [196]).

of life in the 1.5 kg group relative to 11.4 gm.dl^{-1} in the term baby (Fig. 1.30).

The reason for this earlier and greater fall in the premature baby is not clear, but presumably it is related to an even shorter red cell survival time than in the term baby as well as the relatively larger volume of blood sampled for laboratory testing. The fact that the fall in Hb results mainly from a decrease in red cell mass has been shown using 51Cr-labelled red cells, rather than a dilutional effect of increasing plasma volume.

The reason for lower red cell survival is not exactly known, although metabolic differences

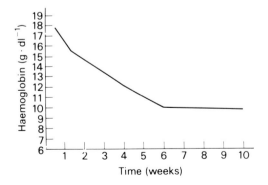

Fig. 1.30 The relation between haemoglobin concentration and age from birth in a group of infants weight less than 1.5 kg. (Reproduced with permission from [197]).

such as increased glucose consumption exist and increased glycolytic enzymes seem to confer greater susceptibility to injury and earlier destruction. Also, the fetal red cell with its relatively larger size and greater degree of wall rigidity is less compliant and possibly more likely to be damaged in small vessels. Several other factors may also be responsible for the susceptibility of fetal red cells to oxidant damage, including reduced levels of methaemoglobin reductase and catalase and reduced levels of membrane sulphadryl groups.[197] The increased permeability of the cell membrane to Na+ and K+ predisposes erythrocytes of the newborn to damage by any adverse osmotic environment.

Red cell production is mediated through the effect of tissue oxygen tension on the output of the hormone erythropoietin which is made in the liver in the fetus rather than in the kidney as in the adult. This erythropoietic activity is controlled endogenously by the fetus. The hormone is detectable in cord blood at high levels and these may be further increased in infants exposed to hypoxia and infants who are born small for their gestational age. Infants with cyanotic congenital heart disease very rarely develop anaemia of prematurity. These infants continue to produce erythropoietin during the first weeks after birth and thus do not show any decline in marrow activity.

After birth levels of erythropoietin fall rapidly until between eight and 12 weeks of life when erythroid activity recommences. However, both term and preterm babies can produce the hormone if necessary, because anaemic newborn babies develop a reticulocytosis above the normal range. A gradual rise in plasma erythropoietin occurs which generally coincides with a decline in Hb concentration below 11 gm.dl^{-1} and the return to full active erythropoiesis occurs at similar minimum Hb levels, even in infants with widely differing values at birth.[198]

In the healthy infant, the lower limit of normal Hb falls by about 1 gm.dl^{-1} per week and values of 8 gm.dl^{-1} or less at any age require explanation but not necessarily correction. The preterm baby resumes active erythropoiesis earlier in post natal life than the term infant. Factors which influence the magnitude of the physiological anaemia include the nutritional status of the infant and supplies of vitamin E, folic acid and iron which may be inadequate in the face of a rapid increase in growth later in the first year of life. The use of oral iron supplements does not prevent the early anaemia of prematurity and indeed, unless there has been perinatal blood loss or repeated sampling, the anaemia is not associated with a low serum iron. However, late anaemia will occur without supplementary dietary iron after the first 5–6 months of life.

tion of 2–4 mg.kg^{-1}.day starting some time in the first 2–4 months of life depending on birthweight, or they will develop iron deficiency anaemia by the time they have doubled their birthweight.[199] Rapid growth outstrips the iron available from normal stores or dietary sources.[200]

Fetal haemoglobin

Before birth, fetal haemoglobin (HbF$\alpha_2\gamma_2$) globin chains accounts for 90–95 per cent of all Hb production and is the major haemoglobin of fetal life. After 35 weeks gestation, the maximum rate of synthesis declines and at term accounts for 50–60 per cent of haemoglobin production. The eventual replacement of fetal by adult haemoglobin is strictly controlled and is related to postconceptual age and is uninfluenced by the timing of the birth.

The most important factor which regulates oxygen affinity with haemoglobin is the presence of the low molecular weight phosphorylated compounds such as 2,3-diphosphoglycerate (2,3-DPG) in the red cell.[201] Adult Hb combines well with 2,3-DPG causing a marked reduction in oxygen affinity. Fetal Hb has far less affinity for 2,3 DPG. The higher levels of fetal Hb in the newborn, which interact with 2,3-DPG less well, are the reason for the higher haemoglobin affinity for oxygen. The consequence of this is a shift in the oxygen dissociation curve to the left (equivalent to adult blood of pH 7.6) and thus markedly favouring transport of oxygen from the maternal to the fetal circulation. The level of red cell 2,3-DPG increases with fetal maturity and at term the concentration in the red cell is the same as that of the adult. Neonatal blood has an oxygen carrying capacity at least 1.25 times that of adult blood. Fetal blood has a P50 (partial pressure of oxygen at which Hb is 50 per cent saturated) 1 kPa (8 mmHg) lower than that of adult blood. This factor, together with the increased oxygen affinity, afford some protection for the baby under the conditions of relative hypoxia experienced during the birth process or afterwards. After birth, the oxygen dissociation curve gradually shifts to the right as concentrations of HbA increase, so that oxygen delivery to the tissues may actually increase in spite of a falling Hb.

Oxygen delivery also depends on cardiac output and changes in alveolar ventilation, and allow a gradual increase in oxygen delivery to the tissues in neonatal life.

Blood volume

The blood volume of an infant with a normal haemoglobin is estimated to be 80–85 ml.kg^{-1} body weight. For the premature baby a higher figure, perhaps as much as 100 ml.kg^{-1} may be the case. The blood volume of the newborn is more variable than that of an older infant, depending on the magnitude of the placental transfusion. Because of this wide variation, difficulties are created if blood replacement intraoperatively or otherwise is to be based on a percentage of blood volume.

If the cord is clamped within a few seconds of birth there will be a lower blood volume than if cord clamping is delayed until pulsations in the cord have ceased. Because the placental vessels contain approximately 100 ml of blood at term, the blood volume of the infant can be increased by up to 60 per cent under conditions, such as delayed clamping of the cord or placing the infant below the level of the placenta, which favour blood flow from the placenta to the baby. The volume of blood in the placenta is unchanged during the last ten weeks of gestation, so the preterm baby may receive a relatively larger percentage increase in his blood volume. Although the haematocrit is the same in all babies whenever

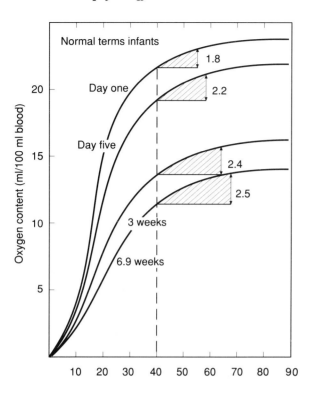

Fig. 1.31 The changing relationship between oxygen content and oxygen tension during the first weeks of life. Although total carrying capacity falls due to the falling haemoglobin level, the amount unloaded in the tissues increases (hatched section) due to the shift in the dissociation curve with a reduced O_2 affinity of haemoglobin. The amount unloaded is displayed as the volume of oxygen released as the PO_2 falls from the point at which the haemoglobin is 95 per cent saturated to 40 mmHg. In actual fact the haemoglobin may often be more than 95 per cent saturated (i.e. PaO_2 >60–70 mmHg). (Redrawn from [202])

clamping of the cord takes place, in those in which clamping is delayed, haematocrit values are as high as 65 per cent after 48 hours, compared with the normal of 45–48 per cent.

In the first four hours after birth there is a rapid fall in plasma volume as fluid shifts from the vascular to extravascular compartments. In infants whose initial blood volume is high there is a greater fall at this time. After four hours then blood volume increases, but even after three days there are still significant differences in blood volume and haematocrit between early and late clamping. From 24 hours to the end of the first week plasma volume remains constant and it has been suggested that an alternative method of calculation based on the more constant plasma volume may be more precise. The plasma volume is generally accepted as 5 per cent of body weight (50 ml.kg^{-1}) and so total blood volume can be regarded as 50 + haematocrit (ml.kg^{-1}).

Coagulation

Several aspects of the coagulation mechanism are defective in the neonate as compared with the adult. The infant is at risk from bleeding, not only because of reduced platelet function or reduced plasma coagulation factors but also because of the susceptibility to acute infections or metabolic disorders associated with disseminated intravascular coagulopathy.

It is widely stated that premature infants have increased vascular fragility – perhaps caused by inadequate connective tissue support of capillaries, although there is no firm evidence to support this.

Platelet counts even in the premature baby are in the same range as for normal adults, but there is evidence that all newborns have a mild transient defect in platelet function. This is without a great deal of clinical significance. Primary platelet aggregation is followed by release of serotonin and adenosine diphosphate, after which secondary aggregation occurs and this is irreversible. Neonatal platelets have lower than normal levels of serotonin and may also be mildly deficient in adenine nucleotides. The platelet defect is accentuated by high levels of unconjugated bilirubin, by phototherapy or by maternal ingestion of aspirin.

Isolated thrombocytopaenia is not common in healthy infants or even low birthweight babies, but a low platelet count is a very common finding in sick small babies and may be one of the most important pointers towards the diagnosis of sepsis in this age group. This type of thrombocytopaenia can be mediated by megakaryocyte damage, endotoxin damage, increased removal by the spleen or disseminated intravascular coagulopathy.

The levels of plasma proteins are usually normal at birth, although there may be a deficiency of certain plasma proteins involved in the coagulation process; for example plasminogen and antithrombin III levels at term are both half of adult levels and preterm babies have 25 per cent of adult values. Synthesis of the vitamin K-dependent factors, II, VII, IX and X by the liver is suboptimal until adult levels are attained after the age of two months. Newborns have grossly deficient stores of vitamin K at birth and deficiency will follow, especially in breastfed babies, since levels of vitamin K are low in human milk and the bacterial flora of breastfed infants probably contribute to a lower level of vitamin K. By the second or third day of life, levels may drop to as low as 5–20 per cent of the adult level, before rising later in the first week of life secondary to the production of vitamin K by the microflora of the colon. Minimal levels of clotting factors are seen in the second or third days of life, at which time the prothrombin time may be very prolonged.

This fall after birth and the risk of spontaneous bleeding (haemorrhagic disease of the newborn) or increased surgical bleeding may be partly prevented by the administration of 1 mg vitamin K parenterally. Nowadays this is given routinely and has eliminated the classic form of the condition.[203] Vitamin K does not fully correct the clotting deficiencies in the neonate, as defective synthetic capacity of the production of coagulation factors by the liver continues for the first weeks of life. Preterm babies continue to have poor prothrombin activity even after vitamin K, because of their greater hepatic immaturity. The prothrombin time (PT) and partial thromboplastin time (PTT) are prolonged in preterm infants. The thrombin time (TT) is also prolonged, possibly because of the presence of breakdown products of fibrin which may have heparin-like activity. Severe deficiency in vitamin K-dependent factors may also occur in infants of mothers taking antiepileptic drugs such as phenytoin during pregnancy and in babies after gut sterilization by antibiotics. Proteins produced by the liver but which are not vitamin K-dependent, such as factor V and fibrinogen, are in the normal range at birth. There is no transplacental passage of clotting factors so a deficiency of any one of them is detectable from cord blood taken at birth.

The fibrinolytic enzyme system is also relatively underdeveloped in the neonate. The plasminogen level is low at term and is even lower in the preterm baby.

Haemoglobin levels

The preoperative haemoglobin level should be at least 10 gm.dl^{-1}, although higher levels in the newborn are to be expected. Levels below 10 gm.dl^{-1} are not usually a contraindication to anaesthesia and surgery, but need to be investigated. Anaemia is most commonly caused by blood removal for investigations, especially in the preterm, though haemorrhage from the umbilical vessels or placenta or fetomaternal haemorrhage may be the cause. Haemolysis and failed red cell production are also possible factors. Even with microanalyses of blood samples, as much as 2–3 ml blood loss per day may result, which over a few days is a considerable blood loss for a very small baby. The decision to transfuse a baby is usually based on the clinical state of the infant and haemoglobin level and the aim should be to raise the Hb level to 13 g.dl^{-1}. Even at an early age, pallor, feeding difficulties, dyspnoea, tachypnoea, tachycardia, diminished activity and poor weight gain are all signs of anaemia.[204,205] Current practice in infants is to assume that a level less than 13 g.dl^{-1} is indicative of anaemia in the first 24 hours of life.[206] and for babies with respiratory distress Hb levels should be maintained around 13 g.dl^{-1} (haematocrit of 40).[207]

Transfusion of blood components is essential in many clinical disorders in the surgical newborn. Prior to transfusion careful consideration must be given to the specific blood component required, the nature of the pathological process for which it is being given, postnatal physiological adaptation taking place and the potential for deleterious effects from the transfusion.

Whole blood should be used when there is hypovolaemia secondary to massive acute blood loss. It should not be used in infants who are normovolaemic who only require an increase in red cell mass. In these cases transfusion is with red cells only. To reconstitute whole blood, red cells can be mixed with fresh frozen plasma.

The blood can be transfused at a rate of 15 ml hourly. To avoid overloading the circulation it is common practice to give frusemide 1 mg.kg^{-1} i.v. towards the end of the transfusion. If possible, a preoperative transfusion should be given at least 48 hours before surgery so that 2,3-DPG levels are normal by the time of surgery. All blood, except fresh donor blood, should pass through at least a 40 μ filter before transfusion.

The advantages of transfusion are not absolutely clear-cut though Stockman[208] transfused a small cohort of neonates who were felt to be gaining weight below their expected rate; in the more severely anaemic neonates (Hb <7.5g.dl^{-1}) there was significant improvement in weight gain. RBC transfusions in infants with bronchopulmonary dysplasia decreased their oxygen utilization; this would not have been predicted by haemoglobin levels alone.[209] The red cell volume has been shown to correlate better with the resting cardiac output in anaemic pretern infants than either a low haemoglobin or haematocrit,[210] suggesting that this parameter may be a better guide in assessing the need for transfusion. In practice, most units transfuse babies with Hb levels below 10 g.dl^{-1}, especially if the reticulocyte count is less than 2 per cent.

The use of exogenous recombinant erythropoietin (r-HuEPO) to stimulate endogenous erythropoietin in premature infants and thereby decrease the number of RBC transfusions required has been assessed. Early reports suggest that its administration is safe and offers a feasible alternative to erythrocyte transfusion in symptomatic anaemia of prematurity.[211] Trials currently being conducted in premature infants may provide more definitive guide-lines for erythropoietin use in the future.

Blood transfusion is not without risks, including infection with viruses such as hepatitis, HIV and cytomegalovirus (CMV).

The likelihood of acquiring CMV is related to the infant's birth weight, serological status (CMV antibody negative) and the volume of CMV antibody positive blood received. Transfusion acquired CMV may be asymptomatic or rarely produce significant morbidity or mortality in infants <1200 gm. In view of the potential serious consequences in these infants the following indications for the use of CMV seronegative blood products (not FFP) are suggested:[206]

1. Low birth weight (< 1250 gm) neonates born to seronegative mothers in centres with a documented high incidence of transfusion-acquired infection in neonates;[212]
2. Low birthweight infants (born to seronegative or seropositive mothers) who require granulocyte transfusions;
3. Neonates undergoing ECMO;
4. Infants infected with HIV type I.

Transfusion will also shift the O_2 dissociation curve to the right and reduce the oxygen affinity of Hb. The period of depressed red cell production will be prolonged and the haemoglobin will fall to an even lower level before reactivation of erythropoiesis.

Cross-matching

The viability of red cells in citrate-phosphate-dextrose (CPD) adenine storage is approximately 80 per cent after five weeks but, because of increase in the number of microaggregates, decrease in 2,3-DPG and increase in potassium concentration with age, blood for transfusion to neonates should be as fresh as possible. Metabolic problems such as citrate binding causing hypocalcaemia, hypomagnesaemia and hyperglycaemia followed by rebound hypoglycaemia are occasionally seen with exchange transfusion. The use of heparinized blood has been suggested for the newborn, but this blood must be used within 12 hours and much is wasted. Red cells with optimal additive (SAGM) appears to be safe for use in newborns. Blood must be cross-matched for all major surgery and for operations where a blood loss of 10 per cent or more of the blood volume is anticipated. This includes most neonatal operations.

A positive sickle test in a mother is an indication for electrophoretic studies of the baby's blood. The introduction of neonatal screening programmes for the very early detection of the disease and subsequent close medical supervision including the use of prophylactic penicillin has allowed a great reduction in infant mortality.[213] At birth, and for the first 8–12 weeks of life, infants are protected from the problems of sickling because of high levels of HbF. Vaso-occlusive crises are rarely seen before six months of age, though fulminant pneumococcal septicaemia and acute splenic sequestration may occur earlier. Oral penicillin prophylaxis is started not later than four months of age in a dose of 62.5 mg twice daily.[214]

Babies may be born with a very high haematocrit either because of active, increased intrauterine erythropoiesis because of placental insufficiency or maternal diabetes or by red cell transfusion from the mother, twin to twin, or because of delayed clamping of the cord. The blood of all infants with a central venous haematocrit of 65 per cent or more will also be markedly hyperviscous.[215] Symptoms such as hypotonia, lethargy, vomiting, hypoglycaemia, hyperbilirubinaemia and respiratory distress may be delayed until the haematocrit rises further during the first 48 hours of life. Symptoms may also be caused by sludging and thrombus formation in the peripheries, affecting mainly the brain, kidneys and bowels (Fig 1.32).

Those babies with symptoms from polycythaemia

and hyperviscous blood should be treated so that immediate and late neurological symptoms can be relieved. A central haematocrit of 55 per cent is considered a safe level and a partial exchange transfusion of whole blood with equal volumes of fresh frozen plasma is undertaken. The volume of the exchange is calculated thus:

$$\text{Total blood volume} \times \frac{(\text{observed Hct} - \text{desired Hct})}{\text{observed Hct}}$$

Polycythaemic babies that do not have symptoms are not usually exchange transfused, but are nursed with care, attention being paid to keeping the baby warm and well hydrated to prevent any sludging in the peripheral circulation.

Haemorrhagic disorders

The cause of any haemorrhagic disorder in the newborn must be sought preoperatively and

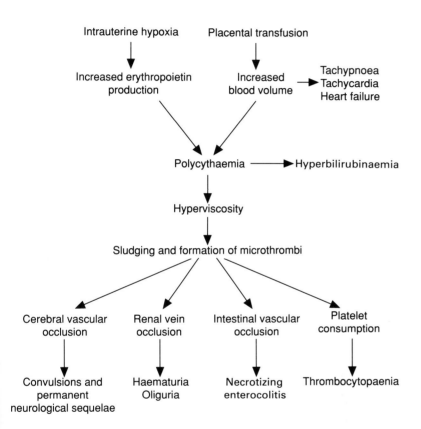

Fig. 1.32 Pathogenesis of polycythaemia and clinical manifestations of hyperviscosity in the newborn infant. (Reproduced with permission from [216])

Table 1.18 Commonly tested haemostatic factors with normal values (venous) in the first 72 hours. (Reproduced with permission from[218])

Factor		Preterm (30–36 wks)	Term
II	% of normal adult values	30–65	40–65
V	%	50–100	50–100
VII	%	20–50	40–70
VIII	%	60–120	70–150
IX	%	10–30	15–55
X	%	10–45	20–55
XI	%	10–50	15–70
XII	%	20–50	25–70
XIII	%	50–100	50–100

treated, and clotting defects are particularly common in low birthweight infants and those with low gestational age.[217] Both term and preterm infants may have levels of clotting factors well below normal adult levels in the first few days of life because of hepatic immaturity. These may have clinical significance especially in newborns who require surgery, though healthy newborns do not

Table 1.19 Commonly used haemostatic screening tests with normal values in the first 72 hours. (Reproduced with permission from [218])

Screening test	Preterm (30–36 wks)	Term	Adult
Prothrombin (PT)/seconds (I, II, V, VII, X)	13–23	13–17	13–16
Thrombotest (TT) % (II, VII, IX, X)	15–50	15–60	80–100
Partial Thromboplastin Time (PTT)/seconds (I, II, V, VII, IX, X, XI, XII)	35–100	35–70	35–45
Thrombin time/seconds	12–24	12–18	10–14
Reptilase time/seconds	18–30	18–24	18–22
Platelet count $\times$ 10^9.l^{-1}	100–350	150–400	150–400
Fibrinogen concentration gm.l^{-1}	1.2–3.8	1.5–3.5	1.5–3.5

Table 1.20 Investigation of acquired coagulation disorders

	Acquired disorder		Liver dysfunction	Vitamin K deficiency
History	Shock/DIC	Sepsis	Jaundice	Diet, diarrhoea antibiotics, malabsorption, obstructive jaundice
Bleeding	Generalized		Generalized	Generalized
Laboratory screening tests:				
PT	Increased	Increased	Increased	Increased
PTT	Increased	Increased	N or increased	Increased
Platelets	N or decreased	Decreased	N or decreased	N
Fibrinogen	Decreased	N or decreased	N or decreased	N
FDP*	Increased	N or increased	N or increased	N
Laboratory specific factors:				
V	Decreased	N or decreased	Decreased	N
VII	N	N	Decreased	Decreased
VIII	Decreased	N or decreased	Increased	N
IX	N or decreased	N or decreased	Decreased	Decreased
X	Decreased	N or decreased	Decreased	Decreased

*FDP is being replaced in certain laboratories by the measurement of D dimer (XDP), cross-linked fibrin derivatives, formed exclusively by the enzymatic degradation of fibrin and felt to be a more specific indicator in the evaluation of patients with thrombotic disorders

Note:
The effects of the routine use of low doses of heparin (to maintain patency of vascular lines) must be taken into account when coagulation screening tests are measured.

bleed because levels of only 30 per cent of most factors are required for clot formation (Table 1.18).

The process of haemostasis following tissue injury involves the interaction of blood vessels, platelets and coagulation factors. The blood vessel wall is more fragile in the preterm and term baby than in older children and although platelets are present in normal numbers, their function may be impaired, especially membrane reactivity and thromboxane production. Because of this there is less recruitment of other platelets into the expanding haemostatic plug and less local vasoconstriction. There is also immaturity of the mechanisms protecting against increased thrombosis such as the fibrinolytic mechanism and other agents such as antithrombin III which neutralizes activated clotting factors. The commonest cause of bleeding in the newborn is trauma during delivery, though a congenital coagulopathy may first show with bleeding from the umbilical stump (Table 1.19).

Prophylactic treatment with vitamin K_1 is still routine in most countries so that haemorrhagic disease of the newborn caused by reduction in the levels of the vitamin K-dependent factors (II, VII, IX and X) is now uncommon. Hydantoin derivative anticonvulsants impair vitamin K activity and babies born to epileptic mothers taking these drugs during pregnancy may develop haemorrhagic disease due to deficiency of vitamin K. Bleeding will stop within 2–4 hours of administration of the vitamin. Water-soluble forms of the vitamin may cause haemolysis so that the natural form such as phytomenadione (Konakion), should be given in a dose of 1 mg (Table 1.20).

Metabolism and pharmacokinetics

Metabolism

Liver function

Before birth, most of the functions of the liver are performed by the placenta or the maternal liver, but after birth, the baby's liver must take on its major role in body homoeostasis. The liver at birth weighs 4 per cent of the total body weight compared to 2 per cent in the adult, but even so, there is considerable instability as enzyme functions develop. Glucose homoeostasis is particularly affected and other aspects of liver function such as the major biotransformation processes of oxidation, reduction, hydrolysis and conjugation may be poorly developed at birth, particularly in prematurity, but others such as the synthesis of albumin and coagulation factors are relatively normal. Hepatic microsomal enzyme systems involving cytochrome P-450 activity are approximately half that found in adults, but the proportion of the isoenzymes changes as the baby develops. For example, hydroxylation of phenobarbitone is low at birth, but actually exceeds adult values at three weeks of age, but theophylline cleared by a demethylation pathway does not reach adult values of clearance until after two months of age. Phase I reactions which convert a substance to a more polar metabolite are generally reduced, particularly in preterm babies. Phase I metabolites are often less active or inactive and may be easily excreted. The ability to oxidize and to reduce substrates is the most affected and phase II processes such as conjugation are severely limited at birth. However, liver enzyme systems do mature rapidly after birth and function at adult levels very early in the neonatal period, usually by three months of age.

Most of the amino acids essential for rapid growth of the fetus are supplied via the placenta. After birth, those amino acids which cannot be metabolized must be supplied in the diet and thus represent essential amino acids at this stage. For example, the last enzyme in the trans-sulphuration pathway for cystine synthesis is absent in the human fetal liver and thus cystine is an essential amino acid to the human neonate. It is readily available in breast milk (Table 1.21). Albumin synthesis in the liver begins at 3–4 months' gestation and increases towards term.

Alpha-feto protein (AFP) is an α_1-globulin synthesized by the yolk sac and the fetal liver, with maximum production at about the 13th week of fetal life. Although the source of the AFP in amniotic fluid is unknown, raised levels are a reliable detector of open neural tube defects of the fetus. Maternal serum levels of AFP are less reliable, although levels 2.5 times normal give a detection rate of 88 per cent for anencephaly and

Table 1.21   Essential amino acids

Adult	Infant
Isoleucine	*All those required by adult, plus:*
Leucine	Histidine
Lysine	Proline
Methionine	Alanine
Phenylalanine	Cystine
Threonine	
Tryptophan	
Valine	

79 per cent for open spina bifida. There is little correlation between AFP levels from amniotic fluid or serum, which suggests that the mechanisms involved in its production are independent of each other. If it is detectable in the serum of babies after the neonatal period, it may be a sign of hepatoma or teratoma.

A major function of the liver is to metabolize bilirubin from the breakdown of red cells and cytochromes and to excrete water soluble conjugated bilirubin in the bile. Because glucuronide conjugation, one of the main methods of detoxification in the liver, is low at birth, the conjugation of bilirubin is very inefficient. The proportion of conjugated bilirubin is slightly less in the neonate than in the adult, but more significant is the fact that only 20 per cent of the bilirubin is found as the diglucuronide in the baby, the rest being the mono form. The second molecule of bilirubin is bound less freely than the first. This represents much less efficient conjugation reflected in the low activity of the hepatic uridine diphosphoglucuronyl transferase system. It is likely that the rapid maturation of this enzyme system in both term and preterm neonates is a birth-related process, possibly due to the disappearance of *in utero* suppressing agents. Adult levels of activity are attained after about 70 days. The activity of the glucuronyl transferase system can be stimulated by the administration of phenobarbitone and requires 2–5 days of treatment for this to be effective. On the other hand some drugs such as sulphonamides displace bilirubin from albumin which may increase the concentration of unbound lipid-soluble bilirubin.

Jaundice

Jaundice of the unconjugated hyperbilirubinaemia type is very commonly seen even in the normal newborn and is unique to that time of life. The incidence is higher in Asian and Chinese babies and in those who are ill or premature. The liver enzymes associated with the conjugation of bile, particularly glucuronyl transferase, have a low activity in the first weeks of life; there is also a greatly increased bilirubin load. This larger load results from both increased enteric reabsorption of unconjugated bilirubin, but also from the rapid breakdown of macrocytic red cells which have a shortened life in the newborn causing double the adult rate of bilirubin production. An additional source of bilirubin may be from the increased resorption of red cells from haematomas caused by birth trauma. A high haemoglobin from placental transfusion increases the incidence of jaundice (up to 32 per cent with late clamping of the cord). Neonatal jaundice usually appears on the second or third days of life and peaks on the third or fourth day. In the term newborn, physiological jaundice is characterized by a progressive rise in serum unconjugated bilirubin from 34 μmol.l^{-1} (2 mg.dl^{-1}) to a peak of more than 100 μmol.l^{-1} (6 mg.dl^{-1}) up to 210 μmol (12 mg.dl^{-1}) and thereafter declines, at first rapidly and subsequently more slowly to reach the adult value of 17 μmol.l^{-1} (1 mg.dl^{-1}) at the tenth day of life. The pattern of jaundice varies with prematurity and ethnic origin; Asian and Chinese babies have more severe and more prolonged jaundice.

The uncoupling of bilirubin from albumin is accelerated by hypoxaemia, acidaemia, hypoglycaemia, sepsis, a very rapid rise of free bilirubin and immaturity. The preterm baby, even if healthy, has a greater incidence of jaundice with up to 28 per cent of babies having values of bilirubin around 250 μmol.l^{-1} (14 mg.dl^{-1}). Jaundice becomes clinically apparent when serum bilirubin rises above 85 μmol.l^{-1} (5 mg.dl^{-1}). They have low total protein levels and defects both in the binding activity of the albumin and in the binding capacity of albumin for bilirubin. This situation is worsened by hypoxia, acidosis, sepsis and drugs such as sulphonamides. In many preterm infants below 1000 g, serum levels of *direct* bilirubin may rise because of intrahepatic cholestasis with slow excretion of bilirubin from the gut.

Lipid soluble unconjugated bilirubin is a tissue poison and the danger of a high level of unconjugated bilirubin is the irreversible damage it may inflict on the cells in the basal ganglia, midbrain and brainstem known as kernicterus. This is manifest in later life by extrapyramidal cerebral palsy, deafness and mental subnormality. If the infant dies, at post mortem intense yellow staining is seen in the subthalamic nuclei, basal ganglia and the 8th nerve. At a cellular level dense yellow inclusion bodies which represent bilirubin-membrane complexes are present in all affected cells. All jaundiced babies tend to be sleepy, but those with bilirubin encephalopathy become very lethargic, develop a high-pitched cry and often suffer from convulsions. The critical level in term infants at which neurological signs appear has never been really established, but they rarely occur if the serum bilirubin levels remain below 340 μmol.l^{-1} (20 mg.dl^{-1}), however levels in the range of 205–340 μmol.l^{-1} (12–20 mg.dl^{-1}) are associated with neurodevelopmental delay in the first year of life. Lower levels can cause damage in the preterm, especially if they are acidotic, hypoxic, hypoglycaemic or hypoalbuminaemic. Because of these different factors, particularly differences in the binding of bilirubin to albumin and to cells and whether the blood–brain barrier is intact, it is quite impossible to produce confident guidelines for the management of jaundice particularly in the preterm (Fig. 1.33).[219]

Jaundice may also, of course, have a pathological basis which requires investigation. Increased red cell destruction is the most common cause from factors such as bacterial infection or ABO incompatibility and congenital anaemias. A raised serum bilirubin with a conjugated component of 20–80 per cent and bile pigments in the urine is always pathological even if the total bilirubin is low (80 μmol.l^{-1} – 5 mg.dl^{-1}). Pathology includes a hepatitis syndrome and disorders of the main intrahepatic and extrahepatic bile ducts. Suspected biliary atresia should be diagnosed and surgically corrected as soon as possible before irreversible liver damage occurs. Although the cause of biliary atresia is unknown it seems that a sclerosing inflammatory process affects previously formed bile ducts at first extra- and then intrahepatic. If surgery is to be successful the intrahepatic bile ducts must be patent out to the porta hepatis. The Kasai procedure constructs a hepaticoportoenterostomy with a Roux-en Y loop of jejunum. Cholangitis is a common complication and if the operation does not succeed death from cirrhosis is usual in the second year of life without a hepatic transplant.[220]

Prolonged total parenteral nutrition (TPN) in infancy, particularly if no enteral feeding is possible, leads to chronic liver damage, cholestasis, conjugated hyperbilirubinaemia with jaundice and eventual cirrhosis of the liver. The incidence increases with prematurity and the time that TPN is required. The situation is likely to be exacerbated by sepsis and hypoxia.[221] All premature infants receiving TPN should have tests of liver function on a weekly basis. The causes of TPN-related liver damage are not clear, but may include an unbalanced supply of amino acids, lack of trace elements, toxaemia and hypoxia.

Phototherapy has become accepted worldwide as the simplest and most effective way of handling unconjugated hyperbilirubinaemia.[222] Bilirubin, when exposed to light in the blue wavelength (425–475nm), is transformed into less lipophilic pigments that can be easily excreted without further conjugation and this is the predominant effect of phototherapy. Actual photodegradation of bilirubin only accounts for a small amount of the bilirubin dealt with by phototherapy. Light in the blue range penetrates the skin, causing photoisomerism of bilirubin molecules mainly in extravascular tissues. The photoisomers diffuse into the blood to be excreted in the bile where they revert to bilirubin. This process may mean that rebound will occur in babies with intestinal stasis or obstruction. The formation of more stable photoisomers is a slower process, but these are efficiently excreted.[223]

Phototherapy has largely removed the need for exchange transfusion which often required several attempts, was expensive in terms of equipment, blood and personnel, and was not without morbidity, even mortality. With phototherapy there is a predictable non-linear correlation of the duration of therapy which is necessary with the particular level of plasma bilirubin before treatment. There is a greater proportionate decline in levels with higher initial bilirubin levels until at 100 μmol.l^{-1} (5.9 mg.dl^{-1}) no further decline occurs. The same clinical effect can be achieved with half the light intensity if double the surface area is exposed to light.

Phototherapy is usually more effective the smaller and more premature the infant. If the jaundice is severe from haemolysis normal lamps may be insufficient to control the bilirubin levels and special blue lamps may be required.

During phototherapy increased fluid administration is essential to offset the increased insensible water loss and stool water loss. 20–60 per cent increases are necessary – the higher levels if the baby is preterm – with further increases if radiant heat or high intensity therapy are used. Eye protection is routine, because even with closed eyes there is a possibility of damage to an infant retina during therapy. Phototherapy bleaches the skin so clinical

Serum bilirubin (mg · dl⁻¹)	Birth weight	<24 h	24–28 h	49–72 h	>72 h
<5					
5–9	All	Phototherapy if haemolysis			
10–14	<2.5 kg	Exchange if haemolysis	Phototherapy		
	>2.5 kg	Exchange if haemolysis		Investigate if bilirubin >12 mg	
15–19	<2.5 kg	Exchange		Consider exchange	
	>2.5 kg	Exchange		Phototherapy	
20 and +	All	Exchange			

☐ Observe ▨ Investigate jaundice

Use phototherapy after any exchange

Fig. 1.33 The management of hyperbilirubinaemia in newborn infants. Guidelines are based on serum bilirubin concentration, birthweight, age and clinical status of the patient. In the presence of (1) perinatal asphyxia, (2) respiratory distress, (3) metabolic acidosis (pH 7.25 or below), (4) hypothermia (temperature below 35C), (5) low serum protein (5 gm.dl⁻¹ or less) (6) birthweight below 1.5 kg, or (7) signs of clinical or CNS deterioration: treat as in next higher bilirubin category. (Reproduced with permission from [224]).

judgement on the severity of jaundice cannot be applied. Bilirubin values are taken 12 hourly from capillary blood samples.

Carbohydrate metabolism

The liver plays a vital role in carbohydrate metabolism, which includes: the storage of carbohydrate as glycogen; the synthesis of glucose by the process of gluconeogenesis; the conversion of carbohydrate to fat; and the release of glucose from glycogen. There is rapid synthesis of glycogen by the liver as fetal life comes to an end (from 36 weeks).

Studies by Aynsley–Green[225] show that blood sugar levels in the fetus, though lower than maternal levels, are in the range of adult normoglycaemia. The development of fetal liver and pancreatic function ensures that a high insulin–glucagon ratio exists which favours anabolism with the 6G7 formation of glycogen, protein and adipose tissue. Fetal insulin certainly plays a vital role in regulating fetal glucose concentration by uptake from umbilical vessels.

The carbohydrate reserves of the normal newborn are relatively low (about 11 gm.kg⁻¹ body weight) and one third of this is available from liver glycogen. The low birthweight baby has proportionately lower carbohydrate reserves. Energy is derived from the use of fat and protein as well as carbohydrate. The amount and availability of each 'fuel' depend on constraints imposed by immaturity of metabolic pathways, caused by lack of specific enzymes or hormones in the first few days of life. The lower the birth weight, the poorer is the carbohydrate tolerance because of deficient insulin response. Thus the poor control of glucose metabolism in the preterm baby is caused partly by immaturity of the liver and also by a lack of gluconeogenic substrates due to inadequate fat stores and low total protein. In such infants, feeding within four hours of birth is essential, especially as the developing brain is affected adversely if nutrition is poor between weeks 26 and 40 of postconceptual age. Until the 35th week the mechanism of swallowing is inadequate and nasogastric or nasojejunal feeding is usually required. Total or partial parenteral nutrition may be necessary for low birthweight babies in whom the enteral route is impossible. Glucose is the main energy source during the first few hours after delivery and the blood sugar falls rapidly with an increase in plasma glucagon levels due to catecholamines and increased sympathetic activity during the birth process (Fig 1.34).

Gluconeogenesis is not functional at the time of delivery, but is rapidly activated within eight hours of birth. The newborn glucose production is 4–6 mg.kg^{-1}.min, initially from glycogenolysis and later from gluconeogenesis. The high glucose demand is related to the high brain mass of the newborn (12 per cent) compared to 2 per cent in an adult. At this stage liver and muscle glycogen stores fall[226] but later metabolism of fat and free fatty acids (FFA) become significant. Blood sugar levels in the normal term baby average 2.7–3.3 mmol.l^{-1} (50–60 mg.dl^{-1}). For a low birth weight infant, 2.2 mmol.l^{-1} (40 mg.dl^{-1}) is an average random finding.

Hypoglycaemia

A biochemical definition of hypoglycaemia has been very difficult partly because levels of blood sugar can go very low indeed and still be clinically unrecognized. The concept of asymptomatic hypoglycaemia is based on the finding of low glucose levels in infants in whom no overt signs of abnormality can be found, particularly common in infants of diabetic mothers (IDM).[227] It may be that lipolysis, which starts soon after birth and produces free fatty acids and ketone bodies, provides sufficient substrates for energy metabolism by several tissues including the brain. (Sann[228] has even suggested the use of intravenous lipid, especially medium chain triglycerides, to induce glucose production by stimulation of gluconeogenesis and ketogenesis in high risk infants.) In asymptomatic hypoglycaemia premature and SGA infants, and possibly in the IDM (where endogenous glucose production in relation to glucose utilization is already insufficient), it is generally considered insufficient to rely

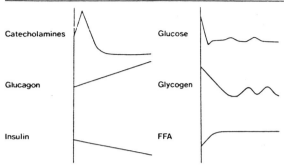

ALTERATIONS IN HORMONES AND METABOLIC FUELS FOLLOWING BIRTH

Fig. 1.34 Metabolic events associated with delivery. At delivery, the neonate greatly increases plasma catecholamine concentrations. Possibly as a result of this surge and other factors, plasma glucagon concentrations also increase whilst insulin decreases. These changes are important because of the abrupt cessation of maternally derived glucose, resulting in a greatly decreased plasma glucose concentration. The hormonal adjustments stimulate glycogen and free fatty acid mobilization. (Reproduced with permission from [226])

on possible alternate substrates and adequate enteral or parenteral glucose should be supplied in appropriate amounts. Hypoglycaemia in the term baby has been defined as 1.6 mmol.l^{-1} (30 mg/100 ml) or less, and in those of birthweights below 3 kg it is 1.1 mmol.l^{-1} (20 mg.dl^{-1}) in the first three days of life. However, on the basis that in fetal life blood sugar levels are considerably higher, a more conservative definition of hypoglycaemia of 2.2 mmol.l^{-1} (40 mg.dl^{-1}) is nowadays taken.[229] After term, levels should always be above 2.2 mmol.l^{-1} and if found to be below this they must be corrected (Table 1.22).

Unless the levels are very low, the hypoglycaemic baby may be asymptomatic, although symptoms such as tremors, ('jittery') apnoea, cyanosis, apathy, hypotonia, hypothermia and convulsions are all well described. The possibility of hypoglycaemia must be anticipated to prevent avoidable brain damage; 25–50 per cent of babies with symptomatic hypogly-

Table 1.22 Plasma glucose concentrations in normal term (mmol.l^{-1})

Age (h)	Hypoglycaemia	Intermediate	Normoglycaemia	Intermediate	Hyperglycaemia
0–6	0–1.4	1.4–2.2	2.2–5.6	5.6–6.9	>6.9
6–24	0–1.7	1.7–2.5	2.5–5.6	5.6–6.9	>6.9
>24	0–2.2	2.2–2.8	2.8–5.6	5.6–6.9	>6.9

caemia develop neurological sequelae. Permanent neurological damage with mental retardation and spasticity is a result of severe and prolonged hypoglycaemia of the newborn and even moderate hypoglycaemia may have an adverse neurological outcome.[231,232] At very low blood sugar levels, cerebral autoregulation of blood flow ceases and flow then changes together with peripheral blood pressure which may be low. Neural damage may follow disturbances in neurotransmitters at the synapses.

Babies very likely to become hypoglycaemic include the premature and infants small for gestational age (SGA) with poor deposits of fat and glycogen, infants of diabetic mothers and those asphyxiated at birth.[233] Very premature infants born before fat and glycogen deposits have been laid down may become hypoglycaemic at any time during the first week or two of life, especially if they are severely ill or if their calorie intake is inadequate. In SGA infants (less than 2.5 kg at term) the peak incidence of hypoglycaemia is usually found between 24 and 72 hours of age. At this stage glycogen stores have fallen whilst the infant, particularly if breastfed, may still be on a hypocaloric intake. There may be increased energy demands if the baby is nursed below the neutral thermal environment range of temperature. Hypoglycaemia may be transient or persistent, and involve one or more of the basic mechanisms of lack of glycogen stores, inability to synthesize glucose and excessive insulin secretion.

Infants of diabetic mothers (IDM) have high insulin levels and may become hypoglycaemic within a few hours of birth with the risk lasting for up to 48 hours. Since their homoeostatic mechanisms are usually working well, such infants seldom come to harm unless they are very ill, e.g. with sepsis, or the mother was on sulphonylurea drugs. IDM also have an increased incidence of respiratory distress syndrome, polycythaemia and thrombotic disorders especially renal vein thrombosis, cardiomegaly secondary to asphyxia, hypoglycaemia, hypocalcaemia or intraventricular septal hypertrophy.[227] Infants with severe birth asphyxia may become hypoglycaemic shortly after resuscitation.

Hypoglycaemia may, of course, be a symptom of some other condition such as glycogen storage disease, abnormalities of the hypothalamic–adrenal axis or adenoma of the pancreas. Hypoglycaemia commonly occurs in infants on i.v. nutrition; infiltration of the peripheral infusion or decreases in the intravenous glucose concentration readily lead to rebound hypoglycaemia. An unusual complication of glucose infusion via an umbilical catheter can induce a hyperinsulinaemic, hypoglycaemic state when the catheter tip is at the level of the 8th to the 11th vertebrae. The infusion may enter the pancreatic circulation via the coeliac and superior mesenteric arteries with resultant hyperinsulinism. Repositioning the catheter to below the body of the 3rd lumbar vertebrae corrects this hypoglycaemic refractoriness.[234]

By performing estimations with BM-Test strips (or Dextrostix) and/or laboratory blood sugar determinations every 4–6 hours in the first three days of life for SGA babies and others at risk, most cases of asymptomatic hypoglycaemia will be detected. Reagent strips may underestimate the degree of hypoglycaemia and any value below 2.2 warrants a blood glucose determination. If possible, early feeding should be undertaken; where this is not possible an infusion of 10 per cent dextrose should be set up at a rate of 75–100 ml.kg^{-1}.24h^{-1}. If the hypoglycaemia is unrelieved, the dextrose should be changed to 15 per cent. If more immediate correction is required, 1–2 ml.kg^{-1} of 25 per cent dextrose should be given promptly. However, such boluses are likely to lead to rebound hypoglycaemia and should be avoided where possible. All intravenous fluids for infants should include dextrose.

If these measures fail to improve the hypoglycaemia the use of glucagon may be considered. Glucagon is used as a continuous infusion of 0.5–1 mg.24h^{-1} (up to 2 mg.24h^{-1}). This is found to be particularly useful in SGA infants with resistant hypoglycaemia, possibly associated with pancreatic dysmaturity. It has been successfully used in infants with hypoglycaemia resistant to dextrose infusions supplying glucose at > 6.5 mg.kg^{-1}.min.[235] Glucagon 0.1–0.3 mg.kg^{-1} may also be given intramuscularly in infants with good glycogen stores; the i.m. route may be useful if venous access is difficult to obtain. If the usual methods do not control the hypoglycaemia, steroids (prednisone 1 mg.kg^{-1} 8-hourly) or ACTH (four units 12-hourly) should be administered.

It is important to give concentrated dextrose solutions slowly to avoid reflex hypoglycaemia from the insulin released by the infusion. The need for repeated administration of such solutions is an indication for a line into a central vein.

Persistent symptomatic hypoglycaemia may be caused by the Beckwith-Wiedemann syndrome of postnatal gigantism, macroglossia and umbilical hernia or, rarely, by beta-cell nesidioblastosis. This latter condition causes a high insulin level and responds to subtotal pancreatectomy. Histology shows aberrant beta cells in small groups of two to six separate from the islets, spread throughout the pancreas. Continued hypoglycaemia with this condition is very often the cause of mental retardation.

Hyperglycaemia

Though not as common as hypoglycaemia there are many recent reports of hyperglycaemia (blood sugar greater than 7 mmol.l^{-1} (120 mg.dl^{-1}) occurring, particularly in lowbirth weight infants. This is partly due to a greater awareness, but also to the desire to maintain a normal blood sugar greater than 2.2 mmol.l^{-1} (40 mg.dl^{-1}) at all times and thus a more liberal approach to the administration of fluids. Hyperglycaemia, with levels as high as 44 mmol.l^{-1} (800 mg.dl^{-1}) is extremely damaging to brain cells, is a probable cause of intraventricular haemorrhage and will cause excessive water and electrolyte loss by osmotic diuresis, contributing to an increased morbidity and mortality. There is also a possible association of transient postoperative neurological deficit after cardiac surgery performed under hypothermic circulatory arrest with high intraoperative blood sugar levels[236] and increased morbidity and mortality in infant primates given dextrose solutions after periods of cerebral ischaemia.[237] There is a significant trend towards increasing blood sugar levels with decreasing birthweight associated with glucose infusions and parenteral nutrition.[238] Hyperglycaemia is also associated with the administration of aminophylline and theophylline for apnoea of prematurity. Sepsis should be suspected in an infant in whom hyperglycaemia develops at a glucose intake that has been previously well tolerated.

Commonly used fluid regimes such as 5 per cent dextrose together with the response to the stress of surgery results in many patients becoming progressively hyperglycaemic in the perioperative period. The hyperglycaemia is initiated by catecholamine release during surgery and is maintained in the postoperative period by glucagon secretion and inhibition of insulin production. These biochemical changes can at least be partially obtunded by standard doses of opioids or inhalational agents.[239] Unnecessary glucose should be avoided especially for those at risk of cerebral hypoxia or ischaemia. For preterm babies a constant infusion during anaesthesia should be maintained at a level to meet the predicted metabolic needs, i.e. never more than 12 g.kg^{-1}.24 hrs^{-1}.[240] Certainly blood glucose levels must be very carefully monitored and if high levels persist an insulin infusion of 0.05–0.1 unit.kg^{-1}.hr^{-1} should be started.

Calcium

Calcium is vital for the function of membranes, for coagulation and for bone growth. Homoeostasis of calcium is influenced by serum phosphate, parathyroid hormone, vitamin D and calcitonin, but relies on a balance between intake in the diet, calcium taken into bone and urinary excretion. The fetus acquires most of its calcium stores in the last 12 weeks of gestation and at birth the calcium and phosphate levels are higher than in the mother. There is active transport of calcium ions from the mother to the fetus and the phosphate is high because of the relative hypoparathyroidism of the fetus.

As expected, low birthweight babies have deficient stores of calcium, so hypocalcaemia is common in preterm babies in the first days of life.

After birth, plasma phosphate levels rise because of low GFR and parathyroid hormone deficiency which takes over 48 hours to rise to detectable levels. The high plasma phosphate depresses the serum Ca^{2+} level. Additional factors which may cause hypocalcaemia at birth are poor conversion of vitamin D to its active metabolite and poor absorption of calcium from the small and large intestine. High levels of glucocorticoids also depress serum calcium.

Hypocalcaemia

Hypocalcaemia is commonest in the first two days of life in sick babies. It is possibly due to immaturity of the parathyroid glands, although it may appear at 5–7 days in babies fed on cow's milk, which has a high phosphate content.

Hypocalcaemia may develop during an exchange transfusion with acid–citrate–dextrose. It is common in premature infants and 50 per cent may have a serum calcium below 2 mmol.l^{-1} (8 mg.dl^{-1}) in the first few days of life. Newborns with smaller calcium stores will tolerate large transfusions of citrated blood or blood products less well and show transient decreases in ionized Ca^{2+} and falls in blood pressure.

The signs of hypocalcaemia – which are mainly non–specific neurological signs such as irritability or failure to synchronize with a ventilator or, rarely, tetany or convulsions – are manifestations of a low ionized Ca^{2+} level, not necessarily fully reflected in total serum levels. The proportion which is protein bound can be estimated from the albumin level.

Treatment of hypocalcaemia is imperative and urgent if the total calcium level falls below 1.5 $mmol.l^{-1}$ or if the ionized calcium level falls below 0.7 $mmol.l^{-1}$. It is wise to treat ionized calcium levels below 0.95 $mmol.l^{-1}$. If convulsions occur, calcium should be given without waiting for the results of serum calcium estimations (1 $ml.kg^{-1}$ of 20 per cent calcium gluconate). In the absence of convulsions, hypocalcaemia should be treated by continuous infusion of a dilute (2 per cent) solution of calcium gluconate at a rate of 5 $mg.kg^{-1}.h$. Because calcium solutions are irritant, they should not be given into scalp veins, where tissue necrosis may occur. Indeed, calcium solutions more concentrated than this should not be given via any peripheral vein. Calcium is also incompatible with sodium bicarbonate.

Other metabolic disorders

Hypomagnesaemia may occur in association with hypocalcaemia, following exchange transfusion or following administration of diphenylhydantoin to the mother for the treatment of toxaemia of pregnancy. Treatment with 1 per cent magnesium sulphate intravenously should not exceed 5–10ml at a rate of less than 1 $ml.min^{-1}$.

Inborn errors of metabolism occasionally require attention in the neonatal period. Galactosaemia may cause hypoglycaemia and others such as hyperglycinaemia may cause acidosis. It is important to detect cases of phenylketonuria and maple syrup urine disease in order to take corrective measures to allow mental development to proceed normally.

Pharmacokinetics

Drugs

There are marked differences between the disposition of drugs in the newborn and in the older child or adult: after one dose of a drug the plasma concentration persists at a higher level for a longer time in the newborn and preterm than in older children. The major factors involved in the handling of drugs are their bioavailability, pharmacokinetics and therapeutic actions: absorption, distribution, detoxication and excretion. These processes are markedly affected by gestational age, the weight for dates and general condition of the baby.

Absorption

In the newborn there is relative achlorhydria and slow gastric emptying which is even slower in preterm babies. Transit through the intestines is slow, though there is a relatively large mucosal surface area. Water-soluble drugs such as tetracyclines, chloramphenicol and penicillin are well absorbed after oral administration and in fact ampicillin may be better absorbed in the small baby than in the adult. Absorption after intramuscular injection may be variable because of the smaller muscle mass, reduced local blood flow and a limited capacity for muscular contraction. Because the skin of the baby is less well keratinized certain drugs such as theophylline can be administered percutaneously.[241]

Distribution

Distribution is affected by many factors such as tissue mass, blood flow, lipid solubility, permeability and protein binding. The neonate has a very high total body water and extracellular fluid volume, giving a greater proportion of the body weight as water, although the extent of this varies from baby to baby depending on, for example, the volume of the placental transfusion. There are smaller fat deposits than in the adult and the blood–brain barrier is less well developed. The markedly increased sensitivity of the newborn to the respiratory depressant effects of the opioid analgesics may be a result not only of greater quantities of the drug crossing the blood–brain barrier but also of the increased sensitivity of specific receptors in the brain related to poorer myelination. This also means that greater concentration of drugs such as antibiotics will reach the CSF by systemic administration. Lipid soluble drugs such as diamorphine readily cross the blood–brain barrier with a rapid equilibration between the blood and the brain. Because cerebral blood flow is relatively higher in the newborn, concentration of drugs in the brain may be higher.

Plasma protein binding is lower in the newborn, so the free fraction of any drug is significantly higher; up to 2.5 times that of the adult. Albumin binding is more likely to be altered by the presence of other substances in the plasma such as bilirubin or by acidotic changes. The consequence is a higher free fraction of drug in jaundiced or acidotic babies. This change in binding may be a more important factor than an actual reduction in the concentration of plasma proteins. The receptor sites for drugs in newborns may have less affinity for drugs than in older people and this may explain why there is less clinical effect with for example diazepam for a given plasma level in a newborn.

Detoxication

Detoxication takes place in the liver and relies mainly on the mechanisms of oxidation (e.g. barbiturates undergo side-chain oxidation as part of the detoxication process) and conjugation, usually with glucuronic acid. Such is the fate of morphine, salicylates, adrenal steroids, chloral hydrate, chlorpromazine and chloramphenicol. Because the enzyme activity involved in the metabolism of these drugs is poor in the early days of life, it is better to avoid their use where possible. Inefficient glucuronidation of chloramphenicol may lead to a build-up of its blood levels, resulting in the 'grey' syndrome of cardiovascular collapse with its typical grey appearance.

As metabolic pathways become activated with improvement in liver function the half-life of drugs does decrease, but at a rate which is varied and usually unpredictable. It is therefore mandatory to monitor the levels of drugs with toxic side effects, such as digoxin or gentamicin.

Excretion

The neonatal GFR is only 30–40 per cent of the adult value, although adult levels are attained in the first year of life. Thus drugs excreted unchanged by the kidneys will have a prolonged action because of the delayed excretion. Drugs such as digoxin and gentamicin treated in this way must have serum levels monitored carefully after several days of administration.

Thus, the combination of absorption rates which are relatively slower and long elimination half-lives for most drugs means that newborns show less fluctuation in plasma concentrations and may allow drug doses to be given less frequently than to older children (Table 1.23).

Pharmacokinetics of inhalation agents

Uptake and distribution

The uptake of inhalation anaesthetics is faster in neonates and infants than in older children and adults for several reasons. First, the ratio of alveolar

Table 1.23 Plasma elimination half-lives in hours for newborns and children. (Reproduced with permission from [242])

Drug	Preterm infants	Term infants	Children
Caffeine*	31–132	26–231	2–4
Carbamazepine	–	–	6–18
Cefotaxime	3.0–5.7	2–3.5	–
Diazepam*	–	–	14–22
Digoxin	60–120	40–100	28–40
Gentamicin	3.5–16.1	2.3–5.9	1.2
Indomethacin*	12–51	–	–
Morphine		6–12	2
Netilmicin	4–5.5	3.8–5.5	–
Phenobarbitone	60–200	41–120	37–73
Phenytoin*	60–130	10–100	2–30
Theophylline*	12–35	–	15–5

*Eliminated by 'dose-dependent' (Michaelis-Menten) kinetics at usual therapeutic concentration. Elimination half-life varies markedly

ventilation to functional residual capacity (FRC) is around four times greater in neonates than adults, so that the ratio of expired to inspired anaesthetic concentration approaches unity more rapidly (Fig. 1.35).

The rise in alveolar concentration will also depend on the blood-gas solubility coefficient of the agent used, the alveolar concentration of less soluble agents rising more rapidly than that of more soluble ones. Age-related differences in blood-gas solubility coefficients have been demonstrated for most inhalation anaesthetic agents,[244–5] solubility in placental or neonatal blood being lower than in adult blood. The reasons for this difference in solubility are not entirely clear, though it seems likely that they are related to the effects of haematocrit, the presence of haemoglobin F and different plasma concentrations of cholesterol, fatty acids and plasma proteins.

Although the high cardiac output of the neonate should theoretically retard the uptake of inhalation anaesthetic agents, a larger percentage of the cardiac output is distributed to the vessel-rich group of tissues (brain, heart and splanchnic bed) so that equilibration in these tissues is relatively rapid. Brain mass in the neonate is relatively large compared to the adult, whilst muscle and fat mass is small. Tissue-blood partition coefficients are also significantly lower in neonates and infants[246] so that tissue extraction is also relatively rapid. In the initial

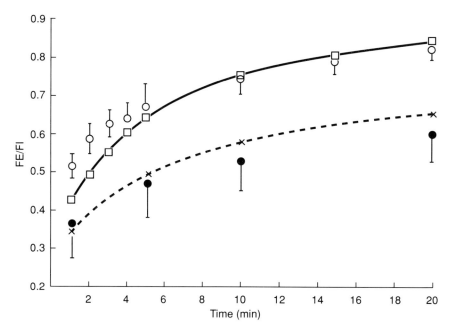

Fig. 1.35 Predicted versus observed F_E/F_I (expired/inspired fraction) for halothane in infants and adults. Predicted F_E/F_I values are those generated by a computer program of anaesthetic uptake and distribution. In infants minute ventilation averaged 1.9 l; in adults minute ventilation was 6.9 l. The inspired fraction of halothane was 0.5% in both cases. (Reproduced with permission from [243].)

uptake phase of anaesthesia the arterial-to-venous anaesthetic tension difference will be great and this also hastens uptake. These age-related differences are more marked for agents with a relatively high blood-gas solubility such as halothane than for insoluble ones like nitrous oxide.

Maintenance requirements

Age-related differences in minimum anaesthetic concentration (MAC) of several anaesthetic agents have now been demonstrated[247] (Fig. 1.36).

During the early neonatal period, the response to pain is attenuated. The reasons for this are not entirely clear, but may be related to the relatively high levels of progesterone, beta endorphins and other endogenous opioids found at birth, to differences in the permeability of the blood–brain barrier or to age-related changes in blood-gas solubility. Whatever the reason, anaesthetic requirements gradually increase during the first few months of life, with the highest MAC values being found at around six months of age. Thereafter MAC gradually decreases with increasing age.[248–50]

Elimination

The relatively high alveolar ventilation in relation to FRC together with the high percentage of cardiac output distributed to vessel-rich groups leads to a more rapid elimination of inhalation anaesthetic agents in neonates. Although renal and hepatic clearance mechanisms are immature, they

probably play an insignificant part in excretion of inhalation agents. The limited mass of muscle and fat has advantages in the later phases of recovery, since the quantity of anaesthetic taken up by these vessel-poor groups is also limited.

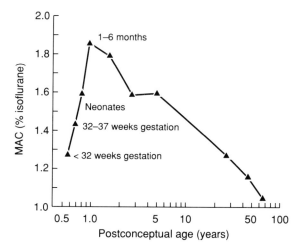

Fig. 1.36 The MAC of isoflurane and postconceptual age. Values for postconceptual age were obtained by adding 40 weeks to the mean postnatal age for each age group. The MAC of isoflurane in preterm neonates is significantly less than in full-term neonates and older infants 1 to 6 months of age ($P < .005$). (Reproduced with permission from [247].)

Cardiovascular effects

The commonly used inhalation agents all have a dose-dependent depressant effect on blood pressure as in adults, with halothane acting primarily by reduction in cardiac output and isoflurane mainly by reduction in systemic vascular resistance. Since cardiac output in the neonate is more rate-dependent than in the adult, the hypotensive effect of halothane can be reversed by atropine,[251] though ejection fraction and left ventricular end diastolic volume remain measurably depressed. In neonates with potentially patent foramen ovale and ductus arteriosus or congenital heart disease with actual intracardiac shunting, the reduction in systemic vascular resistance caused by isoflurane may be a factor in the magnitude of any right-to-left shunt.

The relatively high percentage of cardiac output distributed to vessel-rich tissues and differences in solubility outlined above lead to higher myocardial concentrations of halothane early in induction in neonates for a given inspired concentration. The therapeutic ratio between surgical anaesthesia and myocardial depression is thus reduced. Cook found the therapeutic ratio for halothane in young rats to be about half that in older ones.[252]

Anaesthesia depresses baroreceptor responses more in neonates, particularly if preterm,[253] reducing the compensatory tachycardic response to hypotension and hypovolaemia. Baroreceptor control of heart rate appears to be more depressed in neonates by halothane than by isoflurane.[254]

Ventilatory effects

All volatile anaesthetics produce a dose-dependent depression of ventilation in children, decreasing tidal and minute volume and attenuating the response to carbon dioxide. This has generally been attributed to depression of the respiratory neurones in the medullary centre, though suppression of intercostal muscle activity and paradoxical breathing also play a major part.[255] The highest carbon dioxide levels have been recorded in the smallest infants[256-7] who have fewer type 1 oxidative muscle fibres in the diaphragm and may be prone to ventilatory fatigue. As in adults, induction of anaesthesia in children causes a significant reduction in FRC.[258] The limited respiratory reserve of the neonate has already been discussed on p. 6. Controlled ventilation of the lungs is a virtually universal practice in neonatal anaesthesia.

The ventilatory response to hypoxia is also suppressed by anaesthesia, which may mask a defect in ventilatory control, particularly in infants younger than 41–46 weeks postconceptual age.[259] These infants are at increased risk of postoperative apnoea.

Immunology

Immunity is the ability of an organism to respond to foreign matter by using a variety of mechanisms involving different types of cells and cellular products to destroy or inactivate the foreign substances. The immune system comprises the thymus, spleen, lymph nodes and gut-associated lymphoid tissue together with lymphocytes and their products, accessory cells, lysozyme and complement, etc.

During its development the fetus is normally protected by its environment from infection, so the immune system is only called upon after birth to respond to outside agents and until this time is antigenically 'innocent'. Bacterial colonization of the skin, respiratory tract and gut occurs rapidly after birth[260] not only from the mother but also from a hospital environment, and the baby may become infected by pathological organisms to which he may have impaired resistance. The healthy term newborn has the physical, humoral and cellular immunological mechanisms adequately to challenge a wide variety of antigenic effects, but certain immaturities, particularly in the preterm baby may reduce the efficiency of the immune response. Certainly there is a high incidence of serious infection particularly in the low birthweight group.

The lymphocytes originate from stem cells in the embryo yolk sac endoderm and migrate to the liver and later to the thymus, but by six weeks gestation definitive T and B cell precursors can be found. By 24 weeks of gestation the number of lymphocytes has reached 50 per cent of the adult levels, together with all the subpopulations such as helper, suppressor, cytotoxic and natural killer cells.[261] T cell function is normal at birth and there is no reduction in the ability of the newborn to reject a skin graft, for example. The number of

B cells is similar to an adult's, but there may be a reduction in antibody production in response to exogenous antigen. There are few plasma cells in the fetus which is a sign that normally there is a low level of stimulation by antigen. There is no transport of IgA or IgM so these are absent at birth unless the immune system has been challenged *in utero* by an infection such as congenital rubella, cytomegalovirus or toxoplasmosis. In these cases, the ability of the fetus to produce specific antibody is shown by high levels of antigen specific IgM in cord blood after 24 weeks gestation.[262]

Immunoglobulin lgG passes from the maternal circulation to the fetus by a selective process across the placenta beginning at 12 weeks, though the bulk of the transfer takes place during the third trimester. Cord IgG levels in babies of 28 weeks gestation are approximately 0.04 g.l^{-1} but reach 1.8 g.l^{-1} at term, often exceeding the maternal level. There is a relative lack of IgG$_2$ which reduces the effectiveness of a response to capsular polysaccharides of group B streptococci.[263] After birth the level of IgG falls with a half-life of between 20 and 30 days so there is a relative hypogammaglobulinaemia, lowest between the second and fourth months until the liver function improves. This is rarely of clinical importance except if in preterm babies IgG levels fall to less than 10 per cent of normal.[264] Preterm babies below 32 weeks gestation may benefit from treatment with immunoglobulin, though this is controversial.[265-6] IgA and macrophages which are present in breast milk and are not absorbed through the bowel wall presumably have an important role

in preventing bowel infections.[267]   The primary immune response consisting of the inflammatory response and phagocytosis is impaired in the fetus and newborn, but the clinical significance of this is dubious and is probably related to the lack of specific antibody which reduces the effectiveness of phagocytic cell function. If specific antibody is present, then phagocytosis and bacterial killing are the same as in an adult. The chemotactic response of polymorphonuclear leucocytes is reduced as is opsonization possibly due to lower levels of complement, especially C3 which is the final pathway for complement activation.[268] The febrile response which implies increased metabolic activity and the release of pyrogens from leucocytes is not well developed and the phagocytosis of ingested pathogens may be further reduced in disease states such as RDS or septicaemia. Neonatal serum is particularly poor in opsonizing capacity against β-haemolytic streptococcus.

The preterm baby is particularly at risk from serious infections and although after 24 weeks there is the capacity to synthesize all the factors required for immunity there is an inadequate amount of transferred maternal immunoglobulin.[269] In addition to this, the preterm baby has very thin skin with limited cornification which is easily invaded by bacteria.

Neonatal anaesthesia and intensive care frequently involve invasive manoeuvres such as intubation and vascular access which provide an easy route for micro-organisms.

References

Respiratory physiology

1. Hasan SU, Rigaux A. The effects of lung distension, oxygenation, and gestational age on fetal behaviour and breathing movements in sheep. *Pediatric Research.* 1991; **30**, 193–201.
2. Wallen LD. Developmental physiology of the fetus and newborn and physiologic changes related to birth, cerebral adaptation, and apnea. *Current Opinion in Pedatrics.* 1992; **4**, 200–5.
3. Jansen AH, Chernick V. Development of respiratory control. *Physiological Reviews.* 1983; **63**, 437–83.
4. Han VKM. Neonatal anatomy, physiology and development. *Current Opinion in Pediatrics.* 1990; **2**, 275–81.
5. Hallman M, Arjomaa P, Mizumoto M, Akino T. Surfactant proteins in the diagnosis of fetal lung maturity. I. Predictive accuracy of the 35 kD protein, the lecithin/sphingomyelin ratio and phosphatidylglycerol. *American Journal of Obstetrics and Gynecology.* 1988; **158**, 531–5.
6. Darling RC, Smith CA, Asmussen E, Cohen FM. Some properties of human fetal and maternal blood. *Journal of Clinical Investigation.* 1941; **20**, 739–47.
7. Hellegers AE, Schrueffer JJP. Nomograms and empirical equations relating to oxygen tension,

percentage saturation and pH in maternal and fetal blood. *American Journal of Obstetrics and Gynecology.* 1961; **81**, 377–84.

8. Delivoria-Papadopoulos M, Roncevic NP, Oski FA. Post-natal changes in oxygen transport of term, premature and sick infants. *Pediatric Research.* 1971; **5**, 235–45.

9. Adamson SL, Kuipers IM, Olson DM. Umbilical cord occlusion stimulates breathing independent of blood gases and pH. *Journal of Applied Physiology.* 1991; **70**, 1796–809.

10. Karlberg P, Koch G. Respiratory studies in newborn infants. III. Development of mechanics of breathing during the first week of life. A longitudinal study. *Acta Paediatrica Scandinavica.* 1962; **Suppl. 135**, 121.

11. Teital DF, Iwamoto HS, Rudolph AM. Changes in the pulmonary circulation during birth-related events. *Pediatric Research.* 1990; **27**, 372–8.

12. Velvis H, Moore P, Heymann MA. Prostaglandin inhibition prevents the fall in pulmonary vascular resistance as a result of rhythmic distension of the lungs in fetal lambs. *Pediatric Research.* 1991; **30**, 62–8.

13. Teitel DF, Dalinghaus M, Cassidy SC, Payne BD, Rudolph AM. In utero ventilation augments the left ventricular responses to isoproterenol and volume loading in fetal sheep. *Pediatric Research.* 1991; **29**, 466–72.

14. Vyas H, Milner AD, Hopkins IE, Boon AW. Physiologic responses to prolonged and slow-rise inflation in the resuscitation of the asphyxiated newborn infant. *Journal of Pediatrics.* 1981; **99**, 635–9.

15. Avery ME, Cook CD. Volume-pressure relationships of lungs and thorax in fetal, newborn and adult goats. *Journal of Applied Physiology.* 1961; **16**, 1034–8.

16. Mortola JP. Dynamics of breathing in newborn mammals. *Physiological Reviews.* 1987; **67**, 187–243.

17. Dobbinson TL, Nisbet HIA, Pelton DA. Functional Residual Capacity (FRC) and compliance in anaesthetized, paralyzed children. Part II: clinical results. *Canadian Anaesthetists Society Journal.* 1973; **20**, 322–33.

18. Stocks J, Godfrey S. Nasal resistance during infancy. *Respiration Physiology.* 1978; **34**, 233–46.

19. Wohl MEB, Stigol LC, Mead J. Resistance of the total respiratory system in healthy infants and infants with bronchiolitis. *Pediatrics.* 1969; **43**, 495–509.

20. Sorbini CA, Grassi V, Solinas E. Arterial oxygen tension in relation to age in healthy subjects. *Respiration.* 1968; **25**, 3–13.

21. Mansell A, Bryan AC, Levison H. Airway closure in children. *Journal of Applied Physiology.* 1972; **33**, 711–14.

22. Rigatto H, Kwiatkowkski KA, Hasan SU, Cates DB. The ventilatory response to endogenous CO_2 in preterm infants. *American Review of Respiratory Disease.* 1991; **143**, 101–4.

23. Cohen G, Xu C, Henderson-Smart D. Ventilatory responses of the sleeping newborn to CO_2 during normoxic rebreathing. *Journal of Applied Physiology.* 1991; **71**, 168–74.

24. Ceruti E. Chemoreceptor reflexes in the newborn. *Pediatrics.* 1966; **37**, 556–64.

25. Manning DJ, Stothers JK. Sleep state, hypoxia and periodic breathing in the neonate. *Acta Paediatrica Scandinavica.* 1991; **80**, 763–9.

26. Sekar KC, Duke JC. Sleep apnea and hypoxemia in recently weaned premature infants with and without bronchopulmonary dysplasia. *Pediatric Pulmonology.* 1991; **10**: 112–16.

27. Thoppil CK, Belan MA, Cowen CP, Mathew OP. Behavioural arousal in newborn infants and its association with termination of apnea. *Journal of Applied Physiology.* 1991; **70**, 2479–84.

28. Poets CF, Southall DP. Patterns of oxygenation during periodic breathing in preterm infants. *Early Human Development.* 1991; **26**, 1–12.

29. Beal S, Porter C. Sudden infant death syndrome related to climate. *Acta Paediatrica Scandinavica.* 1991; **80**, 278–87.

30. Rabbette PS, Costeloe KL, Stocks J. Persistence of the Hering–Breuer reflex beyond the neonatal period. *Journal of Applied Physiology* . 1991; **71**, 474–80.

31. Cook CD, Sutherland JM, Segal S, Cherry RB, Mead J, McIlroy MB, Smith CA. Studies of respiratory physiology in the newborn infant. III. Measurements of mechanics of respiration. *Journal of Clinical Investigation.* 1957; **36**, 440–8.

32. Hjalmarson O, Krantz ME, Jacobsson B, Sorensen SE. The importance of neonatal asphyxia and Caesarean section as risk factors for neonatal respiratory disorders in an unselected population. *Acta Paediatrica Scandinavica.* 1982; **71**, 403–8.

33. White E, Shy KK, Daling JR. An investigation of the relationship between the Cesarean section birth and respiratory distress syndrome of the newborn. *American Journal of Epidemiology.* 1985; **121**, 651–63.

34. Robert MF, Neff RK, Hubbell JP, Taeusch HW, Avery ME. Association between maternal diabetes and the respiratory distress syndrome in the newborn. *New England Journal of Medicine.* 1976; **294**, 357–60.

35. Arnold C, McLean FH, Kramer MS, Usher RH. Respiratory Distress Syndrome in second-born versus first-born twins. *New England Journal of Medicine.* 1987; **317**, 1121–5.

36. Collaborative Group on antenatal steroid therapy. Effect of antenatal dexamethasone administration on the prevention of respiratory distress syndrome.

American Journal of Obstetrics and Gynecology. 1981; **141**, 276–87

37. Jobe AH. Preterm factors influencing surfactant deficiency. *International Journal of Technology Assessment in Health Care.* 7: Suppl. 1; 1991, 16–20.

38. Pena IC, Teberg AJ, Finello KM. The premature small-for-gestational-age infant during the first year of life: Comparison by birth weight and gestational age. *Journal of Pediatrics.* 1988; **113**, 1066–73.

39. Thompson PJ, Greenough A, Gamsu HR, Nicolaides KH. Ventilatory requirements for respiratory distress syndrome in small-for-gestational-age infants. *European Journal of Pediatrics.* 1992; **151**, 528–31.

40. Tubman TRJ, Rollins MD, Patterson C, Halliday HL. Increased incidence of respiratory distress syndrome in babies of hypertensive mothers. *Archives of Disease in Childhood.* 1991; **66**, 52–4.

41. Evans NJ, Archer LNJ. Doppler assessment of pulmonary artery pressure and extrapulmonary shunting in the acute phase of hyaline membrane disease. *Archives of Disease in Childhood.* 1991; **66**, 6–11.

42. Corbet AJS, Ross JA, Beaudry PH, Stern L. Ventilation perfusion relationships as assessed by a-ADN$_2$ in hyaline membrane disease. *Journal of Applied Physiology.* 1974; **36**, 74–81.

43. Moses D, Holm BA, Spitale P, Liu M, Enhorning G. Inhibition of pulmonary surfactant function by meconium. *American Journal of Obstetrics and Gynecology.* 1991; **164**, 477–81.

44. Cole VA, Normand ICS, Reynolds EOR, Rivers RPA. Pathogenesis of hemorrhagic pulmonary edema and massive pulmonary hemorrhage in the newborn. *Pediatrics.* 1973; **51**, 175–87.

45. Van Straaten HLM, Gerards LJ, Krediet TG. Chylothorax in the neonatal period. *European Journal of Pediatrics.* 1993; **152**, 2–5.

Retinopathy of Prematurity

46. Avery GB, Glass P. Retinopathy of prematurity: what causes it? *Clinics in Perinatology.* 1988; **15**, 917–28.

47. Fielder AR, Moseley M, Ng Y. The immature visual system and premature birth. *British Medical Bulletin.* 1988; **44**, 1093–118.

48. Betts EK, Downs JJ, Schaffer DB, Johns R. Retrolental fibroplasia and oxygen administration during general anaesthesia. *Anesthesiology.* 1977; **47**, 518–20.

Cardiovascular physiology

49. Rigby ML, Shinebourne EA. Growth and development of the cardiovascular system: functional development. In: Davis JA, Dobbing J (eds) *Scientific Foundations of Paediatrics.* 2nd edn. London: Heinemann Medical, 1981, p. 373.

50. Rudolph AM, Heymann MA. Fetal and neonatal circulation and respiration. *Annual Review of Physiology.* 1974; **36**, 187.

51. Lauer RM, Evans JA, Aoki M, Kittle CF. Factors controlling pulmonary vascular resistance in fetal lambs. *Journal of Pediatrics.* 1965; **67**, 568–77.

52. Campbell AGM, Dawes GS, Fishman AP, Hyman AI, Perks AM. The release of a bradykinin-like pulmonary vasodilator substance in foetal and newborn lambs. *Journal of Physiology.* 1968; **195**, 83–96.

53. Dawes GS. *Foetal and Neonatal Physiology.* Chicago: Year Book Medical, 1968.

54. Gittenberger de Groot AC, Strengers JLM, Mentink M, Poelmann RE, Patterson DF. Histologic studies on normal and persistent ductus arteriosus in the dog. *Journal of the American College of Cardiology.* 1985; **6**, 394–404.

55. Gersony WM. Patent Ductus Arteriosus in the Neonate. *Pediatric Clinics of North America.* 1986; **33**, 545–60.

56. Rabinovitch M, Boudreau N, Vella G, Coceani F, Olley PM. Oxygen-related prostaglandin synthesis in ductus arteriosus and other vascular cells. *Pediatric Research.* 1989; **26**, 330–5.

57. Agata Y, Hiraishi S, Oguchi K, Misawa H, Horiguchi Y, Fujino N, Yashiro K, Shimada N. Changes in left-ventricular output from fetal to early neonatal life. *Journal of Pediatrics.* 1991; **119**, 441–5.

58. Shaddy RE, Tyndall MR, Teital DF, Li C, Rudolph AM. Regulation of cardiac output with controlled heart rate in newborn lambs. *Pediatric Research.* 1988; **24**, 577–82.

59. Van Hare GF, Hawkins JA, Schmidt KG, Rudolph AM. The effects of increasing mean arterial pressure on left ventricular output in newborn lambs. *Circulation Research.* 1990; **67**, 78–83.

60. Parish MD, Farrar S. Force and oxygen consumption in the immature rabbit heart. *Pediatric Research.* 1990; **27**, 476–82.

61. Fisher DJ, Towbin J. Maturation of the heart. *Clinics in Perinatology.* 1988; **15**, 421–46.

62. Shavit G, Sagy M, Nadler E, Vidne BA, Gitter S. Myocardial response to alpha-agonist (Phenylephrine) in relation to age. *Critical Care Medicine.* 1989; **17**, 1324–7.

63. Broughton-Pipkin F, Smales ORC. A study of factors affecting blood pressure and angiotensin II in newborn infants. *Journal of Pediatrics.* 1977; **91**, 113–19.

64. Palmisano BW, Clifford PS, Coon RL, Seagard JL, Hoffmann RG, Kampine JP. Development of baroreflex control of heart rate in swine. *Pediatric*

Research. 1990; **27**, 148–52.

65. Murphy JD, Rabinovitch M, Goldstein JD, Reid LM. The structural basis of persistent pulmonary hypertension of the newborn infant. *Journal of Pediatrics*. 1981; **98**, 962–7.

66. Pfenninger J, Tschaeppeler H, Wagner BP, Weber J, Zimmerman A. The paradox of adult respiratory distress syndrome in neonates. *Pediatric Pulmonology* 1991; **10**, 18–24.

67. Faix RG, Viscardi RM, DiPietro MA, Nicks JJ. Adult respiratory distress syndrome in full-term newborns. *Pediatrics*. 1989; **83**, 971–6.

68. Hansen DD. Pulmonary circulation and pediatric anesthesia. *Current Opinion in Anesthesiology*. 1992; **5**, 387–91.

69. Johns RA. Endothelium-derived relaxing factor: basic review and clinical implications. *Journal of Cardiothoracic and Vascular Anesthesia*. 1991; **5**, 69–79.

70. Ignarro LJ. Biological actions and properties of endothelium derived nitric oxide formed and released from artery and vein. *Circulation Research*. 1989; **65**, 1–21.

71. Frostell C, Tratacci M-D, Wain JC, Jones R, Zapol WM. Inhaled nitric oxide. A selective pulmonary vasodilator reversing hypoxic pulmonary vasoconstriction. *Circulation*. 1991; **83**, 2038–47.

72. Santulli TV. Fetal echocardiography: Cardiovascular anatomy and function. *Clinics in Perinatology*. 1990; **17**, 911–40.

73. Ward RM. Maternal drug therapy for fetal disorders. *Seminars in Perinatology*. 1992; **16**, 12–20.

74. Lin AE, Garver KL. Genetic counselling for congenital heart defects. *Journal of Pediatrics*. 1988; **113**, 1105–9.

75. Nelson RM, Bucciarelli RL, Eitzman DV, Egan EA, Gressner IH. Serum creatinine phosphokinase MB fraction in newborns with transient tricuspid insufficiency. *New England Journal of Medicine*. 1978; **298**, 146–9.

76. Turner-Gomes SO, Izukawa T, Rowe RD. Persistence of atrioventricular valve regurgitation and electrocardiographic abnormalities following transient myocardial ischemia of the newborn. *Pediatric Cardiology*. 1989; **10**, 191–4.

77. Friedman WF. The intrinsic physiologic properties of the developing heart. In: Friedman WF, Lesch M, Sonnenblick EH, (eds) *Neonatal Heart Disease*. New York: Grune & Stratton, 1972: pp. 21–49.

78. Greenwood RD, Rosenthal A, Parisi L, Fyler DC, Nadas AS. Extracardiac abnormalities in infants with congenital heart disease. *Pediatrics*. 1975; **55**, 485–92.

79. Berg KA, Boughman JA, Astemborski JA, Ferencz C. Implications for prenatal cytogenetic analysis from the Baltimore–Washington study of liveborn infants with confirmed congenital heart defects. *American Journal of Human Genetics*. 1986; **39**, A50.

80. Park MK. In: *Pediatric Cardiology for Practitioners*. Chicago: Year Book Medical, 1988, pp. 63–4.

81. Garson A. *The electrocardiogram in infants and older children*. Philadelphia: Lea & Febiger, 1983: p. 404.

82. Park MK. *Pediatric Cardiology for Practitioners*. Chicago: Year Book Medical, 1984, pp. 63–4.

83. Leung MP, Cheung DLC, Lo RNS, Mok C-K, Lee J, Yeung C-Y. The management of symptomatic neonates using combined cross-sectional echocardiography and pulsed Doppler flow study as the definitive investigations. *International Journal of Cardiology*. 1989; **24**, 41–6.

84. Musewe NN. Neonatal heart disease with an emphasis on patent ductus arteriosus. *Current Opinion in Pediatrics*. 1991; **3**, 240–7.

85. Gentile R, Stevenson JG, Dooley T, Franklin D, Kawabori I, Pearlman A. Pulsed Doppler echocardiographic determination of time of ductal closure in normal newborn infants. *Journal of Pediatrics*. 1981; **98**, 443–8.

86. Reller MD, Buffkin DC, Colasurdo MA, Rice MJ, McDonald RW. Ductal patency in neonates with respiratory distress syndrome: A randomized surfactant trial. *American Journal of Diseases of Children*. 1991; **145**, 1017–20.

87. Bell EF, Warburton D, Stonestreet BS, Oh W. Effect of fluid administration on the development of symptomatic patent ductus arteriosus and congestive heart failure in premature infants. *New England Journal of Medicine*. 1980; **302**, 598–604.

88. Green TP, Thompson TR, Johnson DE, Lock JE. Furosemide promotes patent ductus arteriosus in premature infants with the respiratory distress syndrome. *New England Journal of Medicine*. 1983; **308**, 743–8.

89. Fujiwara T, Maeta H, Chida S, Morita T, Watabe Y, Abe T. Artificial surfactant therapy in hyaline membrane disease. *Lancet*. 1980; **1**, 55–9.

90. Charon A, Taeusch HW, Fitzgibbon C, Smith GB, Treves ST, Phelps DS. Factors associated with surfactant treatment response in infants with severe respiratory distress syndrome. *Pediatrics*. 1989; **83**, 348–54.

91. Heldt GP, Pesonen E, Merritt TA, Elias W, Sahn DJ. Closure of the ductus arteriosus and mechanics of breathing in preterm infants after surfactant replacement therapy. *Pediatric Research*. 1989; **25**, 305–10.

92. Clyman RI. Patent ductus arteriosus in the premature infant. In: Taensch HW, Ballard RA, Avery ME, (eds) *Diseases of the Newborn*, 6th edn. Philadelphia: W.B. Saunders Co., 1991; pp. 563–70.

93. Krauss AN, Fatica N, Lewis BS, Cooper R, Thaler HT, Cirrincione C, O'Loughlin J, Levin

A, Engle MA, Auld PA. Pulmonary function in preterm infants following treatment with intravenous indomethacin. *American Journal of Diseases of Children.* 1989; **143**, 78–81.

94. Stefano JL, Abbasi S, Pearlman SA, Spear ML, Esterly KL, Bhutani VK. Closure of the ductus arteriosus with indomethacin in ventilated neonates with respiratory distress syndrome. *American Review of Respiratory Disease.* 1991; **143**, 236–9.

95. Shaw J. Growth and nutrition of the very preterm infant. *British Medical Bulletin.* 1988; **44**, 984–1009.

96. Barst RJ, Gersony WM. The pharmacological treatment of patent ductus arteriosus: A review of the evidence. *Drugs* 1989; **38**, 249–66.

97. Cassady G, Crouse DT, Kirklin JW, Strange MJ, Joiner CH, Godoy G, O'Loughlin J, Levin A, Engle MA, Auld PA. A randomized, controlled trial of very early prophylactic ligation of the ductus arteriosus in babies who weighed 1000g or less at birth. *New England Journal of Medicine.* 1989; **320**, 1511–16.

98. Seri I, Tulassay T, Kiszel J, Machay T, Liptak M, Csomor S. The use of dopamine for the prevention of the renal side effects of indomethacin in premature infants with patent ductus arteriosus. *International Journal of Pediatric Nephrology.* 1984; **5**, 209–14.

99. Yeh TF, Wilks A, Singh J, Betkerur M, Lilien L, Pildes RS. Furosemide prevents the renal side effects of indomethacin therapy in premature infants with patent ductus arteriosus. *Journal of Pediatrics.* 1982; **101**, 433–7.

100. Campbell AN, Beasley JR, Kenna AP. Indomethacin and gastric perforation in a neonate. *Lancet.* 1981; **1**, 1110–11.

101. Wolf WM, Snover DC, Leonard AS. Localized intestinal perforation following intravenous indomethacin in premature infants. *Journal of Pediatric Surgery.* 1989; **24**, 409–10.

102. VanBel F, Guit GL, Schipper J, van de Bor M, Baan J. Indomethacin-induced changes in renal blood flow velocity waveform in premature infants investigated with color Doppler imaging. *Journal of Pediatrics.* 1991; **118**, 621–6.

103. Coombs RC, Morgan MEI, Durbin GM, Booth IW, McNeish AS. Gut blood flow velocities in the newborn: Effects of patent ductus arteriosus and parenteral indomethacin. *Archives of Disease in Childhood.* 1990; **65**, 1067–71.

104. Mardoum R, Bejar R, Merritt TA, Berry C. Controlled study of the effects of indomethacin on cerebral blood flow velocities in newborn infants. *Journal of Pediatrics.* 1991; **118**, 112–15.

105. Colditz P, Murphy D, Rolfe P, Wilkinson AR. Effect of infusion rate of indomethacin on cerebrovascular responses in preterm neonates. *Archives of*

Disease in Childhood. 1989; **64**, 8–12.

106. Hammarman C, Aramburo MJ. Prolonged indomethacin therapy for the prevention of recurrences of patent ductus arteriosus. *Journal of Pediatrics.* 1990; **117**, 771–6.

107. Rennie JM, Cooke RWI. Prolonged low dose indomethacin for persistent ductus arteriosus of prematurity. *Archives of Disease in Childhood.* 1991; **66**, 55–8.

108. Gersony WM, Peckham GJ, Ellison RC, Miettinen OS, Nadas AS. Effects of indomethacin in premature infants with patent ductus arteriosus: Results of a national collaborative study. *Journal of Pediatrics.* 1983; **102**, 895–906.

Nervous system

109. Chemtob S, Beharry K, Rex J, Varma DR, Aranda JV. Changes in cerebrovascular prostaglandins and thromboxane as a function of systemic blood pressure: cerebral blood flow autoregulation of the newborn. *Circulation Research.* 1990; **67**, 674–82.

110. Pryds O, Greisen G, Friss-Hansen B. Compensatory increase in CBF in preterm infants during hypoglycaemia. *Acta Paediatrica Scandinavica.* 1988; **77**, 632–7.

111. Painter MJ. Fetal heart rate patterns perinatal asphyxia, and brain injury. *Pediatric Neurology.* 1989; **5**, 137–44.

112. Rosa FW. Spina bifida in infants of women treated with carbamazepine during pregnancy. *New England Journal of Medicine.* 1991; **324**, 674–7.

113. Jones KL, Lacro RV, Johnson KA, Adams J. Pattern of malformations in the children of women treated with carbamazepine during pregnancy. *New England Journal of Medicine.* 1989; **320**, 1661–6.

114. Hobbins JC. Diagnosis and management of neural-tube defects today. *New England Journal of Medicine.* 1991; **324**, 690–1.

115. Luthy DA, Wardinsky T, Shurtleff DB, Hollenbach KA, Hickok DE, Nyberg DA, Benedetti TJ. Cesarean section before the onset of labour and subsequent motor function in infants with meningomyelocele diagnosed antenatally. *New England Journal of Medicine.* 1991; **324**, 662–6.

116. Dubowitz LMS, Dubowitz V. Clinical assessment of gestational age in the newborn infant. *Journal of Pediatrics.* 1970; **77**, 1–10.

117. Brazelton TB. Neonatal behavioral assessment scale. *Clinical Developments in Medicine.* No. 50. Spastics International Medical Publications. Philadelphia: Lippincott 1973.

118. Tronick EZ, Scanlon KB, Scanlon JW. Protective apathy, a hypothesis about the behavioral organization and its relation to clinical and

physiologic status of the preterm infant during the newborn period. *Clinics in Perinatology*. 1990; **17**, 125–54.

119. Volpe JJ. Neonatal seizures: Current concepts and revised classification. *Pediatrics*. 1989; **84**, 422–8.

120. Mizrahi EM, Kellaway P. Characterization and classification of neonatal seizures. *Neurology*. 1987; **37**, 1837–44.

121. Neonatal seizures (editorial). *Lancet*. 1989; **2**, 135–7.

122. Aso K, Scher MS, Barmada MA. Cerebral infarcts and seizures in the neonate. *Journal of Child Neurology*. 1990; **5**, 224–8.

123. Clancy R, Malin S, Laraque D, Baumgart S, Younkin D. Focal motor seizures heralding stroke in full-term neonates. *American Journal of Diseases of Children*. 1985; **139**, 601–6.

124. Levy SR, Abroms IF, Marshall PC, Rosquette EE. Seizures and cerebral infarction in the full-term newborn. *Annals of Neurology*. 1985; **17**, 366–70.

125. Sarnat HB, Sarnat MS. Neonatal encephalopathy following fetal distress; a clinical and electroencephalographic study. *Archives of Neurology*. 1976; **33**, 696–705.

126. Volpe JJ. *Neurology of the Newborn*. 2nd edn. Philadelphia: W.B. Saunders Co., 1987.

127. Noetzel MJ. Myelomeningocele: Current concepts of management. *Clinics in Perinatology*. 1989; **16**, 311–29.

128. Schwersenski J, McIntyre L, Bauer CR. Lumbar puncture frequency and cerebrospinal fluid analysis in the neonate. *American Journal of Diseases of Childhood*. 1991; **145**, 54–8.

129. Hendricks-Munoz KD, Shapiro DL. The role of the lumbar puncture in the admission sepsis evaluation of the premature infant. *Journal of Perinatology*. 1990; **10**, 60–4.

130. Fielkow S, Reuter S, Gotoff SP. Cerebrospinal fluid examination in symptom-free infants with risk factors for infection. *Journal of Pediatrics*. 1991; **119**, 971–3.

131. Weiss MG, Fonides SP, Anderson CL. Meningitis in premature infants with respiratory distress: Role of admission lumbar puncture. *Journal of Pediatrics*. 1991; **119**, 973–5.

132. Saez-LLorens X, McCracken GH. Bacterial meningitis in neonates and children. *Infectious Disease Clinics of North America*. 1990; **4**, 623–44.

133. Sarff LD, Platt LH, McCracken GH. Cerebrospinal fluid evaluation in neonates: Comparison of high-risk infants with and without meningitis. *Journal of Pediatrics*. 1976; **88**, 473–7.

134. Allan WC. The IVH complex of lesions: Cerebrovascular injury in the preterm infant. *Neurologic Clinics*. 1990; **8**, 529–51.

135. Allan WC, Philip AGS. Neonatal cerebral pathology diagnosed by ultrasound. *Clinics in Perinatology*. 1985; **12**, 195–218.

136. Papile L, Burstein J, Burstein R, Koffler H. Incidence and evolution of subependymal and intraventricular hemorrhage: A study of infants with birth weights less than 1,500 gm. *Journal of Pediatrics*. 1978; **92**, 529–34.

137. Baker LL, Stevenson DK, Enzmann DR. End-stage periventricular leukomalacia: MR evaluation. *Radiology*. 1988; **168**, 809–15.

138. Feldman HM, Scher MS, Kemp SS. Neurodevelopmental outcome of children with evidence of periventricular leukomalacia on late MRI. *Paediatric Neurology*. 1990; **6**, 296–302.

139. Wyatt JS, Edwards AD, Azzopardi D, Reynolds EOR. Magnetic resonance and near infrared spectroscopy for investigation of perinatal hypoxic-ischaemic brain injury. *Archives of Disease in Childhood*. 1989; **64**, 953–63.

140. Reynolds EOR, Wyatt JS, Azzopardi D, Delpy DT, Cady EB, Cope M, Wray S. New non-invasive methods for assessing brain oxygenation and haemodynamics. *British Medical Bulletin*. 1988; **44**, 1052–75.

141. Eyre JA. Neurophysiological assessment of the immature central nervous system. *British Medical Bulletin*. 1988; **44**, 1076–92.

142. Connell J, Oozeer R, deVries L, Dubowitz LMS, Dubowitz V. Continuous EEG monitoring of neonatal seizures: diagnostic and prognostic considerations. *Archives of Disease in Childhood*. 1989; **64**, 452–8.

143. Bridges SL, Ebersole JS, Ment LR, Ehrenkranz RA, Silva CG. Cassette electroencephalography in the evaluation of neonatal seizures. *Archives of Neurology*. 1986; **43**, 49–51.

144. Clancy RR, Tharp BR, Enzman D. EEG in premature infants with intraventricular haemorrhage. *Neurology*. 1984; **34**, 583–90.

145. Lacey DJ, Topper WH, Buckwald S, Zom WA, Berger D. Preterm and very low birthweight neonates: relationship of EEG to intracranial haemorrhage, perinatal complications and developmental outcome. *Neurology*. 1986; **34**, 1084–7.

146. Marret S, Paraain D, Samson-Dollfus D, Jeannot E, Fessard C. Positive rolandic sharp waves and periventricular leukomalacia in the newborn. *Neuropediatrics*. 1986; **17**, 199–202.

147. Takeuchi T, Watanabe K. The EEG evolution and neurological prognosis of perinatal hypoxia neonates. *Brain and Development*. 1989; **11**, 115–20.

148. Legido A, Clancy RC, Berman PH. Neurologic outcome after electroencephalograhically proven neonatal seizures. *Pediatrics*. 1991; **88**, 583–96.

149. Taylor MJ, Murphy WJ, Whyte HE. Prognostic reliability of somatosensory and visual evoked potentials of asphyxiated term infants. *Developmental Medicine and Child Neurology*. 1992; **34**, 507–15.

150. Majnemer A, Rosenblatt B, Riley PS. Prognostic significance of multimodality evoked response testing in high-risk newborns. *Pediatric Neurology*. 1990; **6**, 367–74.

Renal physiology

151. Rudolph AM, Heymann MA, Teramo AW. Studies on the circulation of the previable human fetus. *Pediatric Research*. 1971; **5**, 452–65.
152. Matson JR, Stokes JB, Robillard JE. Effect of inhibition of prostaglandin synthesis on fetal renal function. *Kidney International*. 1981; **20**, 621–7.
153. Arant BS. Developmental patterns of renal functional maturation compared in the human neonate. *Journal of Pediatrics*. 1978; **92**, 705–12.
154. Vanpee M, Herin P, Zetterstrom R, Aperia A. Postnatal development of renal function in very low birthweight infants. *Acta Paediatrica Scandinavica*. 1988; **77**, 191–7.
155. Rudd PT, Hughes EA, Placzek MM, Hodes DT. Reference ranges for plasma creatinine during the first month of life. *Archives of Disease in Childhood*. 1983; **58**, 212–15.
156. Aperia A, Herin P. Electrolyte balance. *International Journal of Technology Assessment in Health Care* (Suppl. 1). 1991; **7**, 90–3.
157. Costarino AT, Baumgart S. Controversies in fluid and electrolyte therapy for the premature infant. *Clinics in Perinatology*. 1988; **15**, 863–78.
158. Daniel SS, James LS, Strauss JJ. Response to rapid volume expansion during the postnatal period. *Pediatrics*. 1981; **68**, 809–13.
159. Stonestreet BS, Bell EF, Warburton D. Renal response in low-birth-weight neonates: Results of prolonged intake of two different amounts of fluid and sodium. *American Journal of Diseases of Children*. 1983; **137**, 215–19.
160. Shaffer SE, Norman ME. Renal function and renal failure in the newborn. *Clinics in Perinatology*. 1989; **16**, 199–218.
161. Rosa FW, Bosco LA, Graham CF, Milstein JB, Dreis M, Creamer J. Neonatal anuria with maternal angiotension-converting enzyme inhibition. *Obstetrics and Gynecology*. 1989; **74**, 371–4.
162. Chavez GF, Mulinare J, Cordero JF. Maternal cocaine use during early pregnancy as a risk factor for congenital urogenital anomalies. *Journal of the American Medical Association*. 1989; **262**, 795–8.
163. Perlman JM, Tack ED. Renal injury in the asphyxiated newborn infant: Relationship to neurologic outcome. *Journal of Pediatrics*. 1988; **113**, 875–9.
164. Adelman RD. The hypertensive neonate. *Perinatal Clinics*. 1988; **15**, 567–85.
165. Leung AKC, Robson WLM. Single umbilical artery: report of 159 cases. *American Journal of Diseases of Children*. 1989; **143**, 108–11.
166. Bidiwala KS, Lorenz JM, Kleinman LI. Renal function correlates of postnatal diuresis in preterm infants. *Pediatrics*. 1988; **82**, 50–8.
167. Leech S, Penney MD. Correlation of specific gravity and osmolality of urine in neonates and adults. *Archives of Disease in Childhood*. 1987; **62**, 671–3.
168. Bush GH. Intravenous therapy in paediatrics. *Annals of the Royal College of Surgeons of England*. 1971; **49**, 92–101.
169. Wilkinson AW, Stevens LH, Hughes ZA. Metabolic changes in the newborn. *Lancet*. 1962; **i**, 983–7.
170. John E, Klavdianou M, Vidyasagar D. Electrolyte problems in neonatal surgical patients. *Clinics in Perinatology*. 1989; **16**, 219–32.
171. Wu P, Hodgman JE. Insensible water loss in preterm infants. Changes with postnatal development and non-ionizing radiant energy. *Pediatrics*. 1974; **54**, 704–12.
172. Hammarlund K, Sedin G. Transepidermal water loss in newborn infants. III. Relation to gestational age. *Acta Paediatrica Scandinavica*. 1979; **68**, 795–801.
173. Shaffer SG, Weismann DN. Fluid requirements in the preterm infant. *Clinics in Perinatology*. 1992; **19**, 233–50.
174. Hammarlund K. Water and heat balance. *International Journal of Technology Assessment in Health Care* (Suppl. 1). 1991; **7**, 85–9.
175. Anand KJS, Sippell WG, Aynsley-Green A. Randomised trial of fentanyl anaesthesia in preterm babies undergoing surgery: Effect on the stress response. *Lancet*. 1987; **i**, 243–8.
176. Anand KJS, Sippell WG, Schofield NM. Does halothane anaesthesia decrease the metabolic and endocrine stress responses of newborn infants undergoing operation? *British Medical Journal*. 1988; **296**, 668–2.
177. Anand KJS, Hansen DD, Hickey PR. Hormonal-metabolic stress responses in neonates undergoing cardiac surgery. *Anesthesiology*. 1990; **73**, 661–70.
178. Anand KJS, Hickey PR. Halothane-morphine compared with high-dose fentanyl for anesthesia and postoperative analgesia in neonatal cardiac surgery. *New England Journal of Medicine*. 1992; **326**, 1–9.

Thermoregulation

179. Bruck K. Temperature regulation in the newborn infant. *Biology of the Neonate*. 1961; **3**, 65–119.
180. Himms-Hagen J. Cellular thermogenesis. *Annual Review of Physiology*. 1976; **39**, 315–51.
181. Jessen K. An assessment of human regulatory nonshivering thermogenesis. *Acta Anaesthesiologica*

Scandinavica. 1980; **24**, 138–43.

182. Jessen K. The cortisol fluctuations in plasma in relation to human regulatory nonshivering thermogenesis. *Acta Anaesthesiologica Scandinavica*. 1980; **24**, 151–4

183. Jessen K. The relation between thyroid function and human regulatory nonshivering thermogenesis. *Acta Anaesthesiologica Scandinavica*. 1980; **24**, 144–50.

184. Engleman DR, Lockhart CH. Comparisons between temperature effects of ketamine and halothane anesthesia in children. *Anesthesia and Analgesia*. 1972; **51**, 98–101.

185. Holdcroft A, Hall GM. Heat loss during anaesthesia. *British Journal of Anaesthesia*. 1978; **50**, 157–64.

186. Nour BM, Boudreaux JP, Rowe MI. An experimental model to study thermogenesis in the neonatal surgical patient. *Journal of Pediatric Surgery*. 1984; **19**, 764–70.

187. Ryan JF. Altered temperature regulation section two: unintentional hypothermia. In: Cooperman LH, Orkin FK (eds) *Complications in Anesthesiology*. Philadelphia: Lippincott, 1982.

188. Hey EN. The care of babies in incubators. In: Gairdner D, Hull D. (eds) *Recent Advances in Paediatrics 4*. Edinburgh: Churchill Livingstone, 1971.

189. Hey EN, Katz G. The optimum thermal environment for naked babies. *Archives of Disease in Childhood*. 1970; **45**, 328–34.

190. Silverman WA, Fertig JW, Berger AP. The influence of the thermal environment upon the survival of newly born premature infants. *Pediatrics*. 1958; **22**, 876–86.

191. Benzinger TH. Heat regulation: homeostasis of central temperature in man. *Physiological Reviews*. 1969; **49**, 671–759.

Haematology

192. Oski FA, Naiman JL (eds) *Hematologic problems in the newborn*, 3rd edn. New York: W.B. Saunders Co., 1982.

193. Huehns ER, Shooter EM. Review: human haemoglobins. *Journal of Medical Genetics*. 1965; **2**, 48–90.

194. Chessells JM. Blood formation in infancy. *Archives of Disease in Childhood*. 1979; **54**, 831–4.

195. Lubin B. Neonatal anaemia secondary to blood loss. In: Perinatal Haematology. *Clinics in haematology*. 1978; **7**(1), 19–34.

196. Davenport HT. *Paediatric Anaesthesia*. London: Heinemann, 1980.

197. Stockman JA, Oski FA. Physiological anaemia of infancy and the anaemia of prematurity. *Clinics in Haematology*. 1978; **7**, 3–18.

198. Stockman JA. Anemia of prematurity: current concepts in the issue of when to transfuse. *Pediatric Clinics of North America*. 1986; **30**, 111–28.

199. Doyle JJ, Zipursky A. Neonatal blood disorders. In: Sinclair JC, Bracken MB, (eds) *Effective Care of the Newborn Infant*. Canada: Oxford University Press, 1992, 425–53.

200. Burman D, Morris AF. Cord haemoglobin in low birth weight infants. *Archives of Disease in Childhood*. 1974; **49**, 382–5.

201. Bellingham AJ, Grimes AJ. Red cell 2,3 diphosphoglycerate. *British Journal of Haematology*. 1973; **25**, 555–62.

202. Delivoria-Papadopoulos M, Roncevic NP, Oski FA. Postnatal changes in oxygen transport of term, premature and sick infants. *Pediatric Research*. 1971; **5**, 235–45.

203. Shapiro AD, Jacobson LJ, Armon ME, Manco-Johnson MJ, Hulac P, Lane PA, Hathaway WE. Vitamin K deficiency in the newborn infant: Prevalence and perinatal risk factors. *Journal of Pediatrics*. 1986; **109**, 675–80.

204. Ross MP, Christensen RD, Rothstein G, Koenig JM, Simmons MA, Noble NA, Kimura RE. A randomized trial to develop criteria for administering erythrocyte transfusions to anemic preterm infants 1 to 3 months of age. *Journal of Perinatology*. 1989; **9**, 246–53.

205. Keyes WG, Donohue PK, Spivak JL, Jones MD, Oski FA. Assessing the need for transfusion of premature infants and role of hematocrit, clinical signs and erythropoietin level. *Pediatrics*. 1989; **84**, 412–17.

206. Blanchette VS, Hume HA, Levy GJ, Luban NLC, Strauss RG. Guidelines for auditing pediatric blood transfusion practices. *American Journal of Diseases of Children*. 1991; **145**, 787–96.

207. Strauss RG, Sacher RA, Blazina JF, Blanchette VS, Schloz LM, Butch SH. Commentary on small-volume red cell transfusions for neonatal patients. *Transfusion*. 1990; **30**, 565–70.

208. Stockman JA, Clark DA. Weight gain: a response to transfusion in selected preterm infants. *American Journal of Diseases of Children*. 1984; **138**, 828–30.

209. Alverson DC, Isken VH, Cohen RS. Effect of booster blood transfusions on oxygen utilization in infants with bronchopulmonary dysplasia. *Journal of Pediatrics*. 1988; **113**, 722–6.

210. Hudson I, Cooke A, Holland BM, Houston A, Jones JG, Turner T, Wardrop CA. Red cell volume and cardiac output in anemic pre-term infants. *Archives of Disease in Childhood*. 1990; **65**, 672–5.

211. Ohls RK, Christensen RD. Recombinant erythropoietin compared with erythrocyte transfusion in the treatment of anemia of prematurity.

Journal of Pediatrics. 1991; **119**, 781–8.

212. Preiksaitis JK. Indications for the use of cytomegalovirus seronegative blood products. *Transfusion Medical Reviews*. 1991; **5**, 1–17.

213. Davies SC, Wonke B. The management of haemoglobinopathies. In: Hann IM, Gibson BES, (eds) *Clinical Haematology*. London: Bailliere, 1991: pp. 361–89.

214. Powars D. Diagnosis at birth improves survival of children with sickle cell anaemia. *Pediatrics*. 1989; **83** (suppl), 830–3.

215. Black VD, Lubchenko LO. Neonatal polycythemia and hyperviscosity. *Pediatric Clinics of North America*. 1982; **29**, 1137–48.

216. Letsky EA. Polycythaemia in the newborn. In: Roberton NRC (ed.) *Textbook of neonatology*. London: Churchill Livingstone, 1992: pp. 719–23.

217. Buchanan GR. Coagulation disorders in the neonate. *Pediatric Clinics of North America*. 1986; **33**, 203–19.

218. Turner TL. Coagulation disorders in the newborn. In: Roberton NRC (ed.) *Textbook of Neonatology*. London: Churchill Livingstone, 1992: pp. 687–95.

Metabolism and pharmakinetics

219. Watchko JF, Oski FA. Bilirubin 2O mg/dl = Vigintiphobia. *Pediatrics*. 1983; **71**, 66O–3.

220. Mieli-Vergani G, Howard ER, Portmann B, Mowat AP. Late referral for biliary atresia: missed opportunities for effective surgery. *Lancet*. 1989; i, 421–3.

221. Pereira GR, Sherman MS, Digiacuimo J. Hyperalimentation induced cholestasis. *American Journal of Diseases of Children*. 1981; **135**, 842–5.

222. Cremer RJ, Perryman PW, Richards DM. Influence of light on the hyperbilirubinaemia of the infant. *Lancet*. 1958; i, 1094–7.

223. Tan KL. Phototherapy for neonatal jaundice. *Clinics in Perinatology*. 1991; **18**, 423–39.

224. Maisels MJ, Gifford K, Antle CE, Leib GR. Jaundice in the healthy newborn infant: a new approach to an old problem. *Pediatrics*. 1988; **81**, 505–11.

225. Aynsley-Green A. Metabolic and endocrine interrelationships in the human fetus and neonate: an overview of the control of the adaptation to postnatal nutrition. In: Lindblad BA. (ed.) *Perinatal Nutrition*. New York: Academic Press. 1988, pp. 162–91.

226. Ogata ES. Carbohydrate metabolism in the fetus and neonate and altered neonatal glucoregulation. *Pediatric Clinics of North America*. 1986; **33**, 25–45.

227. Cowett RM, Schwartz R. The infant of the diabetic mother. *Pediatric Clinics of North America*. 1982;

29, 1213–31.

228. Sann L. Neonatal hypoglycemia. *Biology of the Neonate*. 1990; **58** (suppl. 1), 16–21.

229. Cornblath M, Schwartz R, Aynsley-Green A, Lloyd JK. Hypoglycemia in infants: The need for a rational definition. *Pediatrics*. 1990; **85**, 834–7.

230. Schwartz R. Neonatal hypoglycemia: Back to basics in diagnosis and treatment. *Diabetes*. 1991; **40** (suppl. 2), 71–3.

231. Lucas A, Morley R, Cole TJ. Adverse neurodevelopmental outcome of moderate neonatal hypoglycaemia. *British Medical Journal*. 1988; **297**, 1304–8.

232. Koh THHG, Aynsley-Green A, Tarbit M, Eyre JA. Neural dysfunction during hypoglycaemia. *Archives of Disease in Childhood*. 1988; **63**, 1353–8.

233. Nilsson K, Larsson LE, Andreasson S, Ekstrom-Jodal B. Blood glucose concentrations during anaesthesia in children: effects of starvation and perioperative fluid therapy. *British Journal of Anaesthesia*. 1984; **56**, 375–9.

234. Urbach J, Kaplan M, Blondheim O, Hirsch HJ. Neonatal hypoglycemia related to umbilical artery catheter malposition. *Journal of Pediatrics*. 1985; **106**, 825–6.

235. Carter PE, Lloyd DJ, Duffty P. Glucagon for hypoglycaemia in infants small for gestational age. *Archives of Disease in Childhood*. 1988; **63**, 1264–6.

236. Steward DJ, Da Silva CA, Flegel T. Elevated blood glucose levels may increase the danger of neurological deficit following profoundly hypothermic cardiac arrest. *Anesthesiology*. 1988; **68**, 653.

237. Lanier WL, Stangland KJ, Scheithauer BW, Milde JH, Michenfelder JD. The effects of dextrose infusion and head position on neurologic outcome after complete cerebral ischemia in primates. *Anesthesiology*. 1987; **66**, 39–48.

238. Louik C, Mitchell AA, Epstein MF, Shapiro S. Risk factors for neonatal hyperglycaemia associated with 10% dextrose infusion. *American Journal of Diseases of Children*. 1985; **139**, 783–6.

239. Anand KJS, Hansen DD, Hickey PR. Hormonal-metabolic stress responses in neonates undergoing cardiac surgery. *Anesthesiology*. 1990; **73**, 661–7O.

240. Steward DJ. Hyperglycaemia, something else to worry about! *Paediatric Anaesthesia*. 1992; **2**, 81–3.

241. Evans NJ, Rutter N, Hadgraft J, Parr GD. Percutaneous administration of theophylline in the preterm infant. *Journal of Pediatrics*. 1985; **107**, 307–11.

242. Rylance GW. Neonatal pharmacology In: Roberton NRC (ed.) *Textbook of Neonatology*. London: Churchill Livingstone, 1992, pp.

1193–211.

243. Brandom BW, Brandom RB, Cook DR. Uptake and distribution of halothane in infants: in vivo measurements and computer simulations. *Anesthesia and Analgesia*. 1983; **62**, 404–10.

244. Gibbs CP, Munson ES, Tham MK. Anesthetic solubility coefficients for maternal and fetal blood. *Anesthesiology*. 1975; **43**, 100–3.

245. Lerman J, Gregory GA, Willis MM, Eger EI II. Age and the solubility of volatile anesthetics in blood. *Anesthesiology*. 1984; **61**, 139–43.

246. Lerman J, Schmitt BI, Willis MM, Eger EI II. Effect of age on the solubility of volatile anesthetics in human tissues. *Anesthesiology*. 1986; **65**, 307–11.

247. LeDez KM, Lerman J. The minimum alveolar concentration (MAC) of isoflurane in preterm neonates. *Anesthesiology*. 1987; **67**, 301–7.

248. Gregory GA, Wade JG, Beihl DR, Ong BY, Sitar DS. Fetal anesthetic requirement (MAC) for halothane. *Anesthesia and analgesia*. 1983; **62**, 9–14.

249. Moss IR, Conner H, Yee WFH, Iorio P, Scarpelli, EM. Human B-endorphin in the neonatal period. *Journal of Pediatrics*. 1982; **101**, 443–6.

250. Bayon A, Shoemaker WJ, Bloom FE, Mauss A, Guillemin R. Perinatal development of the endorphin- and enkephalin-containing systems in rat brain. *Brain Research*. 1979; **179**, 93–101.

251. Barash PG, Glanz S, Katz JD, Taunt K, Talner NS. Ventricular function in children during halothane anesthesia: an echocardiographic evaluation. *Anesthesiology*. 1978; **49**, 79–85.

252. Cook DR, Brandom BW, Shiu G, Wolfson BW. The inspired median effective dose, brain concentration at anesthesia, and cardiovascular index for halothane in young rats. *Anesthesia and Analgesia*. 1981; **60**, 182–5.

253. Gregory GA. The baroresponses of preterm infants during halothane anesthesia. *Canadian Anaesthetists Society Journal*. 1982; **29**, 105–7.

254. Murat I, Lapeyre G, Saint-Maurice C. Isoflurane attenuates baroreflex control of heart rate in human neonates. *Anesthesiology*. 1989; **70**, 395–400.

255. Tusiewicz K, Bryan AC, Froese AB. Contributions of rib cage-diaphragm interactions to the ventilatory depression of halothane anesthesia. *Anesthesiology*. 1977; **47**, 327–7.

256. Larsson LE, Andreasson S, Ekstrom-Jodal B, Nilsson K. Carbon dioxide tensions in infants during mask anaesthesia with spontaneous ventilation. *Acta Anaesthesiologica Scandinavica*. 1987; **31**, 273–5.

257. Olsson AK, Lindahl SGE. Pulmonary ventilation, CO_2 response and inspiratory drive in spontaneously breathing young infants during halothane anaesthesia. *Acta Anaesthesiologica Scandinavica*. 1986; **30**, 431–7.

258. Dobbinson TL, Nisbet HIA, Pelton DA. Functional residual capacity (FRC) and compliance in anaesthetized, paralysed children. Part II: clinical results. *Canadian Anaesthetists Society Journal*. 1973; **20**, 322–33.

259. Liu LMP, Cote CJ, Goudsouzian NG, Ryan JF, Firestone S, Dedrick DF, Liu PL, Todres ID. Life-threatening apnea in infants recovering from anesthesia. *Anesthesiology*. 1983; **59**, 1506–10.

Immunology

260. Eriksson M, Melen B, Myrback KE, Winbladh B, Zetterstom R. Bacterial colonization of newborn infants in a neonatal intensive care unit. *Acta Paediatrica Scandinavica*. 1982; **71**, 779–83.

261. Lassila O. Embryonic differentiation of lymphoid stem cells. *Developmental and Comparative Immunology* . 1981; **5**, 403–14.

262. Vanderbeeken Y, Sarfati M, Bose R, Delespesse G. In utero immunization of the fetus to tetanus by maternal vaccination during pregnancy. *American Journal of Reproductive Immunology and Microbiology*. 1985; **8**, 39–42.

263. Christenson KL, Christenson P. IgG subclasses and neonatal infections with group B streptococcus. *Monographs in Allergy*. 1988; **23**, 138–47.

264. LaGamma EF, Drusen EM, Mackles AW, Machalek S, Auld PAM. Neonatal infections. *American Journal of Diseases of Children*. 1983; **137**, 838–44.

265. Cairo M. Neonatal host defence. Prospects for immunologic enhancement during neonatal sepsis. *American Journal of Diseases of Children*. 1989; **143**, 40–6.

266. Kliegman RM, Clapp DW. Rational principles for immunoglobulin prophylaxis and therapy of neonatal infections. *Clinics in Perinatology*.1991; **18**, 303–24.

267. Leventhal JM, Shapiro ED, Aten CB, Berg AT, Egerton SA. Does breastfeeding protect against infections in infants less than 3 months of age? *Pediatrics*. 1986; **78**, 896–903.

268. Adinolfi M, Cheetham M, Lee T, Rodin H. Ontogeny of human complement receptors CR1 and CR3: expression of these molecules on monocytes and neutrophils from maternal, newborn and fetal samples. *European Journal of Immunology*. 1988; **18**, 565–9.

269. Wilson CB. Immunologic basis for increased susceptibility of the neonate to infection. *Journal of Pediatrics*. 1986; **108**, 1–12.

2 The Surgical Neonate

Neonatal intensive care for the infant with a surgical disorder must be seen as one point within the continuum from fetal life, labour and delivery, the identification of an anomaly and transport to a regional centre, the perioperative multisystem care in the neonatal intensive care unit (NICU), through to the discharge and follow-up of the infant and integration into the family system.

Antenatal diagnosis

Ultrasound identification of a fetal anomaly

Ultrasound techniques in their various modes, real time, M-mode, continuous and pulsed wave Doppler ultrasound, have made it possible to study fetal anatomy and function in great detail and have become an integral part of the obstetric management of pregnancy. The estimation of gestational age, evaluation of fetal size and growth, detection of fetal structural abnormalities and abnormalities of extrafetal structures, e.g., the umbilical cord and placenta, and the evaluation of the fetal circulation yield valuable clinical information, enable surveillance of fetal well-being, and in some cases provide an opportunity for intrauterine therapy. Guidelines for the application of all these techniques have not yet been firmly established.

The role of ultrasonography in the identification of congenital anomalies is well established in pregnancies complicated by diabetes, abnormalities of amniotic fluid volume, intrauterine growth retardation, abnormal alpha-feto protein measurement, family history of birth defects or any other history suggestive of a congenital abnormality. The increasing ability of ultrasound to detect fetal abnormalities has led to the identification of disorders in all systems, e.g.:

1. *Renal tract* anomalies including renal agenesis, cystic disease and urinary tract obstruction;
2. *Gastrointestinal tract* abnormalities including abdominal wall defects, gastroschisis and omphalocele; internal anomalies of the GI tract, cleft lip, diaphragmatic hernia, duodenal atresia, meconium peritonitis and sacrococcygeal teratomas.
3. *Central nervous system* abnormalities including neural tube defects, abnormalities of the brain and ventricular size, e.g. microcephaly, hydrocephaly, anencephaly, porencephaly and encephaloceles.
4. Congenital heart defects, skeletal dysplasias, cystic hygromas, solid tumours such as neuroblastoma, Wilm's tumour and hepatoblastoma.

There are, however, a number of caveats about ultrasound; it may only demonstrate non-specific findings suggestive of a congenital anomaly such as intrauterine growth retardation, amniotic fluid volume abnormality or hydrops fetalis; it may fail to identify the full degree of an abnormality or may only determine one part of a multiple anomaly syndrome. What is defined on ultrasound must always be evaluated in the context of the gestational age of the fetus; for example, whilst it is normal to observe herniation of the fetal bowel into the base of the umbilical cord up to 12 weeks gestation, the same finding is more likely to be evidence of an omphalocele at a later gestational age. All of these potential limitations have major clinical and ethical implications which require appropriate multidisciplinary exploration with the parents.[1,2]

Chromosome analysis

The identification of one fetal anomaly will lead to careful sonographic screening for other known associated anomalies. It will also prompt investigation for a genetic or chromosomal disorder because of the increased risk for cytogenetic abnormalities in fetuses with structural anomalies. Fetal karyotyping has been advanced considerably with amniocentesis, cordocentesis and chorionic villous sampling, allowing detection of genetic abnormalities as early as 9–11 weeks of gestation.

Management options

Advances in antenatal detection of anomalies have created a range of management alternatives, including the termination of pregnancy, serial *in utero* evaluation to determine the evolution of an anomaly, consideration of fetal surgery, and planning the timing, site and possible route of delivery for the infant.

Fetal surgery

Fetal surgery has been performed in a number of disorders including obstructive uropathy, congenital diaphragmatic hernia and hydrocephalus. In obstructive uropathy, the small group that could theoretically benefit from *in utero* decompression are those with bilateral hydronephrosis secondary to urethral obstruction with favourable urinary electrolytes and osmolality and no other life-threatening anomalies.[3,4] Prenatal repair of congenital diaphragmatic hernia to prevent compression of the growing lung has been reported,[5] but remains an experimental procedure.[3,6] Ventriculoamniotic shunting for fetal ventriculomegaly has been very disappointing with a 'de facto' moratorium on this procedure now in place.[7]

For several reasons, fetal surgery, although technically feasible, must generally be considered experimental at present: the results have been disappointing, the ethical implications are unclear and many of these disorders have a far worse prognosis when diagnosed *in utero* than when diagnosed postnatally.[8] Those counselling parents should therefore have at their disposal not just the details of what usually happens to a baby with a given condition after birth, but also the increasingly available intrauterine prognosis.

Timing, site and route of delivery

The ability to follow serially the evolution of disorders such as congenital diaphragmatic hernia, abdominal wall defects or hydrocephalus may allow the timing of delivery to be optimized. Occasionally early delivery may be indicated for hydrocephalus which is increasing in size or a gastroschisis which is showing signs of change in the bowel wall thickness or bowel loop distension,[9,10] In general, however, further studies must be done to develop objective selection criteria for early delivery;[11] conservative management of the pregnancy with spontaneous onset of labour and vaginal delivery is usually preferred.

The diagnosis of a fetal anomaly makes the choice of delivery site very important. Infants with anomalies that are known to be amenable to surgery should be transferred, preferably before the onset of labour, to facilities offering the best available resuscitation and delivery room management and subsequent care. There is no consensus, however, on the mode of delivery for a complicated pregnancy, (e.g. the fetus with an abdominal wall defect)[12–14] and most centres reserve caesarean section for standard obstetric indications or occasionally for giant omphaloceles and neural tube defects.[10]

Resuscitation and stabilization of the newborn

The principles of neonatal resuscitation are:

Anticipation and preparedness

The intensity that has characterized antenatal fetal surveillance must be continued into the intrapartum period, as pregnancies complicated by fetal abnormalities have an increased incidence of perinatal asphyxia. It is estimated that 6 per cent of all newborns and up to 80 per cent of infants weighing less than 1500 gm will require some form of resuscitation in the delivery room; thus the availability of appropriate equipment and personnel skilled in neonatal resuscitation must be ensured. Excellent manuals and training videos are now available on this topic.[15,16] Maternal conditions which predispose to birth asphyxia include diabetes, hypertension, fever, heavy sedation, drug dependence or severe concomitant illness. Fetal conditions with increased risk include prematurity, postmaturity, multiple pregnancy, intrauterine growth retardation and isoimmunization. Babies born after antepartum haemorrhage, prolonged labour, abnormal presentation or prolapsed cord are particularly prone to asphyxia.

Appropriate initial assessment

This involves assessment of the elements contained in the Apgar score, in particular, respiratory effort and heart rate (Table 2.1).

An Apgar score should be done at one and five minutes and thereafter at 5-minute intervals until a score of 7 is achieved.

In addition, attention needs to be paid to the infant's temperature for reasons that are discussed later in this chapter. Therefore, the delivery room is kept warm, the isolette or overhead warmer is preheated and the infant is quickly dried of amniotic fluid.

The infant is routinely positioned on his/her back with the head slightly down and the neck slightly extended. Specific positioning may be important in infants with congenital diaphragmatic hernia, glossoptosis or a high gastrointestinal tract obstruction, (i.e. hernia side down, prone or head slightly elevated, respectively). Patency of the airway must be established without delay.

Suctioning is only indicated to clear the upper airway of mucus, blood or meconium. The mouth is first gently suctioned for a few seconds; vigorous suctioning of the posterior pharynx can produce significant bradycardia and delay the onset of respiration. Suctioning under direct laryngoscopy is indicated if meconium is present; the detection of meconium in the amniotic fluid should ideally lead to the mouth, pharynx and nose being suctioned while the infant is still on the perineum. Once the infant has been delivered, the mouth and nose are suctioned to remove meconium from the oro- and nasopharynx. If thin meconium is present and the infant is vigorous and active, no further management is necessary; if the meconium is thick or particulate, the trachea should be intubated and the lower airway suctioned.

Table 2.1   The Apgar score.[17]

Apgar	Sign	0	1	2
Appearance	Colour	Blue, pale	Body pink; extremities blue	Completely pink
Pulse	Heart rate	Absent	<100 beats/min.	>100 beats/min.
Grimace	Reflex irritability	No response	Grimace	Cry, cough or sneeze
Activity	Muscle tone	Limp, flaccid	Some flexion of extremities	Active, well flexed
Respiration	Respiratory effort	Absent	Gasping; slow, irregular	Regular, good lusty cry

The tactile stimulation of drying and suctioning induces effective respiration in most infants; other tactile stimuli include gentle slapping of the soles of the feet (no more than twice) or rubbing the infant's back.[18] Oxygen should be administered by funnel or facemask.

The routine passage of a nasogastric tube to exclude choanal or oesophageal atresia is usually not indicated unless there is a clinical suspicion of these disorders.

Early gastric aspiration is also usually not indicated unless meconium or abdominal distension is present, or in cases of diaphragmatic hernia. Infants requiring positive pressure ventilation with a bag and mask for more than 2 minutes should have an orogastric tube inserted and left in place during ventilation.[18]

Establishment of adequate ventilation

It is critically important to establish adequate chest expansion. If oxygen applied to the face or tactile stimulation is insufficient to stimulate respiration, bag and mask ventilation with inspiratory pressures of 2–3 kPa (20 cmH$_2$O) is initiated. Self-inflating bags cannot attain high oxygen concentrations unless an oxygen reservoir is attached; they may also have a mechanism limiting inspiratory pressure. Inflation bags should have a volume of at least 500 ml[19] (but not exceeding 750 ml) so that inflation pressures can be maintained for a longer period.

Bag and mask ventilation is contraindicated if a gastrointestinal anomaly such as tracheo-oesophageal fistula or diaphragmatic hernia is suspected. In these infants tracheal intubation should be performed if respiration is compromised.

Intubation is also required if bag and mask ventilation has failed to initiate respiration or where immediate assessment indicates that the infant is unlikely to respond to bag and mask ventilation alone. Initial lung inflation pressures up to 3–4 kPa (30–40 cmH$_2$O) may be required; after the first 1–2 breaths lower pressures, ±2 kPa (20 cmH$_2$O), will usually suffice. The chest is observed for symmetry of movement and breath sounds.

Once the heart rate is greater than 100 bpm and spontaneous respiration attained, positive pressure ventilation may be discontinued, dependent on the assessment of respiratory sufficiency. If the tracheal tube is to remain in place following resuscitation,

its position must be confirmed with a chest X-ray as soon as possible.

High concentrations of oxygen, 90–100 per cent, are used in the initial stage of resuscitation in all infants.[18] Whether 100 per cent oxygen in this acute phase of resuscitation in the delivery room in very low birthweight infants is deleterious is not known but the danger of severe hypoxia is greater. As soon as the infant responds in colour and oxygen monitoring is initiated, the fractional inspired oxygen concentration should be decreased appropriately.

The majority of preterm infants less than 28 weeks are intubated in the delivery room either electively in the hope of decreasing the incidence of respiratory distress/atelectasis or with the demonstration of clinical signs of respiratory distress or early apnoea. Preterm infants with surfactant deficiency may need relatively high inflation pressures, greater than 3 kPa (30 cmH$_2$O) to create an adequate functional residual capacity (FRC); in general, lower pressures are initiated and then only increased if cardiorespiratory responses, chest movement, air entry or colour remain unsatisfactory.

When called to the delivery room for an infant who has not established postnatal ventilation, it is important to determine whether the infant is suffering from the prolonged effects of asphyxia that began before or during labour and delivery or whether the infant was initially vigorous at birth and thereafter developed apnoea, cyanosis or bradycardia. Differential diagnosis in the latter situation includes airway obstruction, intrathoracic masses, pneumothorax or congenital abnormalities of the airway, e.g. choanal atresia, macroglossia, laryngeal web, etc.

Naloxone hydrochloride (Narcan) is used for the reversal of respiratory depression in infants in whom there is a history of narcotic administration to the mother within four hours of the delivery. Narcan is only given after assisted ventilation and cardiac output have been established. The dose is 0.1 mg.kg^{-1} either i.v. or via tracheal tube; intramuscular administration is also acceptable.[18] If an effect is elicited an additional dose may be given for more sustained effect. Narcan is contraindicated in the infant of a narcotic addicted mother as it may produce severe, acute withdrawal and seizures in the newborn.

Establishment of cardiac output

If the peripheral pulses are not palpable, or the heart rate felt at the base of the umbilical cord or by auscultation is 60–80 bpm despite adequate assisted ventilation with 100 per cent oxygen, external cardiac massage (ECM) is indicated. ECM with the hands encircling the chest and supporting the back and with both thumbs compressing the middle to lower sternum may be the preferred method of improving cardiac output;[19,20] both the thumb technique or compression by the index and middle finger on the lower sternum are accepted by the American Heart Association (Fig 2.1). The sternum is compressed ½″ to ¾″ at a rate of 120 bpm.

If the heart rate does not improve rapidly with these measures a dose of adrenaline (0.1–0.3 ml.kg^{-1} of 1:10 000) should be administered intravenously.

Adrenaline can also be rapidly administered via the tracheal tube, though blood levels achieved may be very low and further doses up to 1 ml.kg^{-1} (1:10 000) may be necessary.

Bicarbonate may be given for documented or assumed metabolic acidosis of a moderate degree, after effective ventilation has been established. This will require the insertion of an umbilical venous catheter, either 4–6 cm below the liver or through the ductus venosus into the IVC. 1–2 mmol.kg^{-1} of 4.2 per cent solution is given over 3–5 minutes at a rate not exceeding 2 ml.min.$^{-1}$

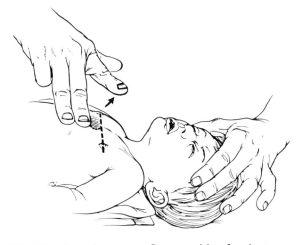

Fig. 2.1 Locating proper finger position for chest compression in infant. Note that the rescuer's hand is used to maintain head position to facilitate ventilation. (Reproduced with permission from [21].)

Evaluation and modification if resuscitation is not succeeding

Evaluation involves consideration of the following if resuscitation is not succeeding:

The tube position
If there is any doubt about the tube position, the child should be extubated and bag and mask ventilation commenced until successful reintubation.

Adequacy of opening pressure
Failure to establish adequate effective ventilation and FRC may be due to insufficient inspiratory pressure or insufficient inspiratory time.[19] Increasing the inflation pressure so as to elicit a respiratory effort and 'Heads' paradoxical reflex, or providing sufficient inspiratory time (at least 1 second) often leads to marked improvement in the FRC.

Presence of a pneumothorax
This is excluded by auscultation, transillumination and where sufficient time is available, by radiographic examination.

Unrecognized hypovolaemia
Hypovolaemia is suspected if the infant remains pale or the pulses remain poorly palpable despite an improvement in the heart rate, or the blood pressure is low and metabolic acidosis persists after the administration of bicarbonate.

Arterial blood pressure (BP) values in normal newborn infants in the first 12 hours of life have been studied[22,23] (Fig 2.23). The availability of oscillometry devices facilitates measurement; although a useful guide, values vary widely with birthweight, gestational age, method of delivery, amount of placental transfusion and the degree of perinatal asphyxia, so that it is difficult to base decisions on a specific BP measurement alone (particularly in extremely low birthweight infants).[24-5]

The central venous pressure is more closely related to neonatal blood volume than arterial BP and monitoring of volume status via an umbilical venous catheter placed in the right atrium or superior vena cava may be very useful in this clinical situation.[24] Volume expansion is achieved with the administration of an appropriate solution, O–negative whole blood or packed cells in the event of blood loss, 5 per cent albumin, fresh frozen plasma or crystalloid solutions at 10–20 ml.kg.$^{-1}$

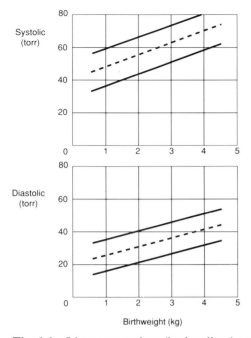

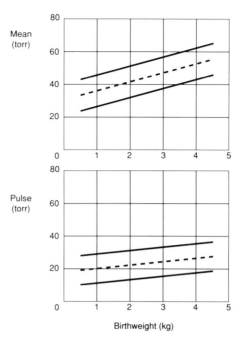

Fig. 2.2 Linear regressions (broken lines) and 95% confidence limits (solid lines) of systolic (top) and diastolic (bottom) aortic blood pressures on birth weight in 61 healthy newborn infants during the first 12 hours after birth. For systolic pressure, $y = 7.13x + 40.45$; $r = .79$. For diastolic pressure, $y = 4.81x + 22.18$; $r = .71$. For both, n = 413 and $P < .001$. (Reproduced with permission from [23].)

Linear regressions (broken lines) and 95% confidence limits (solid lines) of mean pressure (top) and pulse pressure (systolic-diastolic pressure amplitude) (bottom) on birth weight in 61 healthy newborn infants during the first 12 hours after birth. For mean pressure, $y = 5.16x + 29.80$; n = 443; $r = .80$. For pulse pressure, $y = 2.31x + 18.27$; n = 413; $r = .45$. For both, $P < .001$. (Reproduced with permission from [23].)

Acute resuscitation is generally not the time to limit fluid administration unless the infant is in obvious congestive heart failure.

The presence of septic or cardiogenic shock may require the use of inotropic agents, antibiotics or occasionally prostaglandins.

The presence of a malformation

Choanal atresia, diaphragmatic hernia, pulmonary hypoplasia, pleural effusion or some other disorder may be the reason for the failure of routine resuscitative measures. Further clinical and radiographic examination will usually determine these conditions.

Stabilization

Continued support and monitoring is required until the infant is able to maintain independent cardiopulmonary function. In addition attention needs to be specifically paid to the thermal environment, fluid requirements and the biochemi-

cal/metabolic status. In cases of fetal distress or depression at birth, measurement of the umbilical cord gases may help establish the duration of preceding asphyxia; postnatal arterial gases help assess the infant's response to resuscitation measures; measurement of serum glucose must also be part of the postresuscitation assessment as glycogen stores will often have been depleted in a prolonged resuscitation. The possibility of serious bacterial infection should be considered, especially when there is no obvious cause for perinatal asphyxia or failure to initiate respiration.

Discontinuing resuscitation

If 20–30 minutes of appropriate vigorous resuscitation in a term infant fails to generate any respiratory effort it may be appropriate to discontinue resuscitative efforts. The decision is, however, based not only on the failure to generate spontaneous respiration but also on any preceding history of intrapartum difficulties, the detection of anomalies, etc. Apgar score of zero for more than 5 minutes is a very poor prognostic indicator.[26] Resuscitation of an infant with an obvious malformation evident at birth should proceed in a normal manner unless the delivery room team can conclusively determine that the condition is incompatible with life or that a malformation detected prior to delivery has previously resulted in a decision between the parents and multidisciplinary team that aggressive resuscitation would not be utilized. In other situations resuscitation is initiated and the effects of the resuscitation and malformations determined subsequently.

Practical implications of temperature control

The unique problems of temperature control faced by neonates have serious implications for their care, not only in the immediate newborn period in the delivery room but also in the newborn nursery and operating theatre, in resuscitation and in transport. Body temperature only reflects the ability of the neonate to increase heat production enough to match heat loss and gives no information about the metabolic cost of achieving this. Every effort must therefore be made to minimize heat loss in an attempt to keep the baby's metabolic state as near basal as possible.

Evaporative losses in the delivery room can be minimized by drying the baby as soon as possible and in all the above environments, thermal stress is reduced by keeping the baby covered whenever possible. Radiant heat losses occur across incubator walls and between the incubator and the environment so that the effective temperature in an incubator is affected by environmental temperature. Hey has calculated that every 7°C difference between the inside and outside of the incubator lowers the effective temperature in the incubator by 1°C. These losses can be minimized by reinforcing the insulation of the incubator or by clothing the baby. Positive efforts have to be made during resuscitation and in the operating theatre before surgery commences to ensure that babies are not left uncovered in a thermally hostile environment.

In the operating theatre, skin preparation should be performed rapidly with warm fluids and sterile drapes should be applied as soon as possible. The environmental temperature in an operating room will be well below the neutral range even if it is kept as high as staff can tolerate, so that additional sources of heat supply are required. Traditionally, electric or water mattresses have been used but the more recently introduced hot air mattress is safer and more efficient.[27] Exposed visceral surfaces should be covered with warm sterile dressings and intravenous fluids should be warmed before administration. Warming and humidifying the inspired gas delivered to the breathing system is also helpful. Outside the operating theatre environment, the use of overhead radiant heaters is widespread and effective, though these increase insensible fluid losses.

Fluid and electrolyte management

The factors affecting fluid requirements in the newborn include:

- Gestational age/birthweight
- Postnatal age
- Environmental temperature/humidity and method of temperature control
- Insensible water losses
- Renal function
- Underlying pathological condition
- Predisposition to PDA and NEC
- Metabolic rate/degree of activity
- Volume status
- Solute load.

All of these require consideration in fluid and electrolyte management decisions.

Evaluation of water balance

1. Clinical signs:
   - blood pressure
   - heart rate
   - skin turgor
   - mucous membranes
   - fontanelle pressure
   - capillary refill
   - peripheral perfusion
   - core–peripheral temperature gradient

2. Body weight

3. Urine:
   - volume
   - osmolality or specific gravity
   - electrolytes
   - glucose

4. Serum:
   - electrolytes (Na and FENa)
   - glucose
   - osmolality
   - urea, creatinine
   - haematocrit
   - acid base status

(NB: FENa = Fractional excretion of sodium)

Guidelines for intravenous fluid therapy

During the first 1–3 postnatal days body water compartment volumes are permitted to adjust to the extrauterine needs of the newborn; restricting water, sodium and chloride to below estimated expenditure allows isotonic contraction of the extracellular water compartment.[28] Initially 10 per cent dextrose water (or 5 per cent in very low birthweight infants to avoid hyperglycaemia) is used and maintenance amounts of Na, K and Ca added thereafter.

Maintenance requirements in the surgical neonate

Fluid therapy must reflect the dynamic changes taking place postnatally; from the initial low glomerular filtration rate (GFR) phase when the infant is not able to cope with water and electrolyte loads and insensible losses are greatest, to the development of a more predictable state after a few days of life when GFR and fractional excretion of sodium (FENa) vary more appropriately with fluid and electrolyte intake.

Table 2.2   Initial fluid requirements (first day of life: no abnormal losses). (Modified from[28] and [29]).

Birthweight (gm)	*Water (see footnote) ($ml.kg^{-1}.day$)	Na^+ ($mmol.kg^{-1}.day$)	K^+ ($mmol.kg^{-1}.day$)	Ca^2 ($mmol.kg^{-1}.day$)	Glucose ($mg.kg^{-1}.min$)
<1000	100	nil	nil	nil	5%
1000–2000	80	nil	nil	nil	10%
>2000	60	nil	nil	nil	10%

Table 2.3   Maintenance fluid requirements (after first day of life: no abnormal losses). (Modified from [28] and [29]).

Birthweight (gm)	*Water (see footnote) ($ml.kg^{-1}.day$)	Na^+ ($mmol.kg^{-1}.day$)	K^+ ($mmol.kg^{-1}.day$)	Ca^2 ($mmol.kg^{-1}.day$)	Glucose ($mg.kg^{-1}.min$)
<1000	120–160	3–4	1–3	1–2	4–8
1000–2000	100–140	2–3	1–3	1–2	4–8
>2000	80–120	2–3	1–3	1–2	4–8

*footnote: Increase for radiant-heater, phototherapy and according to the evaluation of water balance.

Preoperative requirements

Intravenous fluid therapy is indicated only if absorption by the oral route is inadequate. Preoperative starvation should not exceed four hours. Even in cases of intestinal atresia or obstruction early diagnosis and treatment may prevent long periods of fluid deprivation. Neonates should be kept on their normal feeding regimen until four hours before surgery and can be given clear fluids up to two hours preoperatively.[30] They should be given priority on any operating schedule because if undue delays occur they will become progressively more water and salt depleted. In practice, an intravenous infusion is usually commenced preoperatively in this age group.

Bowel function usually returns fairly quickly after surgery in the neonate and feeds of milk – preferably human – should be established as soon as possible, either orally or via a nasogastric or transanastomotic feeding tube.

Intraoperative requirements

Intraoperative fluid requirements should be based on the maturity of the baby, the length of preoperative fluid deprivation and an estimation of the fluid lost into body cavities. Any fluid given in the injection of diluted muscle relaxants or other drugs should be included in the overall fluid balance. The normal maintenance requirements should be reduced by approximately 30 per cent in the first 24 hours after major surgery because of the antidiuretic response to the stress of anaesthesia and surgery, although infants with abnormal kidneys may not show this response. Postoperative fluid regimens should, however, include appropriate replacement for gastrointestinal losses and increased insensible loss associated with prematurity or the use of overhead heating canopies.

Maintenance requirements for sodium and potassium in the neonate are 3 mmol.kg^{-1}.24h and 2 mmol.kg.$^{-1}$.24 hr respectively, although sodium requirements are halved by the end of the first week of life. It should be remembered that premature babies of under 30 weeks gestation require 5 mmol.kg^{-1} or more, whilst those between 30 and 35 weeks gestation require at least 4 mmol.kg^{-1}.24h.

Fluid and electrolyte disturbances

Primary water disturbances

Normal values
The osmolality ratio between plasma and urine should be 1:1.5. Normal serum osmolality is 270–285 mosm.l^{-1}; although values up to 310 mosm.l^{-1} are still within the normal range, they do require an explanation. Urine osmolality varies with the fluid balance and the range of normal values is between 50 and 600 mmol.l^{-1}.

Abnormal water losses
Increased insensible water loss with prematurity, phototherapy and exposure to radiant heat has been mentioned as has increased urine volume in infants with water-losing renal disease. Perhaps the most critical pure water-losing situation in the newborn occurs with nephrogenic diabetes insipidus, where fluid replacement should be managed by a paediatric nephrologist.

In the presence of excess water loss, either through the skin as in very low birthweight babies, infants under radiant heat canopies or through the bowel, the urine output will fall. If adequate fluid replacement is not given, plasma osmolality will rise because of the limited ability of the neonatal kidney to concentrate the urine. On the other hand, when a high solute load is given, either intravenously or as unmodified cow's milk, plasma osmolality may also rise because of the large amounts of urinary water required in which to excrete the solutes. The loss of saliva in patients with oesophageal atresia seldom causes much disturbance, but duodenal atresia may cause loss of gastric, duodenal, biliary and pancreatic secretions by vomiting.

When obstruction occurs lower down the intestinal tract, both the volume and the complexity of the composition of lost fluid increase. In addition, intestinal obstruction and sepsis are commonly associated with gross abdominal distension, which increases losses of crystalloid and colloid from the vessels in the bowel wall – the so-called third space losses. As well as loss of alimentary secretions, intestinal obstruction is further complicated by starvation. It is reasonable to assume that the chemical composition of the neonate with congenital intestinal obstruction is normal at birth, but the fluid and electrolyte losses outlined above will become increasingly severe the longer diagnosis and treatment are delayed.

Deficit replacement (Table 2.4)

An infant who is clinically dehydrated has probably lost 50–100 ml.kg^{-1} body weight (5–10 per cent). At 5 per cent dehydration there is loss of skin turgor, the fontanelles are slightly depressed and the baby is lethargic. At 10 per cent, the fontanelles and orbits are sunken, peripheral blood flow is poor and the body temperature may be high or low. Dehydration greater than 10 per cent affects the cardiovascular system and circulatory collapse is imminent.

If the deficit is severe, up to 20 ml.kg^{-1} of physiological saline may be given, and its effect judged clinically (improved skin elasticity, reduced pulse rate, decreasing core–peripheral temperature gradient, increased venous pressure and urine output). Children with water-losing renal disease may require 200 ml.kg^{-1} day or more and their sodium intake should be increased if there is combined salt and water loss. In nephrogenic diabetes insipidus water is required in large amounts, with only minimal salt and even giving 0.9 per cent saline can actually increase water losses to cover the excretion of the additional sodium.

Intestinal losses should be replaced with physiological saline, although if a metabolic acidosis is present, some of the sodium may be administered as bicarbonate. It is not usually necessary to give more than 2 mmol.kg^{-1} of sodium bicarbonate in the first instance unless acidosis is severe.

Hypertonic and hypotonic dehydration should be appropriately corrected, the former with 0.18 per cent saline or 5 per cent dextrose, possibly after initial correction of any hypovolaemia with colloid. Care must be taken not to correct the deficiency too quickly or cerebral oedema will follow. Hypotonic dehydration is corrected with physiological saline.

Shock

In states of hypovolaemic shock, blood 20 ml.kg^{-1} body weight, plasma or 5 per cent albumin should be infused rapidly, depending on the Hb and haematocrit. In severe cases, 40 ml.kg^{-1} or more may be needed. This is sometimes the case in states of severe peritonitis. Central venous pressure monitoring is useful in ensuring the optimum right atrial filling pressure.

As dehydration is corrected, the peripheral circulation will improve and core-periphery temperatures will approximate. Indeed, the state of the peripheral circulation is a very sensitive guide to cardiac output and filling pressures in the baby.

The aim in preparation for surgery must be to achieve an optimal clinical state, but there should be as little delay as possible in operating on babies with severe peritonitis or possible gangrenous bowel.

Primary electrolyte disturbances

Sodium

During the first 12–24 hours of life there is no obligatory sodium requirement due to the low GFR and urine volume. Sodium is usually included in therapy after day one to prevent extreme changes in plasma concentration due to the simultaneous changes taking place in water balance. Disturbances in sodium homoeostasis occur frequently

Table 2.4 Contents of commonly used intravenous fluids

Solution	Na$^+$ (mmol·l^{-1})	Cl$^-$ (mmol·l^{-1})	K$^+$ (mmol·l^{-1})	Ca^{2+} (mmol·l^{-1})	Lactate (mmol·l^{-1})	Calories MJ·l^{-1}
0.9% Saline	154	154	—	—	—	—
0.45% Saline in 2.5% dextrose	77	77	—	—	—	0.4
0.18% Saline in 4% dextrose	31	31	—	—	—	0.63
Hartmann's solution	131	111	5.0	2.0	29	—
Half-strength Hartmann's solution	65.5	55.5	2.5	1.0	14.5	—
5% Dextrose	—	—	—	—	—	0.8

in neonatal ICU patients necessitating frequent monitoring of serum levels and adjustment of fluid therapy, especially in low birthweight infants and those infants undergoing surgical procedures.[31]

Hyponatraemia (Na <130 mmol.l^{-1})

Hyponatraemia must always be evaluated in conjunction with an assessment of the extracellular fluid volume status to differentiate water retention/dilutional hyponatraemia, from hyponatraemia secondary to excessive sodium losses or inadequate intake.

In the sick premature these factors may coexist to a greater or lesser extent. Occasionally spurious hyponatraemia is seen in hyperlipidaemic or hyperglycaemic states.

Causes of hyponatraemia include

Water retention/dilutional hyponatraemia This is seen in association with:

1. *Excessive fluid intake:* This is the most common cause of hyponatraemia in the first few days of life as a high fluid intake will readily exceed the neonatal kidney's capacity to excrete a water load. Hyponatraemia may also be seen in infants born to mothers given hypotonic intravenous fluids during labour, particularly toxaemic mothers who have been on salt poor diets.

2. *Oedematous states:* In congestive heart failure, renal failure, liver failure and occasionally in overwhelming neonatal sepsis, a combination of factors may lead to hyponatraemia including increased proximal tubular reabsorption of sodium and water and a decrease in the delivery of filtrate to the distal diluting sites, elevated aldosterone and ADH secretion. Hyponatraemia occurs with a low urine output, moderately high urine specific gravity and osmolality, a low urine sodium and the use of diuretics.

    The use of indomethacin for the treatment of PDA may be associated with hyponatraemia if fluid intake is not adjusted to accommodate the anticipated antidiuretic effect of the drug.

3. *Excess anti-diuretic hormone (ADH) secretion:* This occurs in a number of medical conditions including intraventricular haemorrhage, asphyxial encephalopathy, meningitis, and lung disorders, atelectasis and pneumothorax. Postoperatively a combination of factors may lead to excessive ADH including anaesthesia,

hypotension, pain and the manipulation of the abdominal viscera. This becomes extremely important in surgical patients with third spacing into the peritoneal cavity, such as that seen in infants with NEC, perforation and peritonitis.

The syndrome of inappropriate ADH secretion (SIADH) is suggested by the combination of hyponatraemia, a low urine output, high urine specific gravity and osmolality (>100mosml.l^{-1}) (urine osmolality > plasma osmolality) and increased sodium in the urine (natriuresis secondary to volume expansion). It is often difficult to diagnose SIADH conclusively as sodium losses in the urine may be secondary to decreased renal tubular absorption due to prematurity alone.

The most common sign accompanying hyponatraemia, whatever the cause, is excessive weight gain. The degree of hyponatraemia and the rate at which it occurs determine whether neurological signs such as lethargy, irritability or seizures (due to the rapid osmotically induced swelling of neurons) are also clinically evident.

Hyponatraemia secondary to excessive sodium losses This may occur through the urine via renal tubular dysfunction either due to immaturity (urinary losses up to 10–12 mmol.kg^{-1}.day may be seen) or secondary to hypoxic tubular damage (ATN). Occasionally the salt-losing form of mineralocorticoid deficiency, 21 hydroxylase deficiency is seen in the newborn towards the end of the first week of life in which hyponatraemic dehydration occurs with hyperkalaemia.

Sodium losses may occur through the gastrointestinal tract secondary to surgical fistulae, diarrhoeal disease, or intestinal obstruction.

Decreased Sodium Intake: Inadequate sodium intake after the first few days of life may lead to the slow evolution of 'late hyponatraemia', particularly common in premature infants with pre-existing tubular immaturity and sodium losses in the urine.

Effects and management of Hyponatraemia

When the loss of sodium exceeds that of water, serum sodium and osmolality fall; contraction of the extracellular fluid leads to a decrease in effective blood volume. In general fluid restriction alone will suffice in most instances of hyponatraemia secondary to water retention. If the state of hydration is normal and to be maintained, insensible water loss (IWL) plus urine output is used as a guide to fluid requirements; however, where pre-existing expansion of the extracellular volume is present, IWL alone is preferred with urine volume only replaced when a normal state of hydration is achieved.

The volume status and degree of dehydration determine the rapidity with which hyponatraemia must be corrected. Hypotonic dehydration with prerenal azotaemia requires more rapid correction with normal saline, 3 per cent saline or both. Slower evolving hyponatraemia may be treated by sodium replacement over 24–48 hours.

Treatment should be controlled by serum and urine electrolyte measurements.

The amount of sodium required to restore the sodium content is largely related to the extracellular fluid volume, which is increased in the neonate to approximately 40 per cent of body weight. An amount equivalent to 20 per cent of body weight is commonly added to this to allow for intracellular requirements; this makes up the 'sodium space' of 0.6.

A useful formula for calculating the amount of sodium required to replace a deficit is:

Sodium required =
 (mmol)
    deficit × bodyweight × 'sodium space'
 (mmol.l^{-1})   (kg)

A 3 kg neonate with a sodium deficit of 12 mmol.l^{-1} would thus require 12 × 3 × 0.6 = 21.6 mmol of sodium. Since physiological saline contains 154 mmol.l^{-1}, this deficit would be corrected by infusion of 21.6/154 × 1000 ml = 140 ml physiological saline.

In surgical patients volume expansion with colloid intra- and postoperatively may ameliorate the tendency to SIADH.[32] Standard fluid solutions are used, e.g. 0.2–0.45 normal saline; however, if the patient is dehydrated normal saline may be appropriate depending on the severity and symptomatology of the hypotonic dehydration. If neurological signs are present, the hyponatraemia is gradually corrected to achieve an increase in the sodium of 1 mmol.hr^{-1}.[31]

Hypernatraemia (Na >150 mmol.l^{-1})

Hypernatraemia, common in low birthweight infants in the first few days of life, is seen when:

1. water losses exceed sodium, or
2. excess sodium is administered to an infant.

Hypernatraemia may occur with overhydration, dehydration or a normal intravascular volume status.

1. Free water losses leading to hypernatraemia are particularly common in very low birthweight infants with high insensible water losses in the first few days of life; this is exacerbated by the high evaporative losses in infants nursed under radiant heaters.

   Hypernatraemia may also occur due to urinary losses via osmotic diuresis secondary to glycosuria or aminoaciduria, or when gastrointestinal losses of water occur in excess of sodium. These infants are generally underhydrated.

2. Sodium administered without the requisite free water occurs with saline flushes of lines and following sodium bicarbonate infusion to correct acidaemia. This may precipitate hypercarbia, congestive heart failure and pulmonary oedema. There is also concern that rapid correction of acidosis with bicarbonate leading to hypertonicity may precipitate IVH in the vulnerable vessels of the subependymal germinal matrix of the premature infant.

Potassium

Hypokalaemia (K <3.0 mmol.l)

Hypokalaemia is usually a reflection of a low intake (less than 2 mmol.kg^{-1}.day) or increased losses via the kidney or the gastrointestinal tract. Urinary losses are seen with the use of diuretics and in renal tubular acidosis; gastrointestinal losses are common with diarrhoea or the use of nasogastric suction. The loss of gastric contents results in hypochloraemic alkalosis which may lead to hypokalaemia as hydrogen ions are conserved at the expense of potassium losses.

Hypokalaemia may occur with the induction of alkalosis without any change in total body potassium; this is due to movement of potassium into the cells and may therefore not require treatment if the alkalosis is to be corrected within a short period. However, potassium should be replaced and normal levels maintained in infants with any ongoing losses from gastrointestinal drainage, persistent alkalosis or with the continued use of diuretics and digoxin. The maximum rate of K replacement is 0.5 mmol.kg^{-1}.hr with a maximum concentration of potassium in the peripheral IV of 40 mmol.l^{-1}. Urine output should be at least 1 ml.kg^{-1}.hr.

Cardiac arrhythmias commonly occur when serum potassium levels are low, as for example during cardiac surgery, where more rapid replacement may be required.

Hyperkalaemia (K >7 mmol.l^{-1})

Hyperkalaemia is more often a reflection of the shift of potassium from its normal intracellular position than an abnormality in total body potassium. It is seen most commonly in the immediate newborn period in metabolic acidosis, haemolysis or cellular leak (particularly in extremely premature infants with extensive bruising, CNS or GI bleeding), and in renal failure. Hyperkalaemia in the very low birth weight infant may occur without evidence of impaired glomerular filtration or urine output; the only evidence of renal dysfunction being altered tubular function with increased fractional excretion of sodium.[33] It is always important to ensure that hyperkalaemia is not due to the haemolysis that commonly occurs when blood sampling is performed by heel-stick sampling. A high potassium may decrease with the treatment of acidosis and dehydration, but could also indicate an aldosterone biosynthetic defect such as 21-hydroxylase congenital adrenal hyperplasia.

If the K level is greater than 6 mmol.l^{-1}, the acid–base status, serum calcium (hypocalcaemia will potentiate the effects of hyperkalaemia) and renal function should be assessed. Management is conservative and includes discontinuing K in the intravenous fluids and treating any associated disorder, e.g. acidosis. If the K is greater than 7 mmol.l^{-1} or if renal failure is present, in the presence of early ECG changes (tall, tented T–waves or broadening of the QRS complex) one or more of the following acute measures are indicated to prevent cardiac arrythymias, cardiac arrest or respiratory impairment.

1. Sodium bicarbonate 1–2 mmol.kg.$^{-1}$ over 10 minutes (to shift potassium intracellularly).
2. 10 per cent calcium gluconate 0.1–0.2 ml.kg.$^{-1}$ via slow intravenous push (to counteract the effect of K on the myocardium).
3. If the above measures fail to lower the potassium level and normalize ECG changes, an ion exchange resin should be used, e.g. sodium polystyrene sulfonate (Kayexalate) 0.5–1 gm.kg.$^{-1}$ rectally. Care must be exercised with its use as sodium retention and hypernatraemia may occur.
4. Insulin and glucose infusion are occasionally required: i.v. glucose 0.5 gm.kg.$^{-1}$ over 1–2 hours with 0.2 units soluble insulin per gram glucose (0.1 units.kg.$^{-1}$) (to promote potassium uptake by the cells).

Transport considerations

The objectives of postnatal transport for the newborn with a congenital abnormality requiring neonatal surgery are to continue the stabilization initiated at the hospital of birth and to provide continuous supportive care in transit at a level equivalent to that at the receiving hospital. The combined expertise of the transport team and the regional centre staff are utilized to minimize the risks inherent in any transfer.

Stabilization by the transport team includes:

1. Ventilatory assistance with sufficient safety margin to account for the effects of altitude and the difficulty of detecting or correcting problems in transit, particularly by air transport. This implies the exclusion or treatment of a pneumothorax prior to transfer, the secure fixation of all tubes, the correction of respiratory acidosis or the administration of exogenous surfactant when appropriate.
2. Vascular access to provide fluid, glucose and drug administration.
3. The use of inotropes or volume expanders for cardiovascular instability. Prostaglandin infusion is initiated in suspected duct–dependent congenital heart disease. Metabolic acidosis is corrected with sodium bicarbonate.
4. Temperature control is of critical importance and requires an appropriate transport incubator.
5. Sedation, analgesia and anticonvulsants are used where appropriate.

Special circumstances:

Infants with congenital diaphragmatic hernia should be intubated prior to transfer. Placing the infant with the affected side down may optimize ventilation as the non–dependent lung receives a larger percentage of the tidal volume; low ventilatory pressures may prevent overdistension of the contralateral lung. A large nasogastric tube for abdominal decompression is required.

To improve drainage of the upper pouch, infants with tracheo–oesophageal fistula who are not intubated may be transported prone with the head elevated and a large suction catheter in the upper oesophageal pouch. If possible, mechanical ventilation should be avoided to prevent enlargement of the fistula; inadvertent intubation of the fistula must also be carefully checked.

Infants with an omphalocele or gastroschisis require particular attention to temperature control because of the large surface area of exposed bowel. The defect is covered with sterile, warm, isotonic saline dressing, wrapped with gauze and covered with sterile plastic. Care must be taken not to compress the exposed bowel. A nasogastric tube for decompression is required and intravenous fluids are essential.

An infant with gastrointestinal obstruction should have a nasogastric tube inserted for intermittent suctioning during transfer. In general, the head should be slightly elevated so as to minimize respiratory compromise due to aspiration.

Infants with myelomeningocele require prone positioning to minimize tension on the sac; the defect should be covered with a sterile dressing and moistened with sterile isotonic saline so as to avoid contamination.

Initial assessment of the newborn

Initial assessment includes a detailed history of the pregnancy, labour and delivery, postnatal adaptation and emergence of signs and symptoms. In addition, a full maternal history, inquiry into parental ages, consanguinity, previous reproductive history, family pedigree and maternal exposure to teratogens or viral infections are elicited.

The routine physical examination of the newborn will be briefly described here; this involves the identification and quantification of any illness or anomalies. In succeeding sections devoted to specific organ systems the examination of that specific system will be discussed in further detail.

Assessment of gestational age:

Assessment of the gestational age is based on a number of physical characteristics as well as an assessment of neuromuscular maturity.[34]

The physical signs include the nature of the skin, hair, ear cartilage, breast tissue, external genitalia and plantar creases. The Parkin assessment provides a rapid means of determining gestational age (Table 2.5);[35] this is then correlated with obstetric dating, e.g. the date of the last menstrual period and other indices of fetal growth obtained during pregnancy.

Growth parameters

Once gestational age has been determined the infant's weight, length and head circumference are plotted on standard growth percentile charts[36] (Figs 2.3 and 2.4).

Ideally, growth charts for the population that most closely represents the infant in question should be employed.[37]

Definitions

An infant is defined as appropriate for gestational age (AGA) when the birthweight is within two standard deviations of the mean for the gestational age; infant is one whose weight is less than a small (SGA) two standard deviations from the mean, and a large (LGA) infant is one whose weight is greater than two standard deviations from the mean for that gestational age.

Infants weighing 2.5 kg or less are defined as low birthweight, less than 1500 gm as very low birthweight infants and a further category of extreme low birth weight has been used for those infants weighing less than 1000 gm at birth.

Prematurity is defined as a gestational age less than 37 weeks, term is considered 37–42 weeks, and post-term more than 42 completed weeks.

Physical examination

Routine physical examination includes initial observation of the infant's colour, breathing pattern, morphology, level of activity and responsiveness; recording of vital signs, heart rate, respiratory rate,

Table 2.5 Parkin Assessment and mean gestational ages derived from the total scores of skin colour, skin texture, breast size and ear firmness. (Modified from[35])

Skin texture
Tested by picking up a fold of abdominal skin between finger and thumb, and by inspection

0   very thin with a gelatinous feel
1   thin and smooth
2   smooth and of medium thickness; irritation rash and superficial peeling may be present
3   slight thickening and stiff feeling with superficial cracking and peeling especially evident on the hands and feet
4   thick and parchment-like with superficial or deep cracking

Skin colour
Estimated by inspection when the baby is quiet

0   dark red
1   uniformly pink
2   pale pink, though the colour may vary over different parts of the body; some parts may be very pale
3   pale, nowhere really pink except on the ears, lips, palms and soles

Breast size
Measured by picking up the breast tissue between finger and thumb

0   no breast tissue palpable
1   breast tissue palpable on one or both sides, neither being more than 0.5 cm in diameter
2   breast tissue palpable on both sides, one or both being 0.5 cm–1 cm in diameter
3   breast tissue palpable on both sides, one or both being more than 1 cm in diameter

Ear firmness
Tested by folding of the upper pinna

0   pinna feels soft and is easily folded into bizarre positions without springing back into position spontaneously
1   pinna feels soft along the edge and is easily folded but returns slowly to the correct position spontaneously
2   cartilage can be felt to the edge of the pinna though it is thin in places and the pinna springs back readily after being folded
3   pinna firm with definite cartilage extending to the periphery, and springs back immediately into position after being folded

Score	Gestational age (w)
1	27
2	30
3	33
4	34.5
5	36
6	37
7	38.5
8	39.5
9	40
10	41
11	41.5
12	42

temperature and blood pressure; and examination of all systems.

Skin

The nature of the skin texture is an indication of gestational age as described above; fine, soft lanugo may cover the back and dorsal aspect of the limbs of premature infants, while the skin of the postmature infant is often dry, cracked and peeling with less than normal subcutaneous tissue present. The fingernails are often long and meconium stained in these infants.

In addition alteration in skin colour must be noted. Pallor may indicate anaemia or vasoconstriction, mottling may indicate sepsis or hypothermia. Peripheral cyanosis is commonly seen shortly after birth whereas central cyanosis is always abnormal and requires immediate investigation. Jaundice is evident in the first few days in the skin; the sclera do not show hyperbilirubinaemia

until days after birth. Patches of cutis aplasia occur in trisomy 13 and a number of other genetic disorders.

Skull and facial features:

Abnormalities of facial appearance should be carefully noted as the face is often the clue to the identification of a dysmorphic syndrome. The size, shape and symmetry of the skull and the cranial sutures and fontanelles are noted. The ears are examined for malformations or abnormalities of position; posterior rotation of the ears is a common finding and may be associated with other birth defects. Sinuses anterior to the ear represent remnants of the first branchial cleft. The shape of the nose, asymmetry or paucity of facial movement, the degree of development of the mandible and the size of the tongue are assessed. Macroglossia may be secondary to Beckwith–Wiedemann syndrome or hypothyroidism. Minor degrees of midline cleft

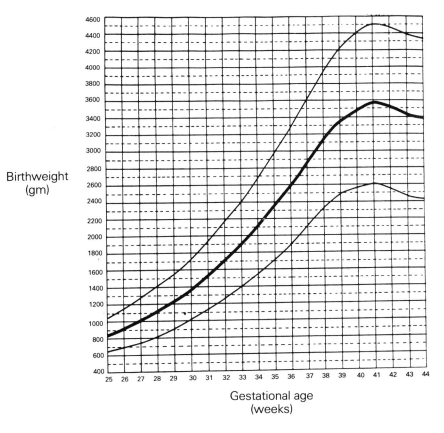

Fig. 2.3 Smoothed curve values for the mean ±2 standard deviations of birthweight against gestational age. (Reproduced with permission from [36].)

palate may be missed unless the mouth is opened; one should also note whether a high arched palate is present. Midline neck masses may be a goitre; lateral neck masses are usually either a cystic hygroma or haemangioma.

Respiratory system

The chest is observed for signs of respiratory distress which may include tachypnoea (respiratory rate greater than 60 within the first day of life,

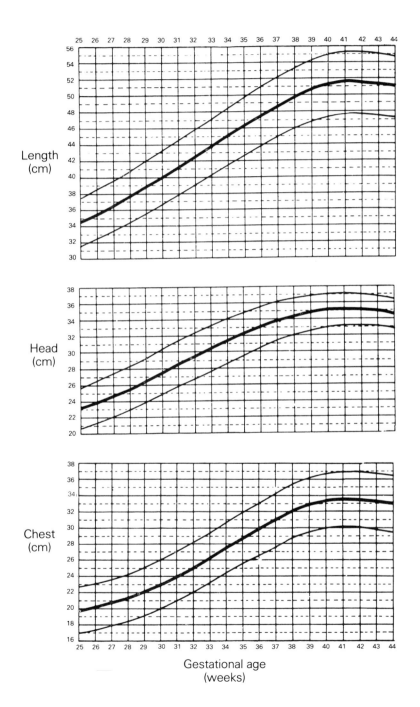

Fig. 2.4 Smoothed curve values for the mean ±2 standard deviations of crown-heel length, head circumference and chest circumference against gestational age. (Reproduced with permission from [36].)

greater than 40 thereafter), retractions, inspiratory stridor, expiratory grunting, flaring of the alae nasi and asymmetry of chest movement. Auscultation of the chest normally reveals bronchovesicular or bronchial breathing; decreased air entry, asymmetry or adventitious breath sounds are important clinical signs of respiratory disease.

Cardiovascular system

Peripheral perfusion is assessed via the capillary refill time and the strength of the pulses. Any difficulty in palpation of the femoral pulses should be followed by measurement of the blood pressure in all four limbs. The maximum cardiac impulse, nature of the heart sounds and the presence of cardiac murmurs are determined.

Abdomen

Any difficulties with swallowing or excess oral mucus require the passage of a nasogastric tube to rule out oesophageal atresia. The abdomen of the newborn is generally flat to slightly distended; if scaphoid in appearance a diaphragmatic hernia should be suspected. If moderate gaseous distension is present it may indicate intestinal obstruction. The abdominal wall and umbilicus should be examined: the umbilicus normally contains two arteries and a vein; a two–vessel cord is often a clue to abnormalities in other systems.

An omphalocele is seen as a midline protrusion with the abdominal contents covered with fetal amniotic membrane; the sac may occasionally rupture with evisceration of the abdominal contents including the liver and intestine.

Gastroschisis is characterized by a defect lateral to the umbilicus with the umbilical cord normally attached to the abdominal wall immediately to the left of the defect; there is no covering sac and small intestine and occasionally liver are visible.

A liver edge may be palpable 2 cm below the right costal margin in many normal infants. A spleen of 1–2 cm below the left costal margin may also be felt in 10–20 per cent of otherwise normal infants. Both lower poles of the right and left kidney may be palpable, the left more easily felt than the right. Enlarged kidneys may indicate underlying hydronephrosis, cystic disease or a tumour. An enlarged bladder may be a sign of a urinary tract outflow obstruction. Patency of the anus must always be determined.

Genitalia

The degree of physical maturity must be accurately assessed prior to designating abnormality of the genitalia. Ambiguity of the genitalia is suggested by the finding of an enlarged clitoris, posterior fusion of the vagina or an empty scrotum. In males it is important to examine for coronal or glandular hypospadias; epispadias is less common. Maldescent or non–descent of one or both testes is determined. Hydroceles are common and require no treatment, whereas the presence of an inguinal hernia may necessitate further management.

The detection of any penile abnormality should prompt observation of the urinary stream to rule out meatal stenosis. A poor stream plus a palpable bladder may be the only indication of posterior urethral valves in a male infant.

In female infants white secretions in the vagina and labia are normal, secondary to fetal stimulation by maternal hormones.

Skeleton

The passive range of motion of all extremities and hips is assessed by flexion and extension of each joint. A malformation should be readily distinguishable from a deformation. Deformations occur as a result of intrauterine constraint on the fetus secondary to decreased amniotic fluid volume or anatomic uterine abnormalities; they may improve with time and positioning; malformations will not be corrected by positioning alone.

Two manoeuvres are performed to exclude congenital dislocation of the hip. The Ortolani reduction test assesses whether the hip is dislocated or subluxated from the acetabulum; a 'clunk' produced by relocation of the femoral head slipping over the acetabulum is the most important finding in a dislocation. The second manoeuvre detects whether the hips are dislocatable (Barlow dislocation test); dislocation is palpable as the femoral head slips out of the acetabulum.

The spine is palpated while holding the infant prone; the presence of bony defects, sacral dimples or tufts of hair may indicate tracts to the spinal cord. Scoliosis can also be detected at this time.

Central nervous system

Throughout the examination the infant is observed for the level of alertness, degree of spontaneous activity, cry, posture, tone and response to stimulation. Tone is assessed by determining the resistance against passive movement by moving the upper and lower limbs through their full range of movement. Tone can also be assessed by the traction response in which the infant is gently and slowly pulled to a sitting position. Numerous reflexes may be evoked including the rooting, sucking, Moro, grasp, placing and automatic walking reflex. Of these, the Moro is the single most significant reflex in terms of detecting neurological abnormality.

Clinical significance of classification of the newborn

At the conclusion of the physical examination the infant is designated as preterm, term or post-term, appropriate, large or small for gestational age. This classification is of major clinical significance as each of these categories carries with it specific risks, e.g. SGA infants are prone to perinatal asphyxia and its complications, meconium aspiration, hypothermia, hypoglycaemia, polycythaemia, thrombo-cytopaenia, pulmonary haemorrhage, necrotizing enterocolitis (NEC) and hypocalcaemia. In addition, the underlying aetiology of the growth retardation may lead to identification of a congenital infection or congenital abnormality.

Common associations in LGA infants include infants of diabetic mothers, infants with Beckwith–Weidemann syndrome or transposition of the great arteries. LGA infants have an increased incidence of perinatal asphyxia, birth trauma, hypoglycaemia, RDS, hyperbilirubinaemia, polycythaemia and hypocalcaemia. Infants of diabetic mothers also have an increased incidence of congenital abnormalities.

Prematurity with its associated risks of respiratory distress, metabolic abnormalities, necrotizing enterocolitis, intraventricular haemorrhage, hyperbilirubinaemia, etc. will complicate the course of an infant with a primary surgical disorder; furthermore the complications of prematurity per se often require surgical intervention.[38]

Approach to infants with congenital anomalies

It is essential that a systematic approach to the clinical identification and management of anomalies is adopted. Whether one or more organ systems are involved there is usually only one specific cause of the disorder. Major congenital anomalies may be either single or multiple (Table 2.6). A single anomaly implies one primary defect or primary embryonic field; multiple anomalies imply the presence of two or more embryonically non–contiguous anomalies and may represent a malformation syndrome, a sequence or an association. A sequence represents the identifiable consequences of an underlying malformation or disruption, i.e. Potter or oligohydramnios sequence caused by renal agenesis or amniotic leakage; an association represents a group of birth defects occurring together more frequently than expected, possibly temporally related to an intrauterine event, e.g. vacterl association.

1. The acronym VATER describes the association of Vertebral, Anal, Tracheo-oesophageal, Renal and Radial anomalies. Cardiac and other Limb anomalies enhance the acronym to VACTERL association.

2. Beckwith–Wiedemann syndrome is one of somatic gigantism, macroglossia, posterior ear pits and creases, hemihypertrophy with hypoglycaemia and polycythaemia.

3. Although sweat chloride by iontophoresis remains the diagnostic test for cystic fibrosis (CF), the recent identification of the CF gene has allowed the identification of a specific mutation (ΔF508) as the single most common mutation in most populations. Thus, in patients homozygous for the ΔF508 a rapid and accurate diagnosis can be made.[39] A number of other mutations have been described and the mutant genotype may be fully characterized in 90 per cent of CF patients.[40]

Normal reference standards for many dysmorphic features allow comparison and quantitation of specific findings. If a specific syndrome is suspected, the features of the patient can be readily compared with a standard reference; however, if the diagnosis is not clear, key physical features are used as starting points in the diagnostic evaluation of the dysmorphic infant. Minor dysmorphic features may be evident in the parents' external appearance. Infants with several minor anomalies have an increased risk of having a major abnormality. In a study of 4305 infants, those with three or more minor anomalies had an almost 20 per cent chance of having a major malformation.[41]

Examination of the placenta is an often neglected aspect of establishing a diagnosis in an infant with dysmorphic features, e.g. a normal sized placenta associated with growth retardation is more likely to be associated with congenital anomalies, whereas a small placenta is more often associated with causes other than congenital anomalies.

Table 2.6 Primary surgical disorders and their common associated abnormalities

Primary surgical condition	Generalized	Specific associations
Oesophageal atresia and tracheo-oesophageal fistula	SGA Prematurity	Congenital heart disease (CHD) Vater assoc. Congenital diaphrogmatic hernia (CDH) Trisomies 18, 21 Imperforate anus
Duodenal atresia	Prematurity ($\pm$ 30%) SGA	Anular pancreas Malrotation, TOF Trisomy 21 Imperforate anus
Jejunal atresia	Prematurity ($\pm$ 25%)	Malrotation Biliary atresia
Ileal atresia	Prematurity ($\pm$ 50%)	Imperforate anus
Multiple atresias	Prematurity	Chromosomal abnormalities, other anomalies common
Colonic atresia		Malrotation Other abnormalities uncommon
Imperforate anus		Low lesions – common assoc. *Vater, Meckels diverticulum Trisomy 21
Malrotation		CDH, anular pancreas CHD, other atresias
Hirschsprung's disease		Uncommon
Omphalocele	Prematurity ($\pm$ 30%) SGA (+/− 20%)	30% assoc. abnormalities *Beckwith–Wiedemann Syndrome Imperforate Anus Trisomies 13, 18, 21 CHD, ileal atresia Meningocele Pulmonary hypoplasia UGT (exstrophy) Skeletal (spinal) defects
Gastroschisis	SGA	<10%
Meconium ileus	*Cystic fibrosis almost certain if not SGA. CF also described with meconium plug syndrome	
Congenital diaphragmatic hernia		Malrotation, occasionally neural tube defects, CHD, omphalocele

The aetiology of most congenital anomalies cannot usually be identified; they may follow Mendelian inheritance traits, but more commonly are chromosomal or multifactorial in origin (including inherited as well as environmental factors) or the cause is unknown. Categorization of a malformation as being due to a single gene defect, chromosomal, multifactorial or teratogenic in origin will direct further investigation; this generally involves a thorough examination of the cardiovascular system with two-dimensional echocardiography, ophthalmological examination, CT scan or ultrasound of the brain, renal ultrasound, spinal x–ray, photographs and chromosome analysis.

It is essential that the neonatal intensive care unit has dysmorphology and genetic laboratory services readily available: an accelerated diagnosis via bone marrow aspiration may be required if a decision to provide surgery is contingent upon chromosomal analysis. The pure malformation syndromes are not generally associated with inborn errors of metabolism and metabolic studies are usually not indicated; similarly the growth retardation of many syndromes is not due to humorally mediated growth deficiency and endocrine studies are not indicated.

It is extremely important that parents have accurate information as to whether the surgical anomaly is single or part of a multiple anomaly pattern, whether any chromosomal abnormality is present and the likely prognosis for that condition, prior to contemplating any surgery. The initial interaction with the parents in the intensive care setting amidst great stress and anxiety does not allow all the genetic aspects of the disorder to be addressed. However, the integration of clinical genetics services with neonatal practice helps to provide immediate genetic counselling with more detailed discussion at a later date.

While future childbearing is not an immediate issue, the recurrence risk for an unknown malformation syndrome could be high if the condition is monogenic. Once a chromosomal disorder is ruled out, a sporadically occurring unrecognized malformation syndrome has a recurrence risk ranging from 0 (based on a fresh mutation for an autosomal dominant disorder) to 25 per cent (based on autosomal recessive inheritance). Much of the progress in the diagnosis of genetic disorders at the DNA level has been in single gene disorders with clear Mendelian inheritance of a characteristic phenotype. The improved understanding of these disorders makes carrier detection and prenatal diagnosis possible in an ever increasing list of disorders. In the future, molecular lesions associated with chromosomal abnormalities and the characterization of the genes and gene defects in the multifactorial diseases will no doubt be identified.[42]

References

1. Lorenz RP, Kuhn MH. Multidisciplinary team counselling for fetal anomalies. *American Journal of Obstetrics and Gynecology*. 1989; **161**, 263–6.
2. Garber AP, Hixon HEC. Prenatal genetic counselling. *Clinical Perinatology*. 1990; **17**, 749–59.
3. Langer JC. Fetal and Neonatal Surgery. *Current Opinion in Pediatrics*. 1991; **3**, 230–9.
4. Crombleholme TM, Harrison MR, Golbus MS, Longaker MT, Langer JC, Callen PW, Anderson RL, Goldstein RB, Filly RA. Fetal intervention in obstructive uropathy: prognostic indicators and efficacy of intervention. *American Journal of Obstetrics and Gynecology*. 1990; **162**, 1239–44.
5. Harrison MR, Adzick NS, Longaker MT, Goldberg JD, Rosen MA, Filly RA, Evans MI, Golbus MS. Successful repair in utero of a fetal diaphragmatic hernia after removal of herniated viscera from the left thorax. *New England Journal of Medicine*. 1990; **322**, 1582–4.
6. Pringle KC. Fetal surgery: Practical considerations and current status: Where do we go from here with Bochdalek diaphragmatic hernia? In: Fallis JC, Filler RM, Lemoine G (eds) *Pediatric Thoracic Surgery*. New York: Elsevier Science Publishing Co. Inc., 1991, pp. 333–42.
7. Evans MI, Drugan A, Manning FA, Harrison MR. Fetal surgery in the 1990s. *American Journal of Diseases of Children*. 1989; **143**, 1431–6.
8. Pringle KC. Fetal diagnosis and fetal surgery. *Clinical Perinatology*. 1989; **16**, 13–22.
9. Bond SJ, Harrison MR, Filly RA, Callen PW, Anderson RA, Golbus MS. Severity of intestinal damage in gastroschisis: correlation with prenatal sonographic findings. *Journal of Pediatric Surgery*. 1988; **23**, 520–5.
10. Langer JC, Bell JG, Castillo RO, Crombleholme TM, Longaker MT, Duncan BW, Bradley SM, Finkbeiner WE, Verrier ED, Harrison MR.

Etiology of intestinal damage in gastroschisis: II Timing and reversibility of histologic changes, mucosal function, and contractility. *Journal of Pediatric Surgery*. 1990; **25**, 1122–6.

11. Lenke RR, Persutte WH, Nemes J. Ultrasonographic assessment of intestinal damage in fetuses with gastroschisis: is it of clinical value? *American Journal of Obstetrics and Gynecology*. 1990; **163**, 995–8.

12. Kirk EP, Wah RM. Obstetric management of the fetus with omphalocele or gastroschisis: a review and report of one hundred twelve cases. *American Journal of Obstetrics and Gynecology*. 1983; **146**, 512–18.

13. Moretti M, Khoury A, Rodriguez J, Lobe T, Shaver D, Sibai B. The effect of mode of delivery on the perinatal outcome in fetuses with abdominal wall defects. *American Journal of Obstetrics and Gynecology*. 1990; **163**, 833–8.

14. Lewis DF, Towers CV, Garite TJ, Jackson DN, Nageotte MP, Major CA. Fetal gastroschisis and omphalocele: is Cesarean section the best mode of delivery? *American Journal of Obstetrics and Gynecology*. 1990; **163**, 773–5.

15. College of Anaesthetists/Royal College of Obstetricians & Gynaecologists Working Party Report. *Resuscitation of the Newborn. Part 1: Basic Resuscitation*. 1990; ISBN 0 902331 41 7.

16. College of Anaesthetists/Royal College of Obstetricians & Gynaecologists Working Party report: *Resuscitation of the Newborn. Part 2: Advanced Resuscitation*. 1990; ISBN 0 902331 48 5.

17. Apgar V, James LS. Further observations of the newborn scoring system. *American Journal of Diseases of Children*. 1962; **104, 419**–28.

18. American Heart Association. *Textbook of Neonatal Resuscitation*. Mesquite, Texas: American Academy of Pediatrics, 1990.

19. Milner AD. Resuscitation of the newborn. *Archives of Disease in Childhood*. 1991; **66**, 66–9.

20. David R. Closed chest cardiac massage in the newborn infant. *Pediatrics*. 1988; **81**, 552–4.

21. Pediatric basic life support. *Journal of the American Medical Association* 1992; **268**, 2251–61.

22. Kitterman JA, Phibbs RH, Tooley WH. Aortic blood pressure in normal newborn infants during the first 12 hours of life. *Pediatrics*. 1969; **44**, 959–68.

23. Versmold HT, Kitterman JA, Phibbs RH, Gregory GA, Tooley WH. Aortic blood pressure during the first 12 hours of life in infants with birth weight 610 to 4220 grams. *Pediatrics*. 1981; **67**, 607–13.

24. Versmold HT. Control of blood pressure and distribution of blood flow. *International Journal of Technology Assessment in Health Care*. 1991; **7**, (Suppl.1); 79–84.

25. Tan KL. Blood pressure in very low birth weight infants in the first 70 days of life. *Journal of Pediatrics*. 1988; **112**, 266–70.

26. Yeo CL, Tudehope DI. Outcome of recusitated apparently stillborn infants: a ten year review. *Journal of Paediatric Child Health*. 1994; **30**, 129–133.

27. Nightingale P, Meakin G. A new method for maintaining body temperature in children. *Anesthesiology*. 1986; **65**, 447–8.

28. Shaffer SE, Norman ME. Renal function and renal failure in the newborn. *Clinical Perinatology*. 1989; **16**, 199–218.

29. Perlman M, Kirpalani H. *Residents Handbook of Neonatology*. St Louis: Mosby Year Book Inc., 1992.

30. Cote CJ. NPO after midnight for children – a reappraisal. *Anesthesiology*. 1990; **72**, 589–92.

31. John E, Klavdianou M, Vidasagar D. Electrolyte problems in neonatal surgical patients. *Clinics in Perinatology*. 1989; **16**, 219–32.

32. Judd BA, Haycock GB, Dalton N, Chantler C. Hyponatraemia in premature babies and following surgery in older children. *Acta Paediatrica Scandinavica*. 1987; **76**, 385–93.

33. Gruskay J, Costarino AT, Polin RA, Baumgart S. Nonoliguric hyperkalemia in the premature infant weighing less than 1000 gm. *Journal of Pediatrics*. 1988; **113**, 381–6.

34. Ballard JL, Novak KK, Driver M. A simplified score for assessment of fetal maturation of newly born infants. *Journal of Pediatrics*. 1979; **95**, 769–74.

35. Parkin JM, Hey EN, Clowes JS. Rapid assessment of gestational age at birth. *Archives of Disease in Childhood*. 1976; **51**, 259–63.

36. Usher R, McLean F. Intrauterine growth of live–born Caucasian infants at sea level: Standards obtained from measurements in 7 dimensions of infants born between 25 and 44 weeks of gestation. *Journal of Pediatrics*. 1969; **74**, 901–10.

37. Arbuckle TE, Sherman GJ. An analysis of birth weight by gestational age in Canada. *Canadian Medical Association Journal*. 1989; **140**, 157–65.

38. Schwartz MZ, Palder SB, Tyson KR, Marr CC. Complications of prematurity that may require surgical intervention. *Archives of Surgery*. 1988; **123**, 1135–8.

39. Kerem E, Corey M, Kerem BS, Rommens J, Markiewicz D, Levison H, Tsui L-C, Durie P. The relationship between genotype and phenotype in cystic fibrosis: analysis of the most common mutation (ΔF508). *New England Journal of Medicine*. 1990; **323**, 1517–22.

40. Korf BR. Genetics: Editorial Review. *Current Opinion in Pediatrics*. 1991; **3**, 1021–3.

41. Leppig KA, Werler MM, Cann CI, Cook CA, Holmes LB. Predictive value of minor anomalies: I. Association with major malformations. *Journal of Pediatrics*. 1987; **110**, 531–7.

42. Antonarakis SE. Diagnosis of genetic disorders at the DNA level. *New England Journal of Medicine*. 1989; **320**, 153–63.

3　Neonatal anaesthesia – basic principles

Preoperative assessment and management

All neonates must be carefully assessed pre-operatively by the anaesthetist. It is usually necessary to explain to the parents what anaesthesia involves for patients in this age group and that a period of intensive care with respiratory support may be necessary for sick babies after major surgery. All babies are accurately weighed on admission and a full history is taken, including the method of delivery and the gestational age, and then a full clinical examination undertaken.

Many congenital defects are multiple and a baby presenting for surgery for one defect could well have others with serious implications for the anaesthetist. One third of patients with oesophageal atresia also have a cardiac defect. 14 per cent of babies with cleft lip and 33 per cent of those with cleft palate have other congenital abnormalities such as the Pierre Robin syndrome of micrognathia and glossoptosis; babies with Down's and Edwards' syndromes may have congenital heart diseases.

The anaesthetist will be alerted to obvious intubation difficulties as seen with Pierre Robin, Treacher–Collins or the Klippel–Feil syndromes.

Fasting

A prolonged fasting time is unnecessary for all children, but particularly so for infants. Prolonged fasting increases the possibility of both hypoglycaemia and dehydration. However, it is important to minimize the residual gastric volume to reduce the risks of oesophageal reflux and pulmonary aspiration of gastric contents. For elective surgery a milk feed may be given up to four hours before surgery and clear fluids such as dextrose up to two hours preoperatively. Clear fluids can be given up to two hours before surgery without increasing the volume of gastric fluid or decreasing its pH.[1] Milk feeds require a longer time since milk proteins precipitate in an acid medium and gastric emptying is somewhat delayed. If surgery is very delayed then maintenance fluids should be given intravenously.

A nasogastric tube should be passed in any sick baby, especially one with intestinal obstruction. Gastric distension is a very common problem in infancy, with acidosis and hypoxaemia as predisposing causes even in babies without intestinal obstruction, and increases the risk of regurgitation. Pulmonary aspiration, elevation of the diaphragm and basal atelectasis may all prejudice normal respiratory function.

Ranitidine (2 mg.kg^{-1} intravenously) both to reduce both residual gastric volumes and to increase the pH of gastric fluid is not used routinely in paediatric practice since the incidence of reflux and aspiration on induction of anaesthesia seems to be very low in small babies.[2]

Oesophageal motility is reduced in the newborn, especially in the lower third, so some degree of reflux occurs continuously. The cardio-oesophageal sphincter mechanism does not develop until the end of the first year. Gastric motility may be low and up to 40 per cent of any feed may still be in the stomach two hours later, depending on the type of fluid (breast milk passes into the intestine more rapidly), the position of the baby (more rapid emptying if the baby is prone) and the fitness of the baby. Gastric emptying times are markedly increased in premature and sick babies. The nasogastric tube should be left to drain freely and the equivalent volume of normal saline should be given intravenously to replace the loss. The tube must be aspirated before anaesthesia and left unclamped.

Too large a nasogastric tube (greater than 8FG) can cause an increase in airway resistance or even respiratory obstruction in infants, as they are obligatory nose breathers.

The aim of preoperative preparation is to bring the baby to the operating theatre in optimum condition after a period of stabilization, in an incubator, when the body temperature is normal, adequate hydration and blood volume ensured and when all the necessary investigations and imaging have been performed. All newborns should come to the operating theatre with an intravenous line established preoperatively and for very sick babies an arterial line is also necessary.

Premedication

Atropine is the only drug commonly used for premedication in neonatal patients.

Newborns rely on their rapid cardiac rate for the maintenance of cardiac input and anaesthetic agents such as halothane or succinylcholine may cause bradycardia with falls in cardiac output. Intubation of the trachea, passage of a nasogastric tube or a nasal temperature probe may provoke a vagal response. Atropine may be given in a dose of 0.02 mg.kg^{-1}, with a minimum dose of 0.1 mg. Traditionally this dose has been administered 30–45 minutes preoperatively by intramuscular injection to coincide with the peak effect of the drug. These doses are very well tolerated and ensure that no bradycardia will occur with intubation or the use of vagally active drugs such as halothane.

The antisialogogue action of atropine (and hyoscine) is rather less important nowadays since inhalational agents are less irritant to the tracheobronchial tree, but their use probably remains more important in small babies than in adults. There is an increased risk of laryngeal spasm on extubation if the patient has excessive tracheobronchial secretions and especially in those who have received halothane. Blockage of a narrow tracheal tube with secretions is also a possibility. If ketamine is to be used as an induction agent, it may be preferable to dry the secretions with atropine premedication. However, excessive drying of secretions is undesirable and atropine may reduce mucociliary function for several hours so that a reduced dose is given to patients with cystic fibrosis or those suffering from dehydration.

Atropine may also be given orally, though the effect may be less certain and a larger dose is usually necessary. Some centres prefer the administration of atropine by intravenous injection during induction of anaesthesia to ensure an immediate and certain action and also avoid the need for a painful injection and the possible discomfort of a dry mouth. There will, of course, be no antisialogogue action at this stage.

Hyoscine, which can cause excitation in the young, is not used in neonatal anaesthesia; its excessive drying action on the mucosa would be undesirable.

Glycopyrrolate in doses of 0.004–0.008 mg.kg^{-1} (maximum 0.2 mg) intramuscularly or intravenously is an alternative to atropine, although its antisialogogue effect is weaker. However, it rarely produces such a marked tachycardia as atropine and is more effective in decreasing the volume and acidity of the gastric contents.

Competence of the cardio-oesophageal junction may be decreased with intravenous atropine. This may be important in patients with gastric emptying problems such as pyloric stenosis or pre-existing reflux which may be exacerbated. However, a large nasogastric tube and gastric washouts should ensure full drainage of the stomach in all such patients. Intramuscular atropine has little effect on lower oesophageal sphincter pressure.

Atropine has been incriminated in the production of febrile convulsions, presumably by inhibiting activity of sweat glands and compromising thermoregulation. Even though other factors such as hypovolaemia may be involved, atropine is best avoided in the pyrexial or toxic patient, or a lower dose should be used, which can be administered intravenously if necessary.

On balance, atropine is the preferred drug for newborns as it causes the most certain vagal block without excessive drying action.

Newborns and infants below one year of age as a rule do not require sedation for premedication. Babies are sensitive to the action of all sedative drugs and their use is limited to very special circumstances. Morphine given to neonates in doses of one third of the adult dose on a weight-for-weight basis significantly reduces the ventilatory response to carbon dioxide and can induce apnoea. However, babies who are to undergo major surgery such as cardiac surgery benefit from sedation as it will reduce irritability, minimize oxygen consumption and promote peripheral vasodilatation during cooling. Morphine 0.2 mg.kg^{-1} is well tolerated and may be beneficial and is used in this dose for the treatment of hypercyanotic attacks in Fallot's tetralogy. The use of EMLA cream will allow a painless insertion of a venous cannula for an intravenous induction if desired.

Vitamin K, 1 mg intramuscularly, should be given to all newborns because of its relative deficiency in the newborn and the immaturity of the liver enzyme systems in synthesizing prothrombin.

The suggested link between childhood cancer and intramuscular vitamin K has been recently challenged by data from the United States, Australia, Britain and Sweden.[3]

Anaesthetic equipment

Adult apparatus is rarely, if ever, suitable for use in neonates, because of its bulky nature and because of the anatomical and physiological differences between the neonate and the adult. Anatomical differences of the face and upper airway affect the design of masks, laryngoscopes and tracheal tubes, whilst the need to minimize resistance and dead space has design implications for breathing systems, connectors and tubes.

The work of breathing, which is higher in the infant than in the adult, is further increased by turbulent gas flow and any added resistance imposed by anaesthetic equipment should be kept to a minimum. At a flow rate of 100 ml.s^{-1}, apparatus resistance (excluding the tracheal tubes) should be less than 0.5 kPa.l^{-1}.s. Since spontaneous breathing techniques are seldom used during anaesthesia in neonates, resistance of equipment is more important during recovery and in weaning from ventilatory support in intensive care. Excessively high resistance during controlled ventilation may cause air trapping.

Apparatus dead space must also be kept low for neonates, though again this factor is not as crucial during controlled ventilation as during spontaneous breathing. Apparatus should be as light as possible and the ability to scavenge expired gas is desirable.

Anaesthetic machines

Although there are no anaesthetic machines specifically designed for neonatal use, one design feature which is useful is the ability to use air in the inspired gas mixture. In preterm infants the administration of high inspired oxygen fractions even for a relatively short period has been implicated in the aetiology of retinopathy of prematurity. When unstable haemodynamics or some other reason prevents the use of nitrous oxide an air/oxygen mixture can be adjusted to give optimal arterial oxygen tension.

Breathing systems

Mapleson D or F systems (Fig. 3.1)

The most efficient semiclosed breathing systems for use with IPPV are those within Mapleson's D or F

classification. Ayre's T-piece, introduced in 1937[4] and modified by Jackson Rees in 1950,[5] is still in common use, especially in the United Kingdom, but various modified Mapleson D systems are also common. The coaxial version, the Bain system,[6] has gained wide popularity. Scavenging is easier with this system, but care must be taken to ensure the fresh gas tubing does not become disconnected.

Although it has been stated for many years that a fresh gas flow (FGF) as high as two and a half times the patient's minute volume is required to avoid rebreathing during IPPV, in practice lower values can be used. As FGF is reduced during IPPV, rebreathing appears first at the end of inspiration, initially only entering the dead space and not affecting alveolar ventilation. This is because carbon dioxide containing expired gas in the expiratory limb of the T-piece is being continuously displaced distally by the fresh gas. Low FGF with rebreathing of dead space gas minimizes heat and water vapour losses from the upper airway as well as reducing cost. Rose and Froese[8] have shown that when low

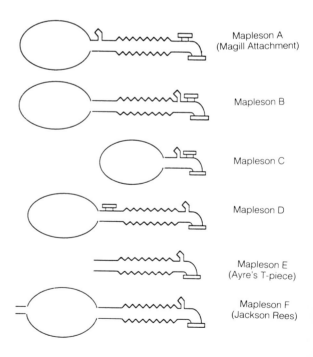

Fig. 3.1   Mapleson breathing systems. (Modified from [7].)

Mapleson A
(Magill Attachment)

Mapleson B

Mapleson C

Mapleson D

Mapleson E
(Ayre's T-piece)

Mapleson F
(Jackson Rees)

FGF is used the alveolar carbon dioxide tension ($PACO_2$) will be relatively independent of minute ventilation, varying more as a function of the degree of rebreathing and hence of FGF rate itself. Normocapnia is therefore maintained even with mild hyperventilation. At higher flows $PACO_2$ varies with minute ventilation in the usual way.

The recommendations for minimal FGF rate during IPPV vary quite widely. Froese and Rose[9] have suggested that with IPPV a FGF of ($1000 + 100$ ml.kg^{-1}) ml.min^{-1} will produce an arterial PCO_2 of 4.9 kPa (50 cmH$_2$O) in children weighing from 10–30 kg, but suggest a minimum FGF of 3 l.min^{-1}. An alternative formula of $15 \times kg \times$ frequency has been suggested[10]. For neonates a FGF of 2–3 l.min^{-1} is sufficient, though continuous monitoring of expired carbon dioxide is particularly important when low FGFs are used. If Mapleson D or F systems are used with spontaneous ventilation in neonates, FGFs of at least 4 l.min^{-1} are required to avoid hypercapnia.

Paediatric circle systems

The two most popular paediatric circle systems are the Bloomquist and Ohio systems.[11] The Ohio circle places the FGF downstream of the unidirectional valve, ensuring constant flow to the patient and minimizing dead space. In the Bloomquist system the direction of gas flow through the carbon dioxide absorber can be changed by reversing the positions of the inspiratory inlet and reservoir bag. A modified adult circle absorber has been described, comprising an interchangeable small canister and tubing together with a low resistance, low dead space valve.[12] The use of a Revell circulator[13] reduces resistance and helps keep undirectional valves open, so that the neonate need not expend energy to open them. The use of circle systems requires a knowledge of alterations in inspired anaesthetic concentration which can occur with changes in FGF.

Ventilators

Many anaesthetists recommend manual ventilation for neonatal anaesthesia, since this allows rapid detection of airway obstruction or disconnection from the 'feel' of the bag. This is particularly helpful during operations such as tracheo-oesophageal fistula, where surgical manipulations may interfere with the airway and air leaks can arise from the trachea. For operations where these problems do not arise, particularly those of long duration, the use of a mechanical ventilator has the advantage of producing predictable carbon dioxide levels as well as freeing the anaesthetist for the administration of drugs and fluids.

There is a limited choice of ventilators suitable for operating room use with the T-piece. Those with a separate source of driving gas are preferable to the older T-piece occluders, since they allow more flexible adjustment of FGF and other parameters. Pressure generators are less likely to cause barotrauma than flow generators and will compensate for leaks in the system to some extent. In the UK, the Penlon Nuffield 200 ventilator with Newton's modification[14] is widely used; in North America the 'bag in bottle' machines are commonly seen. With both these paediatric ventilators, as with all pressure generators, tidal volume will fall in the face of reduction in compliance or surgical retraction of the lung and minute volume will also change with changes in fresh gas flow. With the modified Nuffield ventilator the fixed orifice leak which enables the ventilator to be used for young children makes any airway obstruction more difficult to diagnose, since the consequent rise in airway pressure is small. With "bag in bottle" ventilators the relatively large compression volume will increase the effect of changes in compliance on minute volume.

Face masks

Face masks are not used for long periods in small babies because general anaesthesia almost invariably involves intubation (p. 128). A good fit on the face is probably of even greater importance than very low dead space, which in practice is reduced by streaming effects of the FGF within the mask. The Rendell-Baker mask has the lowest dead space, but may not make a good air seal on the baby's face and a little practice is required in its use. The Rendell-Baker divided airway further reduces dead space.[15] Newer moulded low dead space transparent face masks are very satisfactory (Fig. 3.2). The laryngeal mask airway (LMA)[16] has been used in infants, though particular care must be taken to ensure continued airway patency in this age group.[17] In one case report the LMA was successfully used in a 2.75 kg neonate with Pierre Robin syndrome in whom intubation had proved impossible.[18]

Laryngoscopes

Because of the anatomy of the neonate's upper airway, a straight-bladed laryngoscope is usually

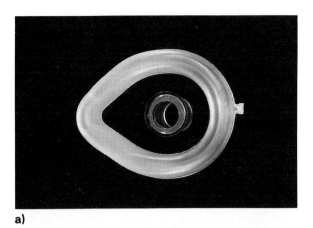

a)

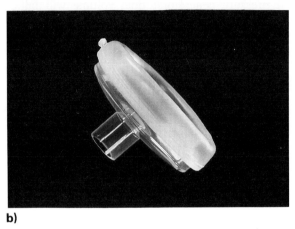

b)

Fig. 3.2   (a and b) Moulded transparent face mask.

preferred, the blade being placed posterior to the epiglottis. There are many different designs of straight-bladed laryngoscopes available (Fig. 3.3).

The Seward and Robertshaw blades are particularly useful for nasotracheal intubation because they allow more room for the introduction of Magill forceps into the mouth than most other blades. The quality of the light source has improved significantly with the introduction of fibreoptics into this field. A modified blade has been described which allows insufflation of oxygen into the pharynx during intubation.[19]

Tracheal tubes

Implantation tested, uncuffed polyvinyl chloride (PVC) tubes have now largely replaced the older rubber tubes in neonates; 3 mm internal diameter

is usual for term babies and 2.5 mm for preterm (under 2 kg). The length to which a tube should be cut for oral intubation depends on the method of fixation. Values given in North American literature often refer to the practice of allowing a length of tube to protrude from the mouth. Tracheal tube lengths commonly required when the tracheal tube connector is strapped to the face as commonly practised in the UK, are shown in Table 3.1. Because of the ease with which inadvertent bronchial intubation can occur, the chest should always be auscultated after intubation to ensure ventilation of both lungs.

Table 3.1   Oral tracheal tube sizes for newborns

Patient's weight (kg)	Tube size (i.d.) (mm)	Tube length (cm)
0.7–1.0	2.5	7.0–7.5
1.0–1.5	2.5	7.5–8.0
1.5–2.0	3.0	8.0–8.5
2.0–2.5	3.0	8.5–9.0
2.5–3.0	3.0	9.0–10.0

Preformed disposable north or south facing tracheal tubes have become increasingly popular in recent years, as they allow the tracheal tube connector to be placed away from the surgical field. Care should be taken when using south facing preformed (RAE pattern) tubes in the presence of a mouth gag, as for palatal surgery, because pressure from the tongue plate can compress the tube.

Reinforced silastic non-kinking tubes are widely used for paediatric neurosurgery (Fig. 3.4).

Cole pattern tracheal tubes (Fig. 3.5) with a shouldered section are made of PVC, but the smallest sizes are unsatisfactory for spontaneous ventilation because of an unacceptably high resistance to breathing caused by turbulent air flow at the shoulder. They are unsuitable for prolonged intubation because fixation is not very firm and there is a tendency for the tube to move further into the trachea, thus dilating the glottis. If the shouldered part rests on the cricoid, the subglottic area will be damaged.[20] Cases have been reported in which continued pressure by the oral tube has caused a cleft in the palate. Other cases have been reported in which accidental dislodgement of the tube has necessitated surgical removal from the oesophagus. However, these tubes are often used for neonatal resuscitation because they are easy

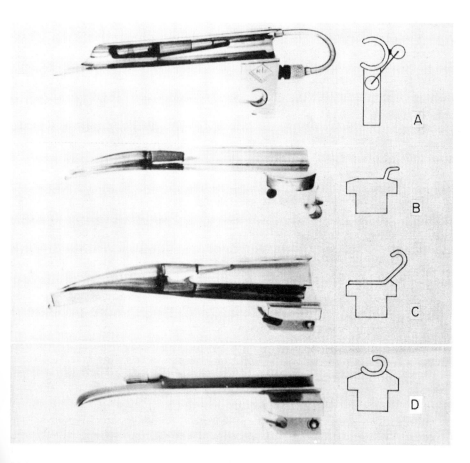

Fig. 3.3 Straightbladed laryngoscopes for infant use: A Anderson-Magill, B Seward, C Robertshaw, D Miller.

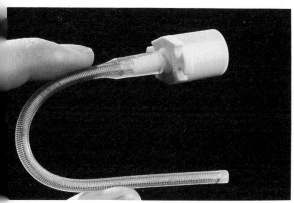

Fig. 3.4 Silastic, non-kinking tracheal tube.

for relatively inexperienced staff to use, and the 2.0 mm tube may be life-saving in an infant with an abnormally small trachea.

Anaesthetic apparatus should be sterilized between cases so that each patient has a clean breathing system. Tracheal tubes and connections are autoclaved and kept sterile until use. If a lubricant is used then this should also be sterile.

Apparatus concerned with intraoperative monitoring and temperature maintenance is discussed on p. 133.

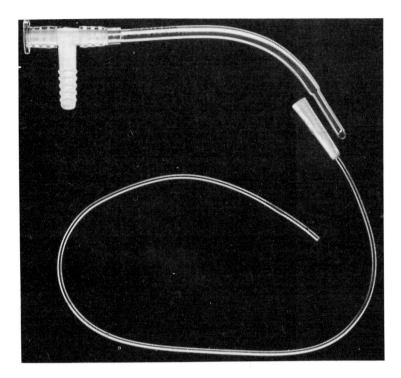

Fig. 3.5   Cole pattern tracheal tube and suction catheter.

Basic techniques

Induction of anaesthesia

The baby is transferred to a prepared operating theatre from the surgical intensive care unit in a heated incubator providing a neutral thermal environment. It is wise to induce anaesthesia for neonates on the operating table itself, prepared with a prewarmed heating pad and warm coverings. The hot air mattress has proved to be a very effective and safe alternative to other types of heated mattress (Fig. 3.6).[21]

The room should be free of draughts and it may be necessary to turn off any air-conditioning. Higher ambient temperatures than 24°C are not recommended, as discomfort of the staff will then become a consideration. The air mattress provides a warm atmosphere around the baby, so excessive room temperatures are no longer necessary. In the operating theatre, maximum heat loss is likely to occur in the period between induction of anaesthesia and the skin incision (Fig. 3.7). It is during

this period that the neonate is most likely to become uncovered; this practice should be kept to an absolute minimum, especially if the baby is premature. At this stage an overhead heater may be used–possibly that from an open type of incubator used to bring the baby from the special care unit. Alternatively, as much of the body as possible, especially the head and limbs, should be covered with warm blankets or insulating plastic sheeting to reduce radiant and evaporative heat losses.

Anaesthesia should not be induced until the surgeon is ready, as the neonate's metabolic response to cold is suppressed once general anaesthesia has been established. Skin preparation by the surgeon should not be prolonged and should preferably be with warm fluid. Drapes should be placed over the baby as soon as possible. Infusion of blood or fluid should be warmed before administration and for prolonged cases the inspired gases should also be warmed and humidified. The baby should be covered with warm blankets as soon as

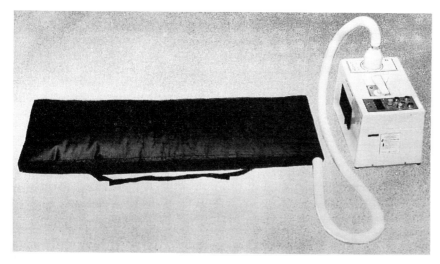

Fig. 3.6 Paediatric hot air mattress.

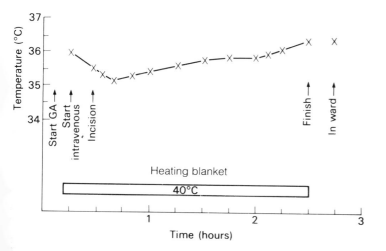

Fig. 3.7 Patient's temperature during surgery for repair of tracheo-oesophageal fistula in a baby aged 14 hours and weighing 2.1 kg.

the operation is finished and should be returned to the ward in a preheated incubator.

Intravenous access should be established before induction of general anaesthesia in neonatal patients. Suitable veins can be found on the dorsum of the hand or at the wrist, on the feet or on the scalp. Metal scalp vein needles are not satisfactory for prolonged use because they tend to cut out of the vein, although they may be easier to insert successfully; 20 and 22 gauge cannulae are available manufactured in polypropylene or Teflon. Teflon is less thrombogenic, but is softer than polypropylene and is more likely to kink unless fixation is meticulous and the arm or leg

is securely splinted. Teflon cannulae are also available in 24 and 26 gauge. Correct holding of the limb is essential for successful venepuncture. If the wrist is squeezed too tightly, blood flow will be interrupted and the veins will collapse; if held too loosely, venous distension will not be achieved. The assistant holding the wrist must also stretch the skin of the hand. After cleansing the skin with spirit, a hole beside the vein is made with a lancet. This is always advisable because otherwise Teflon cannulae buckle over the needle as they are advanced through intact skin. Some anaesthetists prefer to perform the manoeuvre single-handed and distend the vein by squeezing the wrist (or ankle) between the index and middle fingers of the left hand. Optimal venous distension and stretching of the overlying skin are achieved more easily in this way.

After successful venepuncture and careful fixation of the cannula, a three-way stopcock is fitted and the wrist (or foot) secured with a small arm splint. Intraoperative fluids may be given by means of a constant infusion pump, although these are strictly necessary only for intravenous alimentation or for the administration of inotropic agents. Care must be taken to watch for signs of extravasation around the vein when an infusion pump is used. If, as usually happens, intravenous access has been obtained on the preoperative ward the size and position of the cannula must also be carefully checked. In practice, the simplest accurate method of administering intravenous fluids during anaesthesia is by means of a 10 ml syringe and three-way stopcock.

After careful checking of the patency of the intravenous line, attachment of ECG, precordial stethoscope and pulse oximeter and 1–2 minutes of preoxygenation, anaesthesia can be induced by intravenous or inhalational methods. Estimated ED_{50} for thiopentone is reduced in neonates[22] so that induction doses in excess of 3–4 mg.kg^{-1} may lead to delayed recovery. In sick neonates inhalational induction may be safer. Halothane is the least irritant of the currently available inhalational agents, though sevoflurane may prove to be a satisfactory alternative. The minimum alveolar concentration (MAC) of all inhalational agents is significantly reduced in neonates.[23]

Tracheal intubation

Anaesthesia for neonates must involve intubation in the vast majority of cases, even for the most minor operations, since the patency of the airway cannot be guaranteed with a face mask. The respiratory system is also vulnerable to the depressant effects of inhalational anaesthesia and reduction in functional residual capacity (FRC) so that controlled ventilation should be an integral part of the anaesthetic technique. This is only possible using a tracheal tube because the compliance of the chest is lower than that of the abdomen and abdominal distension would tend to occur if assisted ventilation were attempted with a face mask.

The practice of awake intubation of the trachea in the newborn before anaesthesia, which was almost universal in the past, has now largely been replaced by intubation under general anaesthesia. This can be performed quickly and safely by experienced paediatric anaesthetists, and is clearly more humane. A recent study[24] demonstrated a significantly higher incidence of hypoxaemia during awake intubation for congenital pyloric stenosis than with intubation after induction of anaesthesia. Concern has also been expressed about the effect of awake intubation on intracranial pressure (ICP) which can now be measured non-invasively using clinical fontanometry. The rise in ICP which occurs during awake intubation may increase the risk of intraventricular haemorrhage in preterm neonates and those with existing increased ICP or coagulopathy. Awake intubation may be indicated in the presence of severe upper airway obstruction and some anaesthetists still favour its use for neonates with tracheo-oesophageal fistula.

Intubation is usually performed after administration of one of the newer, short-acting non-depolarizing muscle relaxants, since controlled ventilation will be required throughout surgery. The position of the head is crucial for successful intubation – in the infant it should be in a neutral position, with the shoulders lying flat on the operating table.[25]

The anatomy of the infant larynx is such that the best view is usually obtained using a straight-bladed laryngoscope, the tip of which picks up the epiglottis from its posterior surface (Fig. 3.8); however,

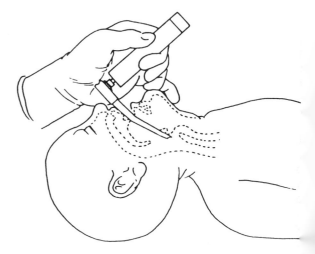

Fig. 3.8 Intubation of the neonate, showing the position of the tip of the straightbladed laryngoscope in relation to the epiglottis.

if the epiglottis is very short, the best view of the larynx may be obtained with the tip of the blade in the vallecula.

The mouth is opened with the index finger of the right hand and the laryngoscope blade is put into it from the right and advanced into the pharynx beyond the glottis, keeping the tongue to the left side of the mouth. The blade is then withdrawn until the glottis is visualized and the vocal cords are seen. A plain Magill tube is gently inserted into the trachea. If firm resistance is met, a smaller tube should be used. The correct size of tube is that which is easily inserted and which has a small air leak around it when positive pressure is applied and is thus not too tight at the cricoid ring. This should be tested by light distension of the lungs with the T-piece bag, when the air leak should be audible. A tube which is too tight may damage the mucosa at the cricoid and cause postoperative oedema and stridor. Ulceration of the mucosa may progress to subglottic stenosis. After auscultation of the chest to confirm that the tip of the tube has not passed into one or other main bronchus, it is firmly secured. An infant airway inserted into the mouth alongside the tracheal tube to splint it will prevent it from kinking. If an oesophageal stethoscope and/or a nasogastric tube are required, these are more easily placed before the oral airway is inserted.

Nasotracheal intubation is rarely used in neonates in the operating theatre except in cases already receiving respiratory support or for whom respiratory support is planned postoperatively. The technique is well established for prolonged airway management, but is technically more difficult to perform because of the need for instrumentation in the mouth with intubating forceps. It is therefore safer to undertake oral intubation first and change to nasal intubation later if required.

The difficult intubation

Neonates may be more difficult to intubate than adults or older children because of the anatomical differences already described. In addition, there are certain conditions which may cause further difficulty: where there is immobility of the cervical spine as in Klippel–Feil syndrome, micrognathia with Pierre Robin syndrome or macroglossia with Hurler's syndrome, laryngoscopy may be very awkward or even impossible. The presence of a cleft palate and an anteriorly placed premaxilla will hinder easy intubation and the blade of the laryngoscope may slip into the cleft. Babies with conditions such as cystic hygroma and haemangiomata of the head and neck with respiratory obstruction may also be very difficult to intubate.

In these situations awake intubation may be required, but if anaesthesia is necessary for an older neonate, inhalational techniques are advisable. Success is best achieved with care and patience. A selection of sterile tracheal tubes down to 2.5 mm internal diameter should always be available. If a 2.5 mm tube will not pass into the trachea, the smallest Cole pattern tube may be required. A choice of straight and curved bladed infant laryngoscopes should be available and also a fairly stiff gum-elastic or similar atraumatic bougie. Laryngoscopy should be performed after preoxygenation; if visualization of the glottis is difficult, its whereabouts can be deduced by seeing bubbles of saliva as the baby breathes in and out. It may be possible to bring the glottis into view by pressing on the front of the neck. In particularly difficult cases it may help to thread the bougie through the tracheal tube and allow it to emerge by 2 cm or so at the tracheal end. The tip of the bougie can then be bent anteriorly and used to guide the tube into the trachea. Occasionally, it may be necessary to use the bougie alone to find the glottic opening. The chosen tracheal tube is then threaded over the bougie into the trachea. If the tracheal tube connector is curved, this is better inserted after the tube is in the trachea and the bougie has been removed, though this can be difficult when small tubes are used.

Respiratory obstruction occurring after induction may be relieved by turning the baby on its side or even prone. Early insertion of an oral airway is less likely to provoke coughing and laryngeal spasm in this age group than in the older child. A nasopharyngeal airway is an alternative, although it carries the risk of epistaxis. When the baby is sufficiently deeply anaesthetized (usually with oxygen and halothane), laryngoscopy and intubation are performed as described above. Muscle relaxants must not be used in any child with airway problems until it has been proved possible to ventilate the lungs using a face mask. Inhalational induction of anaesthesia, especially in the presence of respiratory obstruction, may be aided by the application of a constant distending pressure on the lungs. This is achieved by maintaining a taut anaesthetic reservoir bag.

Use of neuromuscular blocking agents

Suxamethonium

It has been clearly shown that neonates require a larger dose of suxamethonium per kg to produce a given effect than do older children or adults, and that the duration of action is shorter. In a comparatively recent study the ED_{95} in newborns was 620 μg.kg^{-1} compared to 729 in infants, 423 in children and 290 in adults.[26] Since pseudocholinesterase activity in infants is only about half that seen in adults[27] it seems that the increased suxamethonium requirement is probably a result of the increased volume of distribution with a lower concentration reaching the neuromuscular junction. The large extracellular fluid volume also tends to facilitate diffusion away from the neuromuscular junction and may explain the relatively rapid recovery from single doses of suxamethonium-induced paralysis in neonates.[28]

Non-depolarizing blocking agents

Early studies using tubocurarine demonstrated that dose requirements were reduced in neonates, particularly on the first day of life.[29–31] More recently Meretoja has confirmed the fact that infants require significantly less tubocurarine than older children to establish 95 per cent neuromuscular blockade, and has shown that the onset time is shorter.[32] The volume of distribution and elimination half-life of tubocurarine are both increased in neonates[33,34] and protein binding is reduced, with consequently higher levels of free muscle relaxant fraction.[35]

The apparent sensitivity is also seen with the more recently introduced non-depolarizing relaxant vecuronium, where during balanced anaesthesia the ED_{95} has been shown to be 47 μg.kg^{-1} in infants compared to 81 μg.kg^{-1} in children.[36] Recovery time is about twice as long in infants.[37] The infant's sensitivity to vecuronium, however, is unusual in that it extends through the first year of life, whereas with most non–depolarisers it is limited to the neonatal period.[28] Prolonged blockade has also been reported with vecuronium in infants with impaired renal function.[38]

Although studies with atracurium have also shown that the dose response curve is shifted to the left in neonates,[39] the duration of action appears, in contrast to other non-depolarizers, to be shorter.[40] This may in part be due to the Hofmann elimination which this drug undergoes and partly result from greater clearance in neonates. Because the age-related changes in volume of distribution and elimination half-life tend to oppose each other, atracurium-induced neuromuscular blockade appears in practice to change very little with age.[41] There is no evidence that histamine release with atracurium is clinically significant in neonates.

The pharmacokinetic differences between neonates and adults have particular implications when non-depolarizing muscle relaxants are given by infusion. Use of adult algorithms will lead to delayed recovery and for reasons which will be apparent from the paragraphs above, atracurium is likely to be an easier drug to use by this method than vecuronium. Following a bolus dose of 0.4–0.6 mg.kg^{-1} an infusion of 9 μg.kg^{-1}.min provides surgical relaxation. The short-acting non depolarizing relaxant mivacurium, inactivated by enzyme hydrolysis by plasma cholinesterase, is also suitable for administration by infusion, though its use has not yet been widely reported in neonates. Careful monitoring of post–tetanic twitch count (PTC) allows fine tuning of infusion rate. PTC of five or more indicates easily reversible neuromuscular blockade.

The speed of onset of vecuronium in neonates combined with its cardiovascular stability makes it suitable for tracheal intubation, especially when neuromuscular blockade is required for over one hour. The intubating dose is 70–100 μg.kg^{-1}.

As in older patients, acidosis, hypothermia or the presence of antibiotics such as amikacin or gentamicin may prolong the effect of non-depolarising muscle relaxant drugs.

Reversal of neuromuscular blockade

It is important to ensure that any residual neuromuscular blockade is fully reversed and the patient is fully awake before attempting extubation in a neonate. The use of a peripheral nerve stimulator will ascertain that neuromuscular function has returned to near normal before reversal agents are used, but the careful choice of the most appropriate relaxant for each procedure is important.

The conventional dose requirements for atropine (0.02 mg.kg^{-1}), glycopyrrolate (0.01 mg.kg^{-1}) and neostigmine (0.05 mg.kg^{-1}) are the same in neonates as in older children. With careful control and monitoring of neuromuscular blockade, however, adequate reversal can be achieved with lower doses.

Maintenance of anaesthesia

Whilst halothane gives the smoothest induction of the currently available inhalational anaesthetics, isoflurane is frequently used for maintenance because of its superior recovery characteristics. Its lower incidence of arrhythmias, especially in the presence of high circulating levels of adrenaline, and its lesser effect on cardiac output may also be advantages, though at the high heart rates seen in neonates cardiac output is usually well maintained. Halothane hepatotoxicity, which is rarer in children than in adults, has been reported in an 11-month-old child[42] though not in neonates. Pharmacokinetic differences in the neonate are described in Chapter 1. Minimum alveolar concentration (MAC) decreases with age from around six months onwards. It is however lower at birth, particularly in preterm infants.[43] The reason for this apparent sensitivity of the newborn to anaesthetic agents is unclear. It may be related to the higher levels of β-endorphins and progesterone found at birth, increased plasma peptide concentrations, differences in permeability of the blood-brain barrier or age-related differences in blood-gas solubility.

Because the closing volume in the neonatal lung is greater than the FRC, airway closure occurs within normal tidal respiration. Controlled ventilation ensures that adequate alveolar ventilation is taking place and some positive end-expiratory pressure (PEEP) helps to maintain an adequate residual lung volume. Many paediatric anaesthetists still feel it is safer to ventilate neonates by hand, rather than with a mechanical ventilator, except in special circumstances such as cardiac surgery or neurosurgery where a steady state is particularly important. A ventilatory rate of 20–25 per minute is usually employed with pressures of 20–25 cmH_2O. It is usual to obtain a PEEP of about 5 cmH_2O during manual ventilation, thus helping to preserve the FRC.

Inspired gases for neonatal anaesthesia should reach the patient fully humidified at a temperature not less than 33°C. This prevents damage to the mucosal lining of the respiratory tract by dry gases and therefore helps preserve mucociliary function and, possibly more important, minimizes heat loss from the baby. Certainly such gases, fully saturated at body temperature, will influence the thermal balance but there is an increased risk of infection from the humidifiers. The aim is to produce mild hyperventilation – a safe procedure unless the patient is hypovolaemic from dehydration or haemorrhage. Great care must be taken with controlled ventilation in the presence of lung cysts or diaphragmatic hernia because of the risk of tension pneumothorax or with tracheo–oesophageal fistula because of gastric distension. Controlled ventilation is not contraindicated in these conditions, but extra vigilance is required and only gentle ventilation should be employed. For those unused to ventilating newborn babies by hand, a manometer may be incorporated in the breathing system so that the actual pressures applied can be seen.

Maintenance fluids and volume replacement

Details of fluid and electrolyte therapy are described in Chapter 2. Most neonatal surgery is performed within the first few days of life, when maintenance fluid requirements are low and can often be met during surgery by the volume in which drugs are diluted. Abnormal fluid losses such as may occur after relief of urethral obstruction must, however, be replaced, as must the increased insensible losses which are seen in the preterm infant.

Fluid deficit resulting from preoperative fasting should be prevented by preoperative intravenous fluid administration or, failing this, by adjusting the intraoperative fluids appropriately.

Intraoperative 'third space' losses of fluid from the intravascular compartment to the interstitial space vary in magnitude depending on the surgical procedure and are greatest during abdominal surgery where they may be as high as 10 ml.kg^{-1}hr. Opinion is divided about whether to replace these losses with crystalloid or colloid, but whichever fluid is used replacement volumes must be based not only on estimated losses but also on the effect on peripheral perfusion, blood pressure and pulse rate. If crystalloids are used, care must be taken to avoid prolonged administration of hypertonic solutions which may cause hyperosmolality and osmotic diuresis. As far as colloids are concerned, there are few published data on the relative merits of 5 per cent albumin and the available synthetic alternatives. Issues of availability and cost must be balanced against the risk of adverse reactions. The composition of some of the commonly used fluids is outlined in Table 3.2. Because of the low blood volume of the neonate ($50 +$ haematocrit ml.kg^{-1}) blood loss must always be assessed as accurately as circumstances allow.

Because of the relatively high haematocrit at birth, red cell replacement is often not required. The concept of allowable blood loss (ABL) permits dilution to an acceptable minimum haematocrit, usually between 35 and 40 per cent. A number of formulae have been devised to estimate ABL, the simplest being:

$$ABL = Wt(kg) \times EBV \times \frac{[Hm - He]}{[Hm]}$$

where EBV = Estimated blood volume ($50 +$ haematocrit ml.kg^{-1})
where Hm = Measured haematocrit
where He = Lowest acceptable haematocrit

Assuming a lowest acceptable haematocrit of 40 per cent, applying this equation to a neonate weighing 3kg with measured haemacrit of 50 per cent gives:

$$ABL = 3 \times 100 \times \frac{[0.5 - 0.4]}{0.5} = 60 \text{ ml}$$

Whilst this formula is useful in term neonates who are haemodynamically stable without respiratory problems, it should be modified in the presence of reduced cardiac output, reduced oxygen saturation or other factors which affect tissue oxygenation. The formula can also be used to calculate the amount of blood required for a top-up transfusion to a set haemoglobin level. During the period of acceptable blood loss, blood volume must be maintained with colloids or crystalloids. The volume of crystalloid required to maintain adequate circulating volume is 1.5–2 times as great as when colloids are used and may lead to hypoproteinaemia. Colloids, however, may adversely increase the osmotic pressure of the interstitial space if they leak through vessel walls.

The presence of high levels of fetal haemoglobin (HbF) will reduce the oxygen-releasing capacity at the tissues as described in Chapter 1. Preterm infants have lower Hb concentrations and higher HbF fractions than term infants. A haematocrit of less than 30 per cent has been shown to be associated with an increased incidence of postoperative apnoea in infants of under 60 weeks postconceptional age.[44]

When red cell transfusion is required, local availability again often dictates which blood product is given. Plasma-reduced blood with its high haematocrit is unsuitable for rapid transfusion through small cannulae and since whole blood is seldom available, reconstituted products such as SAG-M (Saline, Adenosine, Glucose, Mannitol) often have to be accepted. Whether the infusion of large volumes of these products has any adverse effects on neonates is at present unclear. Massive blood loss may also be associated with loss of platelets and labile clotting factors, when specific replacement therapy with platelet concentrate and fresh frozen

Table 3.2   Contents of commonly used intravenous fluids

Solution	Na$^+$ (mmol·l^{-1})	Cl$^-$ (mmol·l^{-1})	K$^+$ (mmol·l^{-1})	Ca^{2+} (mmol·l^{-1})	Lactate (mmol·l^{-1})	Calories MJ·l^{-1}
0.9% Saline	154	154	—	—	—	—
0.45% Saline in 2.5% glucose	77	77	—	—	—	0.4
0.18% Saline in 4% glucose	31	31	—	—	—	0.63
Hartmann's solution	131	111	5.0	2.0	29	—
Half-strength Hartmann's solution	65.5	55.5	2.5	1.0	14.5	—
10% Dextrose	—	—	—	—	—	1.6

plasma may be indicated. In this situation blood warming also becomes more important. The exciting developments in new synthetic blood products may reduce the hazards of blood transfusion in the future.

The most accurate method of transfusion of blood or fluid in the newborn is by syringe and the volume of fluid injected as diluent for muscle relaxants or other drugs should be included in the total fluid balance.

Monitoring of blood loss is best achieved by weighing small numbers of swabs before they dry out. The experienced anaesthetist should also be able to make an approximate estimate of the blood loss from visual observation of the swabs. Allowance should be made for loss on drapes and the volume of blood contained in the suction bottle should be measured directly. Colorimetric techniques are time consuming and do not allow the anaesthetist to obtain an estimate of blood loss at the time when it is occurring. Urine output may be monitored by the use of adhesive collecting bags, but in major surgery (such as cardiac surgery) catheterization should be performed.

Adequacy of volume replacement during surgery can be assessed by blood pressure, peripheral circulatory state or, in cases of massive blood replacement, by CVP monitoring. A core-peripheral temperature difference greater than $2°C$ is a sensitive sign of a reduced cardiac output, though changes in the gradient are of more use than absolute values.

Extubation

Extubation is carried out when the baby is fully awake (moving all limbs, eyes open) and respiratory effort is judged to be fully adequate in terms of depth, rate and absence of signs of distress such as intercostal recession and nasal flaring. The tube is withdrawn during compression of the reservoir bag so that the infant coughs the moment the tube leaves the trachea. The practice of extubating with a suction catheter down the tube is to be condemned because serious hypoxaemia may occur and there is a risk of aspiration of pharyngeal contents into the lungs as the first respiratory movement is inspiration.

There are many factors involved in poor respiratory function postoperatively, including pulmonary dysfunction such as hypoplasia occurring with diaphragmatic hernia or aspiration in tracheo-oesophageal fistula (see Chapter 1). Of the anaesthetic causes of postoperative respiratory insufficiency, inadequate reversal of the relaxant should be considered first. The dose of relaxant may have been excessive or increments may have been given too late, but the effects of normal doses are intensified in the presence of high concentrations of inhalational anaesthetics or diazepam transferred via the placenta from the mother. Reversal difficulties may be experienced if the patient is hypothermic, acidotic, low in ionized Ca^{2+}, very premature or has a low cardiac output. Such patients may need a period of mechanical ventilation while these abnormalities are corrected. Hypoventilation leads to pulmonary atelectasis, hypoxia, acidosis and circulatory failure.

After careful assessment, the baby is returned to its heated incubator for the journey back to the intensive care unit.

Patient care and monitoring during anaesthesia

Careful and continuous monitoring of the clinical status of the patient is essential during any anaesthetic. Because of the high metabolic rate and reduced respiratory reserve of the neonate, the clinical condition can deteriorate very rapidly and no piece of monitoring apparatus has yet been designed which will replace the meticulously careful, well-trained clinical anaesthetist. There are, however, several devices available which help in patient monitoring and the best are those which make the contact between the anaesthetist and the patient closer rather than more remote. In addition, a number of pieces of monitoring equipment are available which can give the anaesthetist information which cannot be obtained by direct clinical observation. It is also important to monitor not only the patient's well–being but also the function of the increasingly complicated pieces of anaesthetic equipment appearing in operating theatres.

Monitoring equipment must be reliable and easy to use and should not by its size or design adversely affect the characteristics of the anaesthetic breathing system or interfere with the safe conduct of the anaesthetic. Alarms should be fitted where appropriate, although these may fail or give false warnings. Unnecessary bleeps and noises can be distracting both to the surgeon and anaesthetist.

Respiration

In the spontaneously breathing patient, monitoring of the airway and adequacy of respiration is carried out by observation of the movements of the reservoir bag of the breathing system. Almost all neonatal anaesthesia is carried out using controlled ventilation, however, and in this case the movements of the chest wall must be continuously watched. When manual ventilation is used, the anaesthetist can sense gross changes in compliance and resistance of the respiratory system or obstruction of the airway by changes in the 'feel' of the reservoir bag of the breathing system with each breath. When mechanical ventilation is used, such changes cause changes in the airway pressure dial of the ventilator, although these are less easily detected. The use of a precordial stethoscope is also helpful in monitoring inflation of the lungs but can only be used as a continuous monitor for long periods of time if employed in conjunction with a monaural earpiece, since a binaural one becomes painful after a few minutes.

Pulse oximetry and capnographic measurement of inspired and expired carbon dioxide tension are mandatory monitors for all neonatal anaesthesia. Neonatal oximeter sensors are readily available and in general satisfactory. Changes in peripheral perfusion can lead to falls in apparent saturation in the absence of tissue hypoxia, but failure to detect serious hypoxaemia is rare. Because of the shape of the oxygen-haemoglobin dissociation curve, oximetry is not a sensitive method of detecting hyperoxia in preterm neonates at risk from retinopathy of prematurity. Although conventional capnometers can be used in the neonate, the relatively high sample flow rate may cause measurement errors. These can be avoided by shining the infrared signal through a window in a cuvette placed in the breathing system (Fig. 3.9).

Paediatric cuvettes with dead space as low as 2 ml are commercially available.

Despite the value of these monitors it is still wise to perform arterial blood-gas analysis if an absolute assessment of blood-gas status is required. In practice, arterial lines are used in neonatal anaesthesia for major surgery, particularly cardiac surgery, and also for any patient who requires respiratory support postoperatively. It may be difficult to obtain an arterial sample quickly in the operating theatre if an indwelling arterial line is not in place; if a central venous pressure line is available, a sample from this may be a helpful guide to metabolic state and also to the blood gases. Serious arterial hypoxaemia is unlikely to be present if the oxygen tension of the venous sample is above 5.3 kPa (40 mmHg).

In the newborn continuous pressure monitoring can be obtained by catheterization of the umbilical artery. A size 5FG polythene cannula is inserted in infants weighing over 1.5 kg. Cannulae should be radio-opaque and the tip of the cannula should be passed into the descending aorta below the origin of the inferior mesenteric and renal arteries at the level of the L2 vertebra. In the older neonate the radial, brachial or femoral artery can often be cannulated percutaneously using a 22 or 24 standard wire gauge polythene or Teflon cannula. This should be connected to a pressure transducer by means of a short length of narrow-bore tubing and a three-way stopcock. Continuous flushing by means of a slow infusion pump using small volumes of heparinized dextrose or dextrose saline (1000 units of heparin per litre of fluid) minimizes the risk of thrombus formation and cannula blockage. Care

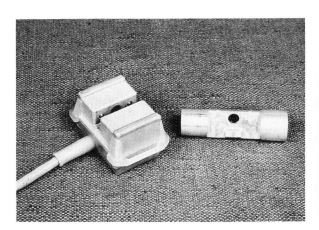

Fig. 3.9 Capnograph with low dead space paediatric cuvette.

must be taken to prevent the inadvertent injection of drugs into the artery. If the artery cannot be cannulated percutaneously, it may be necessary to expose it surgically and insert a similar cannula under direct vision. Although arterial cannulation is often followed by a temporary period of obstruction to blood flow, the incidence of long-term serious complications of radial and brachial artery cannulation in infants is very low.

Heart and circulation

It is more difficult to assess cardiovascular status clinically during anaesthesia than respiration, although useful information can be obtained by careful observation of the peripheral circulation and by keeping a finger on the axillary or femoral pulse. The following apparatus, although essential, should supplement this basic clinical monitoring rather than replace it.

Precordial/oesophageal stethoscope

The precordial or oesophageal stethoscope (Figs. 3.10 and 3.11) provides useful information about the heart sounds and heart rate, and reduction in intensity of the heart sounds may indicate a fall in blood pressure or cardiac output. The chest piece should be sufficiently small to sit comfortably on the neonatal chest and should be securely fixed. The smallest available oesophageal stethoscope (12FG) is sometimes too large to be used in the neonate, although it can be very useful especially when there is difficult access to the chest.

Blood pressure

The conventional measurement of blood pressure by auscultation of the Korotkoff sounds is often unsatisfactory during neonatal anaesthesia, again owing to difficulty of access. The introduction of the automated recording and display of blood pressure and pulse rate from these sounds was a significant advance and there is little excuse for not recording blood pressure regularly in all patients. It should be remembered, however, that accuracy still depends on using a cuff width of 4 cm for neonates. There have been reports of petechial haemorrhages appearing in the arm if measurements are made too frequently, although this problem is lessened with the newer machines whose inflation/deflation time is shorter. Doubts have been cast on the accuracy

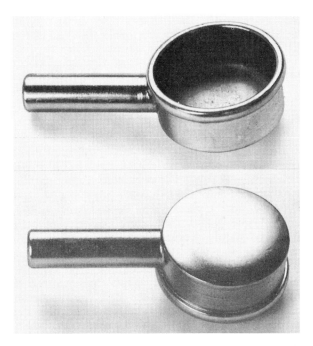

Fig. 3.10 The chest piece of a precordial stethoscope.

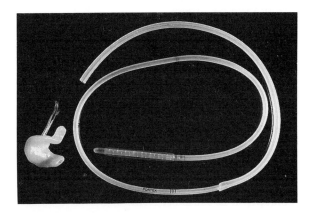

Fig. 3.11 Oesophageal stethoscope with moulded monoaural earpiece.

of these automatic devices in adults when blood pressure is very low and they have an irritating tendency to give zero readings at critical times, when clinical information obtained from palpation of the axillary or femoral pulse is essential.

Other methods of blood pressure measurement include the use of Doppler ultrasound flow meters (which become useless when diathermy is used), amplification of the signal from a microphone placed under the cuff, visual observation of the oscillations produced in an aneroid gauge as the cuff deflates, and oscillotonometry.

Intra-arterial blood pressure monitoring is preferable when continuous monitoring is necessary or when arterial blood samples are required.

Electrocardiogram

The ECG is a good monitor of pulse rate and disturbances of rhythm, although it provides no information about blood pressure or cardiac output. ECG recorders suitable for use in operating theatres should have a high common mode rejection ratio and therefore suppress unwanted signals from other pieces of electrical apparatus. It is useful to have an easily read trace, a rate counter and a freeze capacity on the oscilloscope. Lead 2 is likely to be the most useful for routine monitoring, although lead 3 will produce the most pronounced R waves in cases of right axis deviation. Leads can be placed on the right and left arms or, preferably, on the right upper chest and in the left midaxillary line. A third lead is not always required but sometimes helps to reduce electrical interference and should be placed on the left flank or leg. A disposable back-plate is available with built-in electrodes.

It should be stressed that circulatory failure leading to hypoxic brain damage may occur before the ECG shows significant abnormalities.

Central venous pressure

Central venous pressure (CVP), which reflects right atrial filling pressure, expresses the relationship between peripheral vascular resistance, blood volume and right heart function. Although CVP measurement must be interpreted with caution, it can provide a useful monitor of blood loss or blood replacement in the short term.

The internal jugular vein can be cannulated percutaneously in the neonate without great difficulty, using the technique described by English et al.[45] Using an aseptic technique, the cannula is inserted through the junction of the medial one third and lateral two thirds of the sternomastoid muscle at a point midway between the mastoid process and the sternoclavicular joint, and directed towards the nipple. The vein, which is superficial in the infant, should be entered within 1–2 cm of the point of skin puncture and can be made to fill and be more easily visualized by pressing over the liver. Care should be taken to avoid entering the common carotid artery,

which lies just medial to the internal jugular vein at this point. If the cannula is inserted too far towards the thoracic inlet, puncture of the subclavian artery, the pleura or even the lung may result.

A lower approach to the vein at the apex of the triangle of the two heads of the sternomastoid is also satisfactory, though the incidence of complications is significant with both approaches. The right vein is preferred because the pathway from right jugular vein to SVC is straight, whereas a cannula in the left may not easily cross the midline and may not function well.

If there is need for a constant infusion of a drug such as an inotrope, a second cannula may be inserted into the same vein. After the cannula has been inserted it is essential to make sure that the pressure is in fact venous. Free aspiration of blood must be possible at all times; if it is not, then the cannula should be repositioned. Unsatisfactory position may be the cause of late perforation of the vessel, resulting in hydrothorax. Multilumen cannulae are now often used in preference to multiple cannulations.

The subclavian vein has been safely cannulated by a percutaneous technique in the neonate. A skin incision is made below the clavicle, at the junction of its lateral and middle thirds, and the needle is aimed at a point 1–1.5 cm above the sternal notch. The angle between the needle and the chest is initially about 45°, enabling the needle to pass beneath the clavicle, when the angle is reduced to 15–20°. If the infant has a prominent chest, the hub of the needle must be flattened against it during entry.

A Seldinger technique is very useful for subclavian cannulation and commercially available packs contain a needle, guide wire and venous catheter.

It is not usually possible to pass a central venous cannula percutaneously up the arm of the antecubital fossa in the neonate, although this can be done following surgical exposure.

The central venous cannula may be connected either to a simple water manometer or, via a short length of narrow bore tubing, to a pressure transducer. It should be remembered that 1 mmHg = 1.36 cmH$_2$0.

Left atrial pressure or pulmonary capillary wedge pressure

As a rule, in paediatric patients if cardiac failure occurs, both ventricles fail together and so left and right filling pressures are usually similar.

However, measurement of left atrial pressure is essential following repair of many congenital heart lesions in the neonate because left atrial pressure gives a more reliable indication of blood loss or adequate replacement than right atrial or central venous pressure in this situation – especially after surgery on the mitral valve. Left atrial pressure lines can be inserted under direct vision at the time of operation by the surgeon, but care must be taken to ensure that air is not injected into them because this will be passed into the systemic circulation and may pass into the cerebral vessels. Following non-cardiac operations, pulmonary wedge pressure may be measured using the Swan-Ganz catheter inserted via the right internal jugular or subclavian vein. This measurement is occasionally used to monitor the effect of pulmonary vasodilating drugs in such conditions as congenital diaphragmatic hernia. It is, however, a difficult, invasive and potentially dangerous technique in the neonate and it is seldom used, even in those patients who have crises of pulmonary hypertension.

Temperature monitoring

Temperature should always be measured during neonatal surgery because of the increased suscep-tibility of the newborn to heat loss and because hypothermia significantly increases morbidity and mortality. Nasopharyngeal, oesophageal or rectal temperatures can be most easily monitored and are all reliable although the rectal temperature probe may become displaced during anaesthesia without the anaesthetist being aware of it.

Biochemical estimations

Biochemical estimations are seldom required during neonatal anaesthesia, although estimation of the blood glucose level is valuable in premature or SGA infants. Commercially available testing strips are simple to use and reasonably reliable as long as they are fresh. In the sick, hypoxic, acidotic newborn, levels of serum calcium, sodium and potassium should be measured before surgery; blood gas and acid-base estimations may be needed, especially if cardiovascular or respiratory failure ensues.

Monitoring of theatre equipment

Anaesthetic machines

Anaesthetic machines and related equipment such as suction devices, upon which the patient's life may depend, must be thoroughly checked before anaes-thesia is induced. This check includes inspection of the gas supply and breathing systems, ensuring that pipeline probes are firmly inserted, that cylinders, if used, are full and are operating properly, a check of flow meters and vaporizers, and a test to make sure there are no leaks in the system. Every anaesthetic machine should be equipped with an oxygen-failure alarm and inspired oxygen fraction (FiO_2) should be monitored at all times. Retinopathy of prematurity has been reported in a premature infant whose only exposure to an increased (FiO_2) occurred during surgery.

If a heated humidifier is to be incorporated into the breathing system it should conform to accepted standards of electrical safety and a fail–safe cut-out device should operate in case of thermostat failure. The performance of the humidifier should be monitored by measurement of the temperature of the inspired gas at the patient end of the system.

Mechanical ventilators

Most mechanical ventilators are fitted with airway pressure gauges, volume meters and disconnection and overpressure alarms and for those without these monitors there is a fairly wide range of 'add-on' modules available.

As with anaesthetic machines, all neonatal venti-lators should be fitted with oxygen analysers, particularly since oxygen blenders cannot always be relied upon to deliver the preset FiO_2 accurately.

Heating devices

Because of the increased susceptibility of the newborn to heat loss, additional heat must be provided during anaesthesia and this is conven-tionally achieved by lying the baby on a heated electric or water blanket. These appliances must be electrically safe and must also be accurately monitored. Water mattresses must have an easily adjusted thermostat and a fail-safe cut-out device to prevent the water temperature rising above 42°C in the event of thermostat failure. The temperature difference between the heating unit and the water in the mattress depends on the length of connecting tubing and the circulating flow rate. It is therefore wise to monitor the temperature of the blanket by means of a thermistor probe placed between it and the skin surface of the neonate.

Because there is less risk of burns with hot dry air than with water, the hot air mattress described on p. 126 is probably the safest as well as the most efficient method of providing heat during anaesthesia. Patient temperature should, however, be carefully monitored, as hyperpyrexia can occur during long operations.

Electrically heated blankets can rapidly overheat and cause serious burns and their use should probably be discontinued.

Environmental monitoring

Temperature

It is essential to monitor both the temperature and the rate of air change in the operating theatre during neonatal anaesthesia. The theatre should be draught-free and the temperature should be comfortably warm.

Pollution

The removal of anaesthetic agents from paediatric breathing systems does not present particular problems when mechanical ventilators are used, though scavenging the T-piece during manually controlled ventilation is more difficult.

Although scavenging systems have been described which involve the insertion of collecting devices into the expiratory limb of the reservoir bag, or the modification of the system to include scavenged expiratory valves, these devices alter the basic simplicity of the T-piece, often make it more cumbersome to use and, in some cases, increase the danger of obstruction to expiratory gas flow. A scavenging dish for the anaesthetic T-piece which does not alter its characteristics has been described by Hatch.[46] The dish removes large volumes of contaminated air and, if placed close to the open-tailed bag of the T-piece, provides a safe and convenient scavenger.

Regional anaesthesia

Regional anaesthesia using central or peripheral nerve blocks has now become an established part of neonatal anaesthesia practice and is used wherever possible. Occasionally techniques such as spinal or caudal blocks are used without general anaesthesia, but overall these techniques have become part of general anaesthesia providing the very best possible reduction of intraoperative stress responses and continuing postoperative pain relief. A further major advantage is the preservation of normal control of breathing with a possibility that the risk of postoperative apnoea is reduced for premature and ex-premature infants. There is evidence that where analgesia is provided before the nociceptive stimulus begins on a 'pre-emptive' basis, subsequent analgesic requirements will be reduced and for a given dose be more effective.[47]

The toxicity of local anaesthetic agents such as lignocaine and bupivacaine depends on how rapidly they are absorbed from the site of the block and the total dose of the drug injected. Newborns are generally assumed to be more at risk from the toxic effects because of increased plasma concentrations of the free drug by reduced binding to albumin and glycoproteins. However, because nerve diameter is smaller and many nerves are not yet myelinated, blockade may be more easily achieved with less agent. Doses of 2 mg.kg^{-1} of bupivacaine for a newborn and 3 mg.kg^{-1} for an older child seem to be safe maximum doses giving plasma levels well below toxic levels of 2–4 μg.ml^{-1}.[48] The elimination half-life of local anaesthetic agents is prolonged in newborns so repeated doses of drugs must be administered with great care.

Caudal analgesia

Caudal blockade is routinely used for operations below the umbilicus even in newborns as it has proved to be easy to perform and very safe. The technique can be used in awake infants, e.g. for inguinal herniorrhaphy in high risk cases such as ex-premature infants with residual bronchopulmonary dysplasia. Up to 1 ml.kg^{-1} 0.25 per cent bupivacaine will block at least to T10 because the agent spreads more easily in the lax tissue of the neonatal epidural space. For sacral roots only 0.5 ml.kg^{-1} is the required dose.

The block is performed with the anaesthetized infant in the lateral position with the knees drawn up. If the baby is awake, the prone genupectoral position is preferred. A 22g needle or cannula is used. The lower end of the dura is at S3 in the newborn so a sharp needle should not penetrate far beyond the sacrococcygeal ligament. Continuous techniques using epidural catheters are not used at this level because of the difficulty in maintaining sterility in the area. An alternative is to use a transsacral approach with a 23g scalp vein needle and loss of resistance to air or saline. This is useful in babies with the sacral abnormality that is often associated with anorectal anomaly. For a continuous technique a 19g Tuohy with a 21g catheter can be used and in some cases the catheter can be threaded even as far as the thoracic region. Complications of the technique are very rare, but include dural puncture and intravascular injection. Hypotension secondary to sympathetic block does not occur in small children.

Lumbar epidural analgesia

With the advent of 19g Tuohy needles it is now feasible to perform epidural techniques even in newborns after general anaesthesia.[49] Loss of resistance to air or saline identifies the epidural space which lies approximately 0.8 cm below the skin. Because this distance is so small, *continuous* pressure, rather than intermittent, must be applied to the loss of resistance syringe. A 21g catheter is threaded 3–4 cm into the space and after aspiration up to 0.75 ml.kg^{-1} 0.25 per cent bupivacaine are slowly injected without an initial test dose. Haemodynamic changes are minimal and there is no motor block. Postoperatively bupivacaine concentration is reduced to 0.125 per cent and infused at a rate of 0.1–0.4 ml.kg^{-1}. Unfortunately the technique is somewhat limited by leakage of solution from the epidural space because of laxity of the tissues surrounding the catheter.

Spinal block

Spinal block has recently regained popularity for ex-premature patients at risk from apnoea and respiratory failure undergoing inguinal hernia repair.[50] The smallest stiletted spinal needle available should be used and 0.13 ml.kg^{-1} heavy bupivacaine (5 per cent) injected via L4–5 or L5-S1. Since inguinal herniotomy in these babies may be difficult and time consuming, the short duration of the technique may sometimes be a disadvantage. The block will not cover peritoneal stimulation such as pulling on the hernial sac. Spinal blocks which continue to be practised in certain centres have not been universally adopted for neonatal use.

Epidural opioid analgesia

The administration of opioid analgesics via the epidural space has become routine practice in paediatric anaesthesia. Analgesia is more profound and prolonged and relieves visceral as well as somatic pain. Respiratory depression is rare, but anxiety over this risk prevents extensive use of the epidural route in neonates. Analgesia is achieved with small doses producing more profound and prolonged analgesia than the same doses given parenterally. One dose may last as long as 24 hours.

Preservative free morphine at 10–20 μg.kg^{-1} or diamorphine 20–30 μg.kg^{-1} can be used or a continuous infusion of diamorphine 3 mg in 60 ml 0.125 per cent bupivacaine 0.1–0.2 ml.kg.$^{-1}$ hour is an alternative. Very close monitoring in a high-dependency unit is required.

Peripheral nerve blocks

Blocks such as ilioinguinal/iliohypogastric and dorsal nerve of the penis have been used in newborns for many years and have the advantage of using less local anaesthetic agent and providing a more localized area of anaesthesia.[51] The penile nerves are blocked by injections at 11 and 1 o'clock at the base of the penis deep to Buck's fascia with 0.5–1 ml of 0.25 per cent bupivacaine *without* adrenaline. The results of this block compare favourably with caudal analgesia.

Ilioinguinal and iliohypogastric nerves supply cutaneous innervation of the inguinal ligament and scrotum (L1) and blocking these nerves provides excellent postoperative analgesia for inguinal herniorrhaphy. The nerves lie 1 cm superior and medial to the anterior superior iliac crest deep to the external oblique fascia. 0.5 ml.kg^{-1} bupivacaine is delivered via a short bevelled needle which can be felt to pierce the fascia.

Pain management

Traditionally there has been a reluctance to provide analgesia for newborns either intra- or postoperatively, not necessarily from a callous attitude, but more from an idea that opioid drugs are not safe or that they are not actually required since the nervous system is immature and there is no memory of pain.[52] In some countries babies had been operated on with only relaxant and oxygen 'anaesthesia' or oxygen and nitrous oxide mixtures without supplementation. It is generally accepted for humanitarian reasons that neonates should receive adequate pain relief, both during and after surgery, irrespective of any benefit arising from a reduction in stress response.

Thus the recent view is that pain in children is quite unacceptable, but studies of the use of analgesics in adults and children show that children receive fewer, less frequent and smaller doses of potent analgesics and minor analgesics are given much earlier postoperatively.[53] Pain after major surgery can last for at least 48 hours. The study of Mather and Mackie[54] found that 75 per cent of children were in pain on the day of surgery, 13 per cent in severe pain, and 17 per cent in severe pain on the first postoperative day. The situation for neonates was worse. Purcell-Jones *et al.*[55] reviewed 933 neonates over a five year period at the Hospital for Sick Children, London, to find that only 14 per cent received analgesia postoperatively. A survey of paediatric anaesthetists from the UK found that although 80 per cent believed that neonates feel pain, only, 5 per cent prescribed analgesics to neonates after surgery.[56] These opinions together with reports of respiratory arrest after injudicious use of opioids in neonates, allowed the practice of providing little or no anaesthesia and postoperative analgesia for newborns to be perpetuated. Attention directed mainly towards improvement of survival and outcome reduced that paid to the control of pain.

It is now clearly understood that neonates feel pain and mount an appropriate stress response to pain and surgery.[57,58] Preterm babies undergoing ligation of patent ductus arteriosus were randomized to two groups, one anaesthetized with 50:50 oxygen and nitrous oxide and the other with additional fentanyl 10 μg.kg^{-1}. Major hormonal changes in adrenaline, noradrenaline, glucagon, aldosterone and corticosteroids were significantly greater in the non–fentanyl group. Significantly, catabolic metabolism most, sensitively shown by the urinary 3-methyl histidine/creatinine ratio was greater in the non-fentanyl group and this group appeared to have less postoperative stability. These metabolic studies are clearly an objective way of assessing pain and its harmful consequences and presumably are the way that new agents and techniques will be assessed. Stress responses, if extreme, for example during neonatal cardiac surgery performed under deep hypothermic circulatory arrest, may be difficult to obtund.[59] Poorly obtunded responses may be associated with a higher postoperative mortality, though this remains controversial.[60] Inhalational agents such as halothane may be successful in obtunding some harmful stress responses intraoperatively,[61] but are of no use for postoperative pain relief. The severity of the response appears to be directly proportional to the degree of surgical stress[62] and can also be significantly modified by regional analgesic techniques.[63]

In addition to the metabolic data there is a body of overwhelming evidence that neonates perceive pain even though the subjective and emotional overtones of the older child or adult are lacking. The neonate has the neurological anatomy to perceive pain and the previous argument that lack of myelination made him different is spurious since most nociceptive impulses are involved with unmyelinated peripheral fibres and the central pathways to the thalamus are myelinated by 30 weeks and thalamocortical fibres by 37 weeks.[64] There is some evidence that nerve transmission in response to pain is modified when nerve tissue is immature.[65,66] Cortical activity is well documented even in very preterm babies. Auditory, olfactory tactile and painful stimuli all result in cortical electroencephalographic activity. Physiological variables such as heart rate, respiratory rate, length of time spent crying, falls in oxygen saturation (SaO_2) to levels as low as 50 per cent and subsequent behaviour are all significantly changed in babies undergoing a neonatal circumcision performed with no anaesthesia compared to those having it done with a dorsal nerve of the penis block.[67] Babies anaesthetized for circumcision were more attentive to stimuli, had better orientation, decreased irritability and settled more quickly after they were disturbed.

Intubation of the trachea in awake babies causes a significant decrease in SaO_2 and increase in blood pressure and intracranial pressure.[68] These changes do not occur in anaesthetized babies and similar changes that occur during tracheal suctioning can be obtunded by fentanyl.[69] This is clinically essential for babies with lability of the pulmonary vasculature at risk from postoperative pulmonary hypertensive crisis.

Levine and Gordon[70] showed by voice spectrographic analysis that the type of cry of a newborn baby related to a painful stimulus can easily be distinguished from ordinary crying. Many parents and well-trained nurses can be equally certain.

Endogenous opioids such as β-endorphins are released at birth in response to fetal and neonatal distress and are increased markedly by hypoxia or acidosis or during a difficult delivery[71] These high levels of β-endorphins in the newborn decrease rapidly after 24 hours, but have been cited as the possible reason for a reduced MAC for inhalational agents in this group[23] and for the reduced requirement for analgesia, because an immature blood–brain barrier may allow easier access to neuronal tissue.[72] However, even the high levels found in the CSF of stressed newborns do not reach the levels required for analgesia in the human adult.[73]

Assessment of pain which relies on self-assessment and subjective reporting as well as objective observations is difficult, but nowhere more difficult than with the newborn. Nowadays assumptions are made that manoeuvres such as intubation, needle stick and venepuncture and postoperative pain are as real and as painful for the newborn as for an older child or adult. The lack of specific methods of assessment has contributed to the practice of withholding analgesia. Physiological changes in heart rate, blood pressure and respiratory rate occur and palmar sweating[74] can also be assessed as well as behavioural characteristics such as facial expression,[75] body movements involving active and precise avoidance of pain, changes in behaviour such as withdrawal and increased periods of non-REM sleep and a typical cry which is easily recognized by experienced personnel.

Porter[76] has used vagal tone which is related to the amplitude of respiratory sinus arrhythmia as a predictor of outcome, showing that vagal tone decreases with gestational age and onset of clinical complications with lower vagal tone predicting poor outcome. They show that with increased invasiveness of procedures, vagal tone was reduced in parallel with other behavioural assessments of pain. Vagal tone changes may thus be an objective means of assessment of acute pain in infants.

For older infants it is easier to use a visual analogue scale, but this cannot be taken as the only guide to the severity of pain and others exist such as the Childrens Hospital of Eastern Ontario Pain Scale (CHEOPS).[77] This scale, based on cardiovascular, respiratory and other observations may be too complicated for everyday use and is difficult to apply to the newborn. A simpler system based on a 1–5 scoring for pain and sedation may be more practical (Table 3.3).

Table 3.3 Pain and sedation scoring

	Sedation	Pain
1	Awake	Pain free
2	Drowsy	Comfortable except on moving
3	Asleep, moving spontaneously	Uncomfortable
4	Asleep, responds to stimuli	Distressed but can be comforted
5	Just rousable	Distressed

The case for providing even preterm newborns with adequate anaesthesia and postoperative analgesia is overwhelming, but cautions must be exercised. Neonates are particularly sensitive to the respiratory depressive side effects of the opioids and reports of respiratory arrest and exacerbation of apnoea are well documented.[55] Lynn and Slattery[78] have shown that elimination half-life of morphine in newborns is twice that of the older infant (6.8 hour compared to 3.9) related to a decreased clearance of the drug and may be very prolonged in babies with mild hepatic dysfunction (28 hours in one patient).[79] Large boluses of morphine may produce haemodynamic effects such as hypotension and bradycardia, especially if the baby is hypovolaemic. Fentanyl has been used for intraoperative analgesia since the early 1980s[80] and Keohntop et al.[81] found an elimination half-life of 1 to 16 hours in a group of neonates (mean 5.3 hours), clearly much longer than in adults, with half the babies having a rebound increase as late as 15 hours after the first dose, probably from sequestration and then release of the drug from tissue storage. This means that any newborn given opioid analgesics must be nursed and monitored in a specialized unit for at least 24 hours postoperatively.

Regional anaesthesia is increasingly used in the neonatal period with or without general anaesthesia to decrease the hormonal responses to surgery and to provide full analgesia well into the postoperative period. However, plasma protein binding of agents such as bupivacaine is reduced in newborns and infants and free bupivacaine may approach toxic levels after, for example, caudal usage of 2.5 mg.kg^{-1}[82]. 3 mg.kg^{-1} of lignocaine and up to 2 mg.kg^{-1} of bupivacaine are considered safe doses for newborns and infants.

Current Practice

Adequate anaesthesia for newborns overrides all considerations. 50 per cent oxygen with nitrous oxide is not sufficient anaesthesia with a relaxant and controlled ventilation technique, though pulse oximetry allows a more confident use of higher concentrations of nitrous oxide. Inhalational agents such as halothane or isoflurane are used sparingly in addition in concentrations of 0.5–1 per cent. Up to 10 μg.kg^{-1} of fentanyl given as a bolus will last for at least 2 hours of surgery.[83] Patients who require postoperative respiratory support can be given these large doses, but for those expected to breathe spontaneously after surgery doses of fentanyl should be reduced; 3–5 μg.kg^{-1} together with inhalational anaesthesia will reduce pain without causing respiratory depression. Preterm infants usually need reduced doses. The inhalation agent should be discontinued 10–15 minutes before the end of surgery.

Morphine is less frequently used intraoperatively but is the mainstay of postoperative pain relief for most age groups. Pain relief for newborns and infants must be administered on an individual basis after individual assessment.

Intraoperatively local and regional blocks should be used where possible as the effects usually last well into the postoperative period. In the newborn a local block can take the place of general anaesthesia, for example spinal analgesia or caudal analgesia for hernia repairs or rectal surgery. These are very satisfactory for the ex-premature infant with residual respiratory problems. Local anaesthesia, e.g. bupivacaine 0.25 per cent 0.5 ml.kg^{-1}, if infiltrated into the surgical wound before closure provides significant postoperative analgesia.

Surface pain such as that following circumcision can be controlled with EMLA (Astra Ltd.) cream. It is easily absorbed from thin neonatal skin and cases of methaemoglobinaemia caused by the prilocaine have been reported.[84]

Many large institutions have established an acute pain service involving specific medical and nursing staff concerned with the clinical management of postoperative patients, audit, teaching and research using advanced techniques such as continuous epidural infusions, opioid infusions controlled by the patient (PCA) or by the nursing staff (NCA).[85]

Continuous infusions of morphine have the advantage of avoiding the peaks and troughs of bolus administration and cause no respiratory difficulties in spontaneously breathing term newborns after major surgery if provided with 5–10 μg.kg^{-1} per hour on a continuous basis. It is also possible for a trained nurse to give small boluses of 5–10 μg.kg^{-1} using a pump of the patient controlled analgesia type (nurse controlled analgesia). These techniques should be confined to high-dependency areas where equipment for monitoring, resuscitation and respiratory support is available. Continuous epidural techniques are also used for term babies when indicated with bupivacaine 0.125 per cent 0.1–0.4 ml.kg^{-1}.hr.

Not all babies require postoperative analgesia if they have been adequately anaesthetized, but they do require individual assessment. Local blocks reduce the need for opioid analgesics. Warmth, swaddling and if possible early feeding make the baby more comfortable. If the pain is not judged so severe that morphine is required, then single doses of codeine phosphate 1 mg.kg^{-1} intramuscularly (not intravenously) are effective and do not cause respiratory depression. Paracetamol 15 mg.kg^{-1} is very safe and effective if given orally or via a nasogastric tube or rectally in a dose of 20 mg.kg^{-1} for babies following minor or moderate surgery especially if the baby is at risk from respiratory depression with the use of opioid analgesics. It may also be used later on in the postoperative course after major pain controlled by morphine has passed, for example, after 24–48 hours. If it is used as a 'background' analgesic, then adequate analgesia for major pain can easily be achieved with much lower doses of potent analgesics.

Recovery

All newborns are nursed postoperatively in an incubator in the neutral thermal environment range of temperature. Babies should also be clothed where possible even in incubators since most incubators are not permitted to have maximum temperatures beyond 36°C. Incubator temperatures can vary considerably around the set point and their performance can be improved by the use of servo–controlled devices. These depend, however, on the skin probe remaining properly attached to the baby, not getting wet and not being covered by anything. Overhead radiant heaters improve access to the baby and can also be servo–controlled, but they increase evaporative water loss. The open type of incubator with an overhead heater of a servo type is more satisfactory for access by the medical and nursing staff and by equipment for phototherapy and portable X–rays. It is suitable for larger newborns whose management after complex surgery involves mechanical ventilation, chest drains, arterial and venous lines and a urinary catheter. Very small babies usually need to be in an enclosed type of incubator because they require a high neutral thermal environment. A heat shield within the incubator or a sheet of 'bubble mat' (Sancell) over the baby is additional protection. Servo-control mechanisms theoretically may deprive the physician of the clinical information derived from changes in the infant's skin temperature, but in practice the difference between core and peripheral temperatures is still a good guide to cardiac output, the normal difference being 2°C.

Modern intensive care incubators incorporate alarm systems for temperature of the air and the baby, optional monitors for oxygen concentration and weighing scales so that the baby can be weighed while remaining inside the incubator.

Apnoeic episodes in susceptible infants should be anticipated by nursing the baby using an apnoea alarm. Apnoea mattresses are available which work on the principle that respiratory movements are transmitted to a segmented, airfilled mattress and air movement from one segment to another is detected. These mattresses are successful, although they give many false negative and positive alarms. They may detect struggling as a respiratory movement as well as failing to detect apnoea of up to ten seconds, especially if the alarm is detecting the heart beat because the baby is incorrectly placed.

Transthoracic impedance types of monitor using ECG leads are also successful, though the electrodes may become displaced. A third type of apnoea alarm detects changes in the curvature of the abdominal wall so will alarm with obstructed respiration as well as apnoea.

Pulse oximetry is also a useful form of monitoring postoperatively and provides accurate information down to very low saturations over wide changes in blood pressure, and vasoconstriction.[86] ECG monitoring with a rate counter, soft bleep and alarm system is essential for all sick babies.

Other intensive care monitoring includes: core and peripheral temperatures; arterial pressure either directly with an arterial line or indirectly using an automatic blood pressure measuring device; central venous pressure.

Oxygen therapy (see also p. 218)

Most babies require an increased inspired oxygen concentration postoperatively to maintain oxygen saturations in the normal range, but especially after thoracotomy or major abdominal surgery, after large blood transfusions or if respiratory distress is present. An oxygen headbox of clear plastic is necessary to achieve accurate and steady concentrations of oxygen over 25 per cent in an incubator which is constantly being opened for nursing manoeuvres. The concentration should be measured using an independent oxygen analyser of the fuel cell sensor type. The resultant PaO_2 ($TcPaO_2$) or SaO_2 should be measured. The gases should be fully humidified to about 34°C (at least 95 per cent saturated) using a heated water-bath type of humidifier at a flow of $6 l.min^{-1}$ to prevent accumulation of carbon dioxide within the headbox. A servo-controlled type of humidifier (e.g. Bennett Cascade Mark II) which meets all electrical safety requirements is satisfactory if the temperature probe is close to the baby but not within the incubator. One disadvantage with this type of humidifier is that if the gas flow is increased from a previously steady state, the baby will be exposed to gas hotter than is desirable. The contents of the bowl are usually maintained at a temperature which is 'self–pasteurizing', but the bowl should be exchanged for a sterile one every 24–48 hours. If cold oxygen is used, there will be stimulation of the trigeminal area of the face and an undesirable increase in metabolic oxygen demand.

Ultrasonic nebulizers are not commonly used for the newborn because they produce a very fine cold mist which may overhydrate the baby. They tend to be more expensive and are more difficult to sterilize between cases. If such a humidifier is used a water gain of at least 2 ml.kg^{-1}.h should be included in the fluid balance.

High inspired oxygen concentrations are used as necessary to give as normal a PaO_2 as possible, although not if the low PaO_2 is caused by a fixed intracardiac right–to–left shunt as in transposition of the great arteries (TGA) or pulmonary valve atresia.

Infants below 38 weeks gestational age are at risk from retinopathy of prematurity. The safe level of PaO_2 and the safe duration of exposure are not known, but it is wisest to aim for a value between 9.3–10.7 kPa (70–80 mmHg) or 90–92 per cent oxygen saturation where possible.

Patients with poor pulmonary compliance and/or poor respiratory effort may be dependent on CPAP.

This is easily delivered to newborns and infants using one nasal prong. CPAP via a nasal prong is commonly used to treat moderate to severe apnoea of prematurity. The increased oxygenation and stimulation of chest wall stretch receptors reduce the intensity and frequency of the apnoeic attacks. CPAP pressures greater than 8–10 cmH$_2$O are not recommended and an unsatisfactory clinical and blood gas state (e.g. continuing SaO_2 below 90 per cent or PaO_2 below 6.7 kPa (50 mmHg) on 80–100 per cent oxygen) is an indication for tracheal intubation and further respiratory support. As a rule, babies oxygen–dependent or with apnoea preoperatively will require nasal CPAP for a period of time postoperatively.

Nasal CPAP is also useful after extubation in most babies, especially those with poor lung compliance. After extubation there may be temporary incompetence of the larynx and impaired ciliary function. Pulmonary atelectasis is very common and often CPAP via the nasal prong is required until competence of the glottis is restored and the baby is able to maintain its own lung volumes (see also p. 226).

References

Preoperative assessment and management

1. Lerman JL. Controversies in paediatric anaesthesia. *Canadian Journal of Anaesthesia.* 1988; **35**, S18–S22.
2. Sandhar BK, Goresky GV, Maltby JR, Shaffer EA. Effect of oral liquids and ranitidine on gastric fluid volume and pH in children undergoing outpatient surgery. *Anesthesiology.* 1989; **71**, 327–30.
3. Rennie JM, Kelsall AWR. Vitamin K prophylaxis in the newborn – again. *Archives of Disease in children.* 1994; **70**, 248–51.

Anaesthetic equipment and techniques

4. Ayre P. Endotracheal anaesthesia for babies: with special reference to hare-lip and cleft palate operations. *Anesthesia Analgesia.* 1937; **16**, 330–3.
5. Rees GJ. Anaesthesia in the newborn. *British Medical Journal.* 1950; ii, 1419–22.
6. Bain JA, Spoerel WA. A streamlined anesthetic system. *Canadian Anaesthetists' Society Journal.* 1972; **19**, 426–35.

7. Mapleson WW. The elimination of rebreathing in various semi-closed anaesthetic systems. *British Journal of Anaesthesia.* 1954; **26**, 323–32.
8. Rose DK, Froese AB. The regulation of $PaCO_2$ during controlled ventilation of children with a T-piece. *Canadian Anaesthetists' Society Journal.* 1979; **26**, 104–13.
9. Froese AB, Rose DK. A detailed analysis of T-piece systems. In: Steward DJ (ed.) *Some aspects of Paediatric Anaesthesia.* Amsterdam: Elsevier, 1982, pp.101–36.
10. Hatch DJ, Yates AP, Lindahl SGE. Flow requirements and rebreathing during mechanically controlled ventilation in a T-piece (MaplesonE) system. *British Journal of Anaesthesia.* 1987; **59**, 1533–40.
11. Bloomquist ER. Pediatric circle absorber. *Anesthesiology.* 1957; **18**, 787–9.
12. Rackow H, Salanitre E. A new pediatric circle valve. *Anesthesiology.* 1968; **29**, 833–4.
13. Revell DG. An improved circulator for closed circle anaesthesia. *Canadian Anaesthetists' Society Journal.* 1959; **6**, 104–7.
14. Newton NI, Hillman KM, Varley JG. Automatic ventilation with the Ayre's T-piece. A modification

of the Nuffield series 200 ventilator for neonatal and paediatric use. *Anaesthesia.* 1981; **36**, 22–36.

15. Rendell-Baker L, Soucek DM. New paediatric facemasks and anaesthetic equipment. *British Medical Journal.* 1962; i, 1960–2.

16. Brain AIJ. The laryngeal mask – a new concept in airway management. *British Journal of Anaesthesia.* 1983; **55**, 801–5.

17. Mizushima A, Wardall GJ, Simpson DL. The laryngeal mask airway in infants. *Anaesthesia.* 1992; **47**, 849–51.

18. Denny NM, Desilva KD, Webber PA. Laryngeal mask airway for emergency tracheostomy in a neonate. *Anaesthesia.* 1990; **45**, 895.

19. Todres ID, Crone RK. Experience with a modified laryngoscope in sick infants. *Critical Care Medicine.* 1981; **9**, 544–5.

20. Quiney RE, Spencer MG, Bailey CM, Evans JN, Graham JM. Management of subglottic stenosis: experience from two centres. *Archives of Disease in Childhood.* 1986; **61**, 686–90.

21. Nightingale P, Meakin G. A new method for maintaining body temperature in children. *Anesthesiology.* 1986; **65**, 447–8.

22. Westrin P, Jonmarker C, Werner O. Thiopental requirements for induction of anesthesia in neonates and infants one to six months of age. *Anesthesiology.* 1989; **71**, 344–6.

23. Lerman J, Robinson S, Willis MM, Gregory GA. Anesthetic requirements for halothane in young children 0–1 month and 1–6 months of age. *Anesthesiology.* 1983; **30**, 421–4.

24. Kong AS, Brennan L, Bingham R, Morgan-Hughes J. An audit of induction of anaesthesia in neonates and small infants using pulse oximetry. *Anaesthesia.* 1992; **47**, 896–9.

25. Creighton RE. The infant airway. *Canadian Anaesthetists' Society Journal.* 1994; **41**, 174–6.

26. Meakin G, McKiernan EP, Morris P, Baker RD. Dose response curves for suxamethonium in neonates, infants and children. *British Journal of Anaesthesia.* 1989; **62**, 655–8.

27. Zsigmond EK, Downs JR. Plasma cholinesterase activity in newborns and infants. *Canadian Anaesthetists' Society Journal.* 1971; **18**, 278–85.

28. Goudsouzian NG, Shorten G. Myoneural blocking agents in infants: a review. *Paediatric Anaesthesia.* 1992; **2**, 3–16.

29. Stead AL. The response of the newborn infant to muscle relaxants. *British Journal of Anaesthesia.* 1955; **27**, 124–30.

30. Bush GH, Stead AL. The use of d-tubocurarine in neonatal anaesthesia. *British Journal of Anaesthesia.* 1962; **34**, 721–8.

31. Bennett EJ, Ignacio A, Patel K, Grundy EM, Salem MR. Tubocurarine and the neonate. *British Journal of Anaesthesia.* 1976; **48**, 687–9.

32. Meretoja OA. Neuromuscular blocking agents in paediatric patients: influence of age on response. *Anaesthesia Intensive Care.* 1990; **18**, 440–8.

33. Fisher DM, O'Keeffe C, Stanski DR, Cronelly R, Miller RD, Gregory GA. Pharmacokinetics and pharmacodynamics of d-tubocurarine in infants, children and adults. *Anesthesiology.* 1982; **57**, 203–8.

34. Matteo RS, Lieberman IG, Salanitre E, McDaniel DD, Diaz J. Distribution, elimination, and action of d-tubocurarine in neonates, infants and children. *Anesthesia Analgesia.* 1984; **63**, 799–804.

35. Wood M, Wood AJJ. Changes in plasma drug binding and alpha1–acid glycoprotein in mother and newborn infant. *Clinical Pharmacology and Therapeutics.* 1981; **4**, 522–6.

36. Meretoja OA, Wirtavouri K, Neuvonen PJ. Age-dependence of the dose-response curve of vecuronium in pediatric patients during balanced anesthesia. *Anesthesia Analgesia.* 1988; **67**, 21–6.

37. Kalli I, Meretoja OA. Duration of action of vecuronium in infants and children anaesthetised without potent inhalational agents. *Acta Anaesthesiologica Scandinavica.* 1989; **33**, 29–33.

38. Haynes SR, Morton NS. Prolonged neuromuscular blockade with vecuronium in a neonate with renal failure. *Anaesthesia.* 1990; **45**, 743–5.

39. Meakin G, Shaw EA, Baker RD, Morris P. Comparison of atracurium-induced neuromuscular blockade in neonates, infants and children. *British Journal of Anaesthesia.* 1988; **60**, 171–5.

40. Brandom BW, Woelfel SK, Cook DR, Fehr BL, Rudd DG. Clinical pharmacology of atracurium in infants. *Anesthesia and Analgesia.* 1984; **63**, 309–12.

41. Fisher DM, Canfell PC, Spellman MJ, Miller RD. Pharmacokinetics and pharmacodynamics of atracurium in infants and children. *Anesthesiology.* 1990; **73**, 33–7.

42. Whitburn RH, Sumner E. Halothane hepatitis in an 11-month-old child. *Anaesthesia.* 1986; **41**, 611–13.

43. Lerman J. Pharmacology of inhalational anaesthetics in infants and children. *Paediatric Anaesthesia.* 1992; **2**, 191–203.

44. Welborn L, Hannallah RS, Luban NLC, Fink R, Ruttiman UE. Anemia and postoperative apnea in former preterm infants. *Anesthesiology.* 1991; **74**, 1003–6.

45. English ICW, Frew RM, Piggott JF, Zaki M. Percutaneous catheterisation of the internal jugular vein. *Anaesthesia.* 1969; **24**, 521–31.

46. Hatch DJ, Miles RM, Wagstaff M. An anaesthetic scavenging system for paediatric and adult use. *Anaesthesia.* 1980; **35**, 496–9.

Regional anaesthesia

47. McQuay HJ, Dickensen AH. Implications of nervous system plasticity for pain management.

Anaesthesia. 1990; **45**, 101–2.

48.   Tucker GT. Pharmacokinetics of local anaesthetics. *British Journal of Anaesthesia.* 1986; **58**, 717–31.

49.   Dalens B, Chrysostome Y. Intervertebral epidural anaesthesia in paediatric surgery: success rate and adverse effects in 650 consecutive procedures. *Paediatric Anaesthesia.* 1991; **1**, 107–17.

50.   Harnik EV, Hoy GR, Potolicchio S, Steward DR, Siegelman RE. Spinal anaesthesia in premature infants recovering from respiratory distress syndrome. *Anesthesiology.* 1986; **64**, 95–9.

51.   Yaster M, Maxwell LG. Pediatric regional anaesthesia. *Anesthesiology.* 1989; **70**, 324–38.

Pain management

52.   Lloyd-Thomas AR. Pain management in paediatric patients. *British Journal of Anaesthesia.* 1990; **64**, 85–104.

53.   Swafford L, Allan D. Pain relief in the paediatric patient. *Medical Clinics of North America.* 1968; **52**, 131–6.

54.   Mackie L, Mather J. The incidence of postoperative pain in children. *Pain.* 1983; **15**, 271–82.

55.   Purcell-Jones G, Dormon F, Sumner E. The use of opioids in neonates: A retrospective study of 933 cases. *Anaesthesia.* 1987; **42**, 1316–20.

56.   Purcell-Jones G, Dorman F, Sumner E. Paediatric Anaesthetists' perceptions of neonatal and infant pain. *Pain.* 1988; **33**, 181–7.

57.   Anand KJS, Brown MJ, Causon RC, Christofides ND, Bloom SR, Aynsley-Green A. Can the human neonate mount an endocrine and metabolic response to surgery? *Journal of Pediatric Surgery.* 1985; **20**, 41–8.

58.   Anand KJS, Sippell WG, Aynsley-Green A. Randomised trial of fentanyl anaesthesia in preterm infants undergoing surgery: effects on the stress response. *Lancet.* 1987; i, 62–6 (erratum: *Lancet.* 1987; **1**, 243–8).

59.   Anand KJS, Hansen DD, Hickey PR. Hormonal-metabolic stress responses in neonates undergoing cardiac surgery. *Anesthesiology.* 1990; **73**, 661–70.

60.   Anand KJS, Hickey PR. Halothane-morphine compared with high-dose Sufentanil for anesthesia and postoperative analgesia in neonatal cardiac surgery. *New England Journal of Medicine.* 1992; **326**, 1–9.

61.   Anand KJS, Sippel WG, Schofield NM, Aynsley-Green A. Does halothane anaesthesia decrease the metabolioc and endocrine responses of newborn infants undergoing operation? *British Medical Journal.* 1988; **296**, 668–72.

62.   Anand KJS, Aynsley-Green A. Measuring the severity of surgical stress in newborn infants. *Journal of Pediatric Surgery.* 1988; **23**, 297–305.

63.   Yeager MP, Glass DD, Neff RK, Brinck-Johnsen T. Epidural anesthesia and analgesia in high-risk surgical patients. *Anesthesiology.* 1987; **66**, 729–36.

64.   Truog R, Anand KJS. Management of pain in the postoperative neonate. *Clinics in Perinatology.* 1989; **16**, 61–78.

65.   Jansco G, Kiraly E, Jansco-Gabor A. Pharmacologically induced selective denervation of chemosensitive primary sensory neurones. *Nature.* 1977; **270**, 741–3.

66.   Lawson SN, Nickels SM. The use of morphometric techniques to analyse the effect of neonatal capsaicin treatment on dorsal root ganglia and dorsal roots. *Journal of Physiology.* 1980; **303**, 12P.

67.   Williamson PS, Williamson NL. Physiologic stress reduction by a local anaesthetic during newborn circumcision. *Pediatrics.* 1983; **71**, 36–40.

68.   Friesen RH, Honda AT. Thiema RE. Changes in anterior fontanelle pressure in preterm neonates during tracheal intubation. *Anesthesia and Analgesia.* 1987; **66**, 874–8.

69.   Hickey PR, Hansen DD, Wessel DL, Long P, Jonas RA, Elixon EM. Blunting of stress responses in the pulmonary circulation of infants by fentanyl. *Anesthesia and Analgesia.* 1985; **64**, 1137–42.

70.   Levine JD, Gordon GA. Pain in prelingual children and its evaluation by pain-induced vocalization. *Pain.* 1982; **14**, 85–93.

71.   Moss IR, Conner H, Yee WFH, Jorio P, Scarpelli EM. Human β-endorphin-like immunoreactivity in the perinatal neonatal period. *Journal of Pediatrics.* 1982; **101**, 443–6.

72.   Sanner JH, Woods LA. Comparative distribution of tritium labelled dihydromorphine between maternal and fetal rats. *Journal of Pharmacology and Experimental Therapy.* 1965; **148**, 176–84.

73.   Anand KJS, Hickey PR. Pain and its effects in the human neonate and fetus. *New England Journal of Medicine.* 1987; **317**, 1321–9.

74.   Harpin VA, Rutter N. Development of emotional sweating in the newborn infant. *Archives of Disease in Childhood.* 1982; **57**, 691–5.

75.   Grunau RVE, Craig KD. Pain expression in neonates: facial action and cry. *Pain.* 1987; **28**, 395–410.

76.   Porter F. Pain in the newborn. *Clinics in Perinatology.* 1989; **16**, 549–64.

77.   McGrath PJ, Johnson G, Goodman JT. The CHEOPS: A behavioural scale to measure postoperative pain in children. In: Fields HL, Dubner R, Cervero F. (eds) *Advances in Pain Research and Therapy.* New York. Raven Press. 1985: pp. 395–402.

78.   Lynn AM, Slattery JT. Morphine pharmacokinetics in early infancy. *Anesthesiology.* 1985; **66**, 136–9.

79.   Koren G, Butt W, Chinyanga H, Soldin S, Tan Y-K, Pape K. Postoperative morphine infusion in newborn infants : assessment of disposition characteristics and safety. *Journal of Pediatrics.* 1985; **107**,

963–7.

80. Robinson S, Gregory GA. Fentanyl-air-oxygen for ligation of patent ductus arteriosus in preterm infants. *Anesthesia and Analgesia.* 1981; **60**, 331–4.

81. Koehntop DE, Rodman JH, Brundage DM, Hegland MG, Buckley JJ. Pharmacokinetics of fentanyl in neonates. *Anesthesia and Analgesia.* 1986; **65**, 227–32.

82. Mazoit JX, Denson DD, Samii K. Pharmacokinetics of bupivacaine following caudal anaesthesia in infants. *Anesthesiology.* 1988; **68**, 387–91.

83. Yaster M. The dose response of fentanyl in neonatal anaesthesia. *Anesthesiology.* 1987; **66**, 433–5.

84. Nilsson A, Engberg G, Henneberg S, Danielson K, deVerdier C-H. Inverse relationship between age-dependent erythrocyte activity of methaemoglobin reductase and prilocaine-induced methaemoglobinaemia during infancy. *British Journal of Anaesthesia.* 1990; **64**, 72–6.

85. Lloyd-Thomas AR, Howard RF. A pain service for children. *Paediatric Anaesthesia.* 1994; **4**, 3–16.

Recovery

86. Langton JA, Lassey D, Hanning CD. Comparison of four pulse oximeters: Effects of venous occlusion and cold-induced peripheral vasoconstriction. *British Journal of Anaesthesia.* 1990; **65**, 245–7.

4 Neonatal anaesthesia – specific conditions

Almost all surgery in the neonatal period is performed on an emergency or urgent basis and early diagnosis and treatment in a regional centre are essential if reasonable survival rates are to be achieved. Many conditions, such as bladder exstrophy are rare and it has been shown that mortality and morbidity are improved with treatment in a tertiary referral centre.[1]

Antenatal ultrasound examinations are routine during pregnancy and have achieved a high level of sophistication so that many fetal abnormalities are discovered before birth. Abdominal wall defects, cardiac defects, hydrocephalus, oesophageal atresia, diaphragmatic hernia and hydronephrosis are all readily seen with ultrasound. Such early diagnosis not only raises the possibility of fetal surgery for example for hydrocephalus or urinary tract obstruction which takes place in some centres, but also the question of whether, with some severe defects such as diaphragmatic hernia or hypoplastic left heart syndrome, the pregnancy should be allowed to proceed. It also allows the delivery of the baby at an optimal time for reception in the regional neonatal surgical unit.

Oesophageal atresia

Oesophageal atresia, with or without fistula, occurs in between 1 in 3000 and 1 in 3500 live births. In this condition the main danger to life comes from the risk of aspiration of secretions into the bronchial tree, with subsequent pulmonary infection together with possible spillover of acid gastric juice through the fistula. Although other factors will affect survival, particularly birthweight and the presence or absence of major congenital abnormalities, early diagnosis and treatment before aspiration and contamination of the lungs has occurred, survival rates are improved by good management.

The condition may be diagnosed antenatally, but the diagnosis should be suspected in any case of polyhydramnios and premature labour. At birth the baby is often seen to produce excess saliva which may drool from the mouth. The presence of oesophageal atresia can be confirmed by the inability to pass a 10FG catheter down the oesophagus and into the stomach. If the catheter is too soft, it may coil in the upper pouch and the diagnosis may be missed. If a radio-opaque catheter is used, X-ray confirmation of the length of the blind-ending upper pouch can be obtained. A plain X-ray of the chest and abdomen will also disclose the presence of a fistulous communication between the tracheobronchial tree and the lower oesophageal pouch, as any gas bubble seen in the stomach must have entered through such a communication (Fig. 4.1).

Since the common anomaly is this combination of blind-ending upper pouch and lower pouch fistula (Fig. 4.2), the majority of cases of oesophageal atresia should be diagnosed easily soon after birth.

The use of contrast medium is to be condemned because of the risk of pulmonary aspiration, compounding the pneumonitis and increasing the morbidity and mortality.

If no gas bubble is seen, the most likely diagnosis is atresia without fistula. The rarer occurrence of an upper pouch fistula (Fig. 4.3) is excluded or confirmed by the surgeon at the time of operation by oesophagoscopy of the upper pouch.

If this is done routinely a greater incidence of upper fistula together with a lower is found than was previously suspected.

Perhaps the most difficult diagnosis to make is that of isolated tracheo-oesophageal fistula without

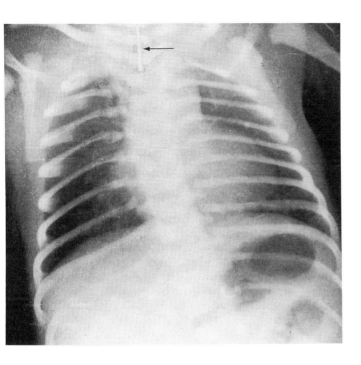

Fig. 4.1 Oesophageal atresia with fistula. X-ray showing opaque catheter in the upper pouch, aspiration pneumonitis and gas in the stomach.

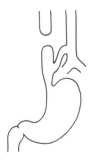

Fig. 4.2 Oesophageal atresia with fistula: the common anomaly (85 per cent incidence).

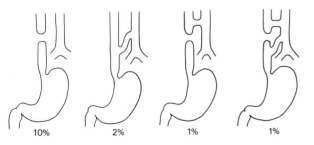

10%   2%   1%   1%

Fig. 4.3 Oesophageal atresia with fistula: the rare anomalies with approximate incidence.

oesophageal atresia. Prominent gaseous distension is sometimes the presenting sign in the newborn but the diagnosis may be delayed for several months, when the infant usually presents with a history of recurrent attacks of chest infection. The differential diagnosis includes cystic fibrosis of the lungs, other causes of repeated aspiration such as incoordinated swallowing or hiatus hernia, and rare lung diseases. In this case diagnosis is usually made with the use of contrast medium by cine-oesophageal swallow. This investigation is performed by an experienced paediatric radiologist and films may be difficult to interpret. Aspiration of feeds into the airway can sometimes be confirmed by the finding of fat-laden macrophages in tracheal aspirate.

Once the diagnosis of oesophageal atresia has been made, steps should be taken to protect the lungs from aspiration. This is most satisfactorily done by the passage of a double-lumen sump tube of the Replogle type into the upper pouch.

Continuous low pressure suction is applied to one lumen and the second lumen entrains air, thus preventing the tube becoming stuck to the wall of the pouch. Alternatively, the upper pouch can be kept empty by intermittent suction. Gastro-oesophageal reflux is discouraged in the upright position but this position does not prevent the collection of mucus in the upper pouch and it may be preferable to nurse the baby prone. A delay of at least several hours with appropriate antibiotic therapy and physiotherapy may be justified before surgery and has been shown to be of particular value where there has already been aspiration and contamination of the bronchial tree before the diagnosis has been made. Provided that there is no increasing abdominal gaseous distension the operation can be performed at the earliest convenient opportunity.

Associated anomalies

Between 30 and 50 per cent of babies presenting with oesophageal atresia have associated congenital abnormalities. The most common are congenital heart disease, particularly Fallot's tetralogy, pulmonary atresia, atrial or ventricular septal defects, patent ductus arteriosus and coarctation of the aorta. Echocardiography is performed routinely on these babies preoperatively. Vascular anomalies and upper airway problems such as laryngo- or tracheomalacia may be present. Severe tracheomalacia is not unusual and may require prolonged intubation or even tracheostomy and the operation of aortopexy is now performed for this condition later in infancy as the condition is associated with 'sudden death' attacks.

Cleft lip and palate may be found in association with oesophageal atresia, as may vertebral, renal and anorectal defects. The VATER syndrome combines vertebral (or ventricular septal defect), anal, tracheal, oesophageal and renal (or radial) anomalies. Plain X-ray of the abdomen may help in screening for some of these defects. The presence of gas in the small bowel, for example, will exclude the possibility of duodenal atresia. Vertebral anomalies may also be detected on plain X-ray.

At least one third of the babies are born prematurely or are of low birthweight. Waterston *et al.* in 1962[2] showed that mortality rose steeply with low birthweight, the presence of other major anomalies and the severity of pneumonia. They described three groups of patients with differing survival rates classified according to these factors. Group A, with lowest mortality (5 per cent), comprised babies of birthweight over 2.5 kg who were well. Group B, with a mortality of 32 per cent, comprised babies weighing 1.8–2.5 kg and those of higher birthweight with moderate pneumonia or congenital anomalies. Group C, with the highest mortality at 94 per cent, comprised babies weighing under 1.8kg and those of higher birthweight with severe pneumonia or congenital anomalies. Nowadays the classification is not so important, as overall mortality is very low even in Group C babies.[3]

Anaesthetic management

Because of the importance of gestational age in relation to mortality, this should be carefully assessed before surgery and steps taken to treat any respiratory distress, hypoglycaemia, etc. Babies who require preoperative mechanical ventilation, for example for hyaline membrane disease or severe apnoea, may require an urgent ligation of the fistula to allow pulmonary ventilation without gastric overdistension. No baby is deemed too sick to undergo this procedure.

Intubation is otherwise carried out as usual in the operating theatre after aspiration of the upper pouch. Because of the high incidence of associated laryngeal abnormality some centres still perform intubation awake in these babies. More usually the babies are intubated after an inhalational or intravenous induction plus a muscle relaxant such as atracurium (0.5 mg.kg^{-1}). When the tracheal tube has been secured in place, the lungs should be gently inflated and careful auscultation of the chest carried out to ensure that adequate air entry is achieved in both lungs. The stethoscope should also be placed over the stomach to check that the anaesthetic gases are not inflating it via the fistula. This is usually situated on the posterior wall of the trachea and is just proximal to the carina.

In the majority of cases the lungs can be adequately inflated without distension of the stomach, but if the position of the tracheal tube is not satisfactory, it is usually because the tip is pointing towards the fistula. It is extremely unusual to intubate the fistula itself, although this has been described. If a significant amount of gas is passing through the fistula, the tracheal tube can be repositioned so that its bevelled edge is pointing in a different direction. Manual ventilation can be adjusted so that in the vast majority of cases the amount of gas passing through the fistula is minimal and pulmonary ventilation is satisfactory. The most important task is to ligate the fistula. When the chest is open, the surgeon can, if adequate inflation of the lungs cannot be achieved, control the leak through the fistula by his finger in the first instance. The normal approach to the fistula and oesophageal pouches is extra-pleural and is worth the additional time this takes because in the event of a subsequent oesophageal leakage no lung soiling will take place.

The practice of performing gastrostomy before thoracotomy has been largely abandoned. The theoretical risk of the enlarging stomach splinting the diaphragm and further impeding respiration is far outweighed by the torrential air leak from controlled respiration if a gastrostomy has been performed before the fistula has been ligated.

The other problem which the anaesthetist is likely to face is surgical retraction during the thoracotomy, which may obstruct ventilation. If the lungs are already stiff with severe pneumonia, it may be difficult to detect complete obstruction, but in most cases the sudden change in pressure required to inflate the lungs is easily detected by the hand. For this reason, manual ventilation is preferred to mechanical ventilation. The use of the precordial stethoscope is extremely valuable in these cases, particularly for the information it provides about the amount of air entering the lungs. It should be positioned over the left side of the chest, or even in the left axilla, well away from the surgical field. Occasionally, the trachea can be seriously damaged during the surgery and large air leaks may occur.

Anaesthesia is maintained with nitrous oxide, oxygen and muscle relaxation with the addition of minimal amounts of an inhalation agent such as halothane. For term babies 2–3 $\mu g.kg^{-1}$ of fentanyl intravenously can be used if the baby is to breathe spontaneously postoperatively. If a decision has been made to ventilate the baby postoperatively more generous doses of fentanyl can be given. Care must be taken not to increase the inspired oxygen fraction above that necessary to prevent hypoxia, especially in the preterm infant particularly at risk from retinopathy of prematurity. Pulse oximetry is used routinely and indirect blood pressure monitoring. Blood should be available for transfusion but with experienced surgical care it is seldom required. Crystalloid or colloid can be administered to cover small blood and evaporative losses to maintain a normal core:peripheral temperature gradient.

The upper pouch should be kept sutured and occasionally tracheobronchial suction is necessary. The Replogle tube is used by the surgeon to identify the upper pouch, but towards the end of the oesophageal anastomosis, the anaesthetist passes a small tube nasally which the surgeon passes through the anastomosis into the stomach to allow early postoperative feeding.

If, for anatomical reasons, primary anastomosis of the two ends of the oesophagus cannot be achieved, a feeding gastrostomy will be performed and continuous suction to the upper pouch or oesophagostomy will be required until a delayed repair such as a gastric or colonic replacement of the oesophagus can be carried out.

Postoperative care

Postoperatively, if the chest is not seriously contaminated and the patient is awake and moving vigorously with no residual effects of muscle relaxation, extubation can be performed. If there is any doubt about the adequacy of ventilation, if the oesophageal anastomosis is tight or if the lungs are seriously contaminated, it is probably wiser to continue controlled ventilation for at least 24 hours.

These babies all need intensive postoperative care; approximately 50 per cent of them will need some period of postoperative ventilation and it is wise in those suffering from severe aspiration pneumonitis, with very low birthweight or life-threatening associated anomaly, to monitor direct arterial and central venous pressure. Oxygen saturation or transcutaneous oxygen tension $TcPO_2$ should be monitored in preterm infants. Chest physiotherapy will be required together with appropriate antibiotic therapy. Intragastric feeding is commenced as soon as possible, either via a transanastomotic feeding tube or by gastrostomy.

Anaesthesia for oesophagoscopy

After primary anastomosis of oesophageal atresia, repeated oesophageal dilatations may be necessary for actual or incipient strictures. Premedication is with atropine and the baby is intubated with either a plain or a preformed tube after induction of anaesthesia and a relaxant such as suxamethonium or atracurium. If anaesthesia is required in an older baby, the use of cricoid pressure after preoxygenation should be considered to prevent aspiration of regurgitated upper oesophageal contents. The T-piece comes down over the baby's chest. A relaxant technique with controlled ventilation is most satisfactory and suxamethonium given intermittently has often been used, though atracurium or vecuronium may be better. The eyes must be protected by taping them shut and heart beat and respiration monitored with a precordial stethoscope. The passage of the oesophagoscope may compress the trachea and obstruct the ventilation. It is wise to hold the tracheal tube in place because the movement of the gastroscope or oesophagoscope can easily displace it. Coughing on the tracheal tube when the oesophagoscope is in place has been responsible for oesophageal perforations, so perfect immobility should be produced throughout.

After the endoscopy the patient is allowed to awaken fully, suction is carefully applied to the pharynx and extubation performed with the infant in the lateral position.

Exomphalos and gastroschisis

Exomphalos is a herniation into the umbilical cord and gastroschisis is a defect of the abdominal wall lateral to the umbilicus, usually on the right side. These conditions are very readily diagnosed antenatally by ultrasonography. The exomphalos sac may be intact or may rupture before, during or after birth with prolapsed abdominal contents coming through it. Gastroschisis, which probably has a different embryological explanation, is an antenatal rupture of the amniotic sac and right-sided because of the obliteration of the right umbilical vein. Further evidence for the two defects being of different origin is the commonly associated thoracic and cardiac anomalies associated only with exomphalos. There is a tendency for the defect to close which may result in partial strangulation of the intestines causing atresias. Prolonged exposure to the amniotic fluid causes the gut to become short and thickened.

Exomphalos, with an incidence of between 1 in 5000 and 1 in 10 000 live births, is more common than gastroschisis, which has an approximate incidence of 1 in 30 000 live births. There is, however, evidence that gastroschisis is becoming more common.

Associated anomalies

Many of these babies are of low birthweight, especially those with gastroschisis. Common anomalies particularly associated with exomphalos are other gastrointestinal or craniofacial anomalies, including hare-lip and cleft palate, or genitourinary anomalies. Severe congenital heart disease may be present and is one cause of the high mortality with this condition (e.g. pentalogy of Cantrell – exomphalos, short sternum, anterior diaphragmatic hernia, left ventricular diverticulum, VSD, pulmonary stenosis). Some patients with exomphalos have a very narrow 'dog type'

chest (Fig. 4.4) with underlying hypoplastic lungs and may die early with respiratory failure or later with cor pulmonale. Exomphalos forms part of the Beckwith–Wiedemann syndrome.

Anaesthetic management

Surgical treatment is usually by excision of the sac when present and complete repair of the anterior abdominal wall usually after this has been stretched manually to enlarge the abdominal cavity. Most anaesthetic problems arise from impaired ventilation if closure of the abdominal wall compresses the intestinal contents, pushing the diaphragm upwards and restricting its downward movement on inspiration. This may occur even with full muscular relaxation.

If the chest is small and the compliance of the lungs is low and this falls further when attempts are made to close the abdomen, it may be wiser to use a silo of silicone rubber (Silastic) for the abdominal contents. There are no good objective methods of determining which patients are best managed with a silo, but a guide to thoracic size is obtained from both clinical examination and chest X-ray appearances. The inadequacy of the abdominal wall may be partly reversed by vigorous stretching of the tissues by the surgeon. The silo augments the abdominal wall temporarily in severe cases and the intestinal contents gradually return to the abdominal cavity during the course of the first few days of life. Tucks are taken from the Silastic to make the pouch progressively smaller. These can be done without anaesthesia, though the final removal of the silo and closure of the abdominal wall requires a full surgical procedure. At any stage, there is a risk that the edges of the silo may tear away from the abdominal wall or may become infected.

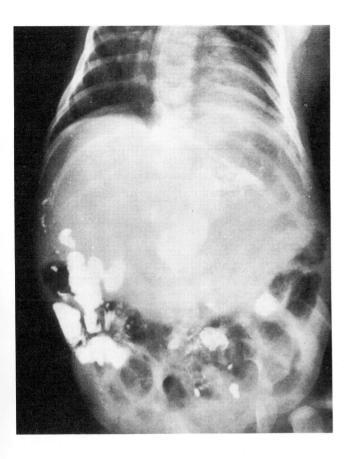

Fig. 4.4   Exomphalos.
X-ray showing the narrow
chest.

Other anaesthetic problems arise from severe fluid and electrolyte disturbances resulting from loss of fluid from the bowel surface and heat loss from the large exposed visceral surfaces.

Postoperative care

Although the mortality from gastroschisis remains fairly high, it has been reduced by advances in surgical and postoperative treatment. If the abdomen has been closed, mechanical ventilation is usually necessary for at least 48 hours because the abdomen becomes even more taut on the second postoperative day. The bowel wall has usually become thickened because of its exposure to amniotic fluid and the onset of peristalsis is often delayed. Continuous intravenous feeding is often required for up to six weeks or so in this condition and this has significantly improved survival rates, although there is a risk that central feeding lines may become infected, leading to septicaemia, particularly from organisms such as candida. Continuous nasogastric suction should be performed during this period and electrolyte and acid-base status regularly checked.

Relatively few cases of exomphalos require postoperative respiratory support and mortality in this condition is due to associated major cardiac or respiratory abnormalities.

Intestinal obstruction

Intestinal obstruction is one of the commonest surgical emergencies in the newborn, amounting to approximately 25 per cent of all neonatal emergency operations. Although the chemical composition of the neonate with congenital intestinal obstruction is normal at birth, delay in diagnosis will cause increasing fluid and electrolyte disturbances. In addition, increasing abdominal distension may lead to respiratory embarrassment and the risk of aspiration. Aspiration pneumonitis has been a common early cause of death, which may occur before other complications have time to arise. The passage of a gastric tube before transfer to a neonatal surgical unit is mandatory. Dehydration, shock and acidosis may complicate the picture, together with the possibility of intestinal perforation and septicaemia due to ischaemic necrosis of obstructed bowel. Finally, the high incidence of associated major congenital anomalies also increases the mortality and morbidity. The fact that a low overall mortality can be achieved in this group of patients is largely related to early diagnosis and treatment.

The possibility of intestinal obstruction should be born in mind in babies presenting with a history of one or more of the following or when there is a family history of such diseases as cystic fibrosis or Hirschsprung's disease.

Maternal polyhydramnios

Polyhydramnios occurs in about 1 per cent of pregnancies and may be due to a variety of fetal anomalies, particularly those related to fetal swallowing. It occurs in approximately 50 per cent of newborns with oesophageal, duodenal and proximal jejunal atresia and in some newborns with ileal or colonic obstruction.[4] Antenatal ultrasound in mothers at high risk for congenital anomalies does not seem to have made a large impact on the low fetal detection rate of intestinal obstruction.[5] The prenatal diagnosis of Hirschsprung's disease and imperforate anus is also unusual as neither of these conditions cause polyhydramnios and colonic distension does not occur until after birth.

Delayed passage of meconium

94 per cent of infants pass meconium within the first 24 hours of life, many in the process of delivery or soon thereafter. By 48 hours, 99 per cent of normal infants have passed meconium; any delay in this process suggests either functional or organic bowel obstruction. A functional ileus is very commonly seen in sick or low birthweight infants. It may be due to prematurity alone (the premature who is not ill usually passes meconium within 24 hours of life) or in association with asphyxia, respiratory distress, acidosis, hypokalaemia, sepsis, maternal narcotic addiction or magnesium sulphate therapy for toxaemia, and occasionally in congenital hypothyroidism. In organic bowel obstruction the delayed passage of meconium is usually accompanied by abdominal distension and vomiting.

Vomiting/Feeding difficulty

Almost all newborn infants regurgitate slightly after feeding; vomiting, however, implies more than mild regurgitation and should be investigated. It may be a sign of a GI tract disorder or secondary to a wide variety of systemic illnesses, including sepsis, meningitis, urinary tract infection, intracranial hypertension, post asphyxia and occasionally inborn errors of metabolism such as the amino acidurias or hyperammonaemia.

That vomiting is due to a primary GI tract disorder is suggested when the vomitus is bile-stained, faeculent or bloody, is excessive or persistent and if more than 15–20 ml of fluid is obtained by gastric aspiration at the time of delivery. Vomiting of bile-stained fluid in the first few days of life indicates intestinal obstruction until proven otherwise. Obstructions proximal to the ampulla of Vater are not associated with bile-stained vomitus.

Primary gastrointestinal tract disorders which cause vomiting include:

Mechanical bowel obstruction

In upper GI obstructions the vomitus is usually bile stained and abdominal distension less marked; in lower GI obstruction the degree of distension is greater while vomiting is normally not bile stained.

Oesophageal atresia with tracheo-oesophageal fistula

This should be suspected in the immediate newborn period whenever there is feeding difficulty with excess oral secretions. When fed, these infants aspirate, cough and choke; they may become cyanotic and develop respiratory distress. The diagnosis is based on the inability to pass a nasogastric tube into the stomach and demonstration of its tip in the airfilled dilated proximal oesophagus on chest X-ray.

Necrotizing enterocolitis (NEC)

In a stressed premature or SGA infant (usually after the institution of oral feeds), vomiting and the passage of blood from the rectum are highly suggestive of NEC.

Gastro-oesophageal reflux

The combination of gastro-oesophageal reflux and oesophageal chalasia (incompetence of the lower oesophageal sphincter) may cause vomiting from birth. This may lead to failure to thrive, aspiration pneumonia and apnoeic or cyanotic episodes.

Swallowing disorders

Feeding difficulties associated with coughing, gagging, regurgitation and aspiration may also result from failure of relaxation of the upper oesophageal sphincter (cricopharyngeal achalasia) or a lack of coordination between the pharyngeal and oesophageal phases of swallowing, as in pharyngeal-cricopharyngeal incoordination.

Diarrhoea

Diarrhoea is not usually a feature in the history of a surgical disorder, but more often a non-specific sign of early infection, either systemic or enteral. When the diarrhoea is persistent, fails to respond to ordinary therapy and is not of proven infectious aetiology, the differential diagnosis includes Hirschsprung's disease, cystic fibrosis or specific malabsorption syndromes.

Intestinal obstruction – signs of GI tract dysfunction

Abdominal distension

This is the single most important sign of GI tract dysfunction. The normal newborn's abdomen is soft, symmetric and slightly rounded. Mild gastric distension is common and if not accompanied by other evidence of disease does not require investigation. If moderate distension is present and persistent it is a reliable, though non specific sign of an underlying pathologic condition (Fig. 4.5). Visible peristalsis may be seen (Fig. 4.6). The first clinical determination is whether the distension is due to air, fluid or an abdominal mass.

Distension due to air

The most common cause of abdominal distension without tenderness is excessive gas within the GI tract due to an adynamic or functional ileus. Many infants swallow large amounts of air during feeding, particularly if the feed is prolonged, as well as during crying or vigorous sucking on a pacifier. Any infant receiving CPAP may collect large amounts of air in the GI tract.

Mechanical obstruction with associated signs of bilious vomiting, abdominal wall resonance, visible peristalsis or delayed passage of stool will lead to greater or lesser degrees of distension depending on the site of the obstruction. Air released by perforation of a viscus is usually accompanied by signs of peritonitis including distension, tenderness, absence of bowel sounds and erythema and oedema of the abdominal wall.

Distension caused by fluid

The fluid causing abdominal distension may be blood, chyle, urine or ascites. Blood is most likely secondary to intra-abdominal haemorrhage following a difficult delivery. Chylous ascites results from thoracic duct obstruction; this may be difficult to diagnose as the fluid is not milky in appearance unless the child has been fed formula containing long chain triglycerides. Ascites from transudation or exudation of fluid into the peritoneal cavity is seen in a number of conditions including Rh haemolytic disease and non-immune causes of hydrops fetalis, congestive heart failure, hypoproteinaemia or peritonitis. Urinary ascites occurs secondary to obstructive uropathy usually associated with posterior urethral valves.

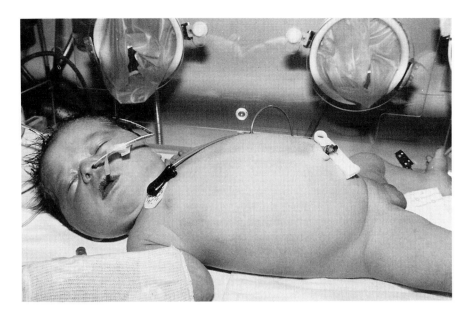

Fig. 4.5 Term infant with abdominal distension.

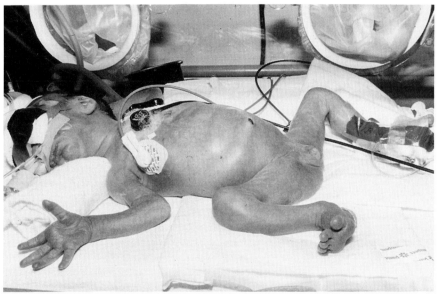

Fig. 4.6 Visible peristalsis in a premature newborn.

Distension due to an abdominal mass

Enlargement of any intra-abdominal organ may lead to abdominal distension; this is usually more localized than the distension caused by gas or fluid. GI masses may be asymptomatic or lead to partial or complete intestinal obstruction. Infants with mid-gut volvulus and malrotation of the colon or, rarely, intussusception, may have an abdominal mass. However, the sign is usually overshadowed by the more obvious signs of intestinal obstruction.

Enteric duplications and cysts are usually mobile on palpation and may lead to intestinal obstruction. Masses of inspissated meconium may occasionally be palpable abdominally in infants with imperforate anus, meconium ileus or Hirschsprung's disease. The mass of hypertrophic pyloric stenosis (epigastric olive) may be felt on rare occasions in the newborn. Birth associated injuries may involve all of the abdominal organs; visceral injuries usually manifest as abdominal distension, lethargy and pallor associated with an abdominal mass or an increase in the size of the liver or spleen resulting from a subcapsular haematoma. A sacrococcygeal teratoma may appear as a large protuberance between the coccyx and rectum. A midline mass in a female infant should raise the suspicion of hydrometrocolpos, particularly if the mass persists after draining the bladder.

GI Bleeding

GI bleeding is common in sick or low birthweight infants in the NICU in whom necrotizing enterocolitis must always be considered. The GI bleeding may range in severity from specks of blood in the stool or the nasogastric aspirate ('coffee grounds'), to massive amounts of bleeding. The amount and character of the blood and any signs of bowel obstruction or hypovolaemia will determine the urgency of investigation of the bleeding.

Causes of GI bleeding include:

1. Necrotizing Enterocolitis (NEC): (see below).
2. *Volvulus and obstructive lesions.* Any obstruction which involves either the venous or arterial blood supply of the gastrointestinal tract will lead to blood in the stools and must be recognized urgently to prevent bowel infarction. Abdominal tenderness suggests either perforation with peritonitis or intestinal infarction.
3. *Trauma* secondary to the presence of an oro- or nasogastric tube in the nasopharynx, oesophagus or stomach. This is usually a superficial injury without other signs and resolves within a few days. Passage of a nasogastric tube may occasionally cause a perforation in the lower pharynx and present with difficulty in swallowing similar to an oesophageal atresia.
4. *Stress* may lead to acute haemorrhagic gastritis or duodenal ulceration with extensive bleeding. This usually responds to saline irrigation; occasionally agents such as cimetidine are used to maintain a gastric pH of 5 or greater.
5. *Generalized bleeding disorders* may occasionally lead to GI bleeding. Haemorrhagic disease of the newborn (HDN) is rarely seen today; DIC with evidence of bleeding from numerous sites is seen in infants with asphyxia, shock or acidosis. Thrombocytopaenia alone without other evidence of DIC does not usually lead to GI bleeding.
6. *Ingestion of maternal blood*, either during delivery or from bleeding from a cracked nipple during breastfeeding, is not infrequently encountered. The blood is red and the infant otherwise well; the diagnosis can be confirmed by the Apt test on the gastric aspirate or stool. (The specimen is mixed with water [1:5], centrifuged and 1 ml [0.25 M] sodium hydroxide added to 5 ml of the supernatant. Brown-yellow colour indicates adult haemoglobin, pink indicates fetal haemoglobin.)
7. *Gastroenteritis* is not usually accompanied by the presence of blood. However, neonatal nursery epidemics due to salmonella and shigella species or enteropathogenic *Escherichia coli*, though uncommon, still occasionally occur. Blood mixed with mucus is found throughout the stool in contrast to blood coating the stool in anorectal conditions.
8. *Anal fissures* are not common in the immediate newborn period, but are seen more commonly in slightly older infants where mucosal tearing secondary to the passage of hard stools occurs. If a fissure is seen in the newborn it is usually secondary to trauma from a thermometer or rectal examination.
9. *Vascular anomalies* with or without obvious haemangiomas on the skin or subcutaneous tissue occasionally lead to GI bleeding.

Radiographic investigation of the GI tract

Plain radiographs of the abdomen are indicated in the newborn with suspected bowel obstruction, an abdominal mass, unexplained abdominal distension, suspected NEC and in the general care of infants in the NICU with placement of umbilical catheters and feeding tubes.

Features to be assessed on the plain film include:

The nature of the gas pattern

The distribution of intraluminal air is dependent upon the postnatal age of the infant: air in the stomach is seen within 15 minutes of birth; by about 3–4 hours the small bowel is visible and the entire GI tract to the rectum will be filled with intraluminal air by 6–8 hours of age. This pattern is delayed in premature or ill infants, in obstructive lesions of the oesophagus without tracheo-oesophageal fistula and in any infant who is not swallowing due to muscular paralysis. The differentiation between small and large bowel is often not possible in radiographs of the neonatal abdomen.

Diffuse gaseous distension is commonly seen in infants with non-obstructive lesions who have swallowed large amounts of air, those with respiratory distress or in infants following resuscitation, particularly with bag and mask ventilation. When bowel loops become elongated or rounded they are more suggestive of intra-abdominal pathology.

The site and degree of mechanical bowel obstruction generally determine the particular pattern of distribution of air; the more proximal and complete the obstruction, the greater the degree of dilatation with air and/or fluid and the easier to determine the anatomic site of obstruction.

Certain characteristic patterns of distension are described, e.g. the 'double bubble' of duodenal atresia, and the 'double bubble' with some distal air in malrotation. However, many low obstructive lesions in the terminal ileum or large bowel may give a non-specific pattern of low bowel obstruction requiring a contrast enema study to determine the site and nature of the obstruction. Midgut malrotation with volvulus occasionally may give the appearance of a low obstructive lesion, particularly if there is severe compromise of the venous drainage of the bowel.

Air fluid levels are seen in both obstructive lesions and in infants with functional ileus. An obstructive lesion that often does not give rise to well defined air fluid levels is meconium ileus, as the thick meconium does not form a straight horizontal layer.

Table 4.1   Causes of high and low bowel obstruction

High bowel obstruction

1   Atresias and stenoses of the stomach (rare), duodenum (common), jejunum and upper small bowel
2   Midgut malrotation with Ladd's bands or volvulus
3   Hypertrophic pyloric stenosis (rare in newborn)

Low bowel obstruction

1   Atresias of terminal ileum and large bowel
2   Meconium ileus (10% of CF present in this manner)
3   Functional immaturity of large bowel in premature infants and IDM (meconium plug syndrome or small left colon syndrome)
4   Hirschsprung's disease
5   Anorectal malformations

Large amounts of free intraperitoneal air give the characteristic 'football' (American) sign on supine radiographs in which free air accumulates as a central lucency in the abdomen; the falciform ligament, highlighted on both sides by air, appears as the seam of the 'football'. Smaller volumes of free air surround and highlight parts of abdominal structures which are normally invisible, e.g. the liver and spleen, the outer surface of the bowel wall, the undersurface of the diaphragm and the umbilical ligaments. Free air is confirmed by horizontal beam radiographs, either a cross table lateral 'shoot through' with the infant supine or with the infant in the left lateral decubitus position.

Intramural gas and portal venous gas are both seen most commonly in necrotizing enterocolitis but rarely may also be seen proximal to any severe bowel obstruction. Portal venous gas might also be related to air entering the venous system during the placement of an umbilical venous catheter. The bubbles of gas in the portal vein can be detected by ultrasound.

Ascites

Ascites appears as a uniform increase in density of the abdomen, particularly in the flank areas with gas-filled loops of bowel floating centrally and anteriorly, on supine and cross-table lateral radiographs, respectively.

Calcification

The site of calcification may either be intestinal or extraintestinal. It is commonly seen in meconium peritonitis following any antenatal perforation; the distribution may be focal or diffuse in nature. Calcification may also occur in congenital tumours, neuroblastomas or teratomas. Renal and biliary stones are very rare in the newborn.

Abdominal masses

A localized area of soft tissue density with displacement of normal bowel is suggestive of an abdominal mass. Plain films, however, are limited in differentiating many abdominal masses and sonography, if done meticulously, will define the site and extent of most masses without having to rely on other cross-sectional imaging modalities.

Contrast studies of the upper GI tract are not usually indicated in infants in whom plain radiographs confirm a complete obstruction. However

ey are extremely important in patients with
artial obstruction (e.g. stenosis, malrotation), in
ny infant with vomiting or feeding difficulties
ven when the bowel gas pattern is normal (e.g.
flux, hiatus hernia, pylorospasm) and in infants
ith suspected aspiration syndromes (e.g., H-type
stula, cricopharyngeal achalasia).

Contrast enemas are indicated in infants in
hom there is suspected low bowel obstruc-
on, malrotation or stricture formation following
ecrotizing enterocolitis.

Duodenal atresia or stenosis requires a contrast
nema to rule out malrotation, volvulus and distal
olonic atresia. In uncomplicated meconium ileus
colon study with water-soluble contrast material
ixed with Mucomyst (acetyl cysteine) is used
relieve the obstruction in an attempt to avoid
rgery. Repeated attempts may be necessary to
roduce complete resolution.

In Hirschsprung's disease the barium enema may
ot be diagnostic in the first few days of life
it is useful in excluding other causes of bowel
obstruction. Barium is not cleared in a delayed
film 24 hours later in Hirschsprung's disease. A
rectal biopsy is mandatory in all suspected cases to
confirm the absence of ganglion cells.

Duodenal atresia

Duodenal obstruction may be due to complete
atresia, stenosis, intraluminal diaphragm or annular
pancreas. The reported incidence is between 1 in
6000 and 1 in 20 000 live births. The stomach and
proximal duodenum dilate rapidly, giving rise to
the classic 'double bubble' on X-ray (Fig. 4.7).

Vomiting usually occurs early and becomes
copious and forceful. If the obstruction is below
the ampulla of Vater, vomiting will become bile-
stained, but many cases of duodenal atresia are
supra-ampullary. Later, hypochloraemic alkalosis,
weight loss and dehydration may occur. Gastric
perforation has been reported.

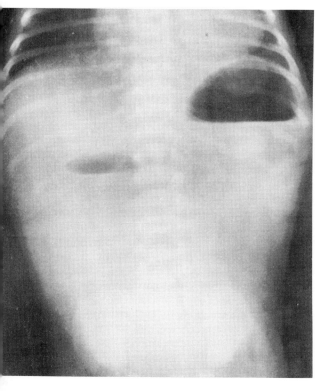
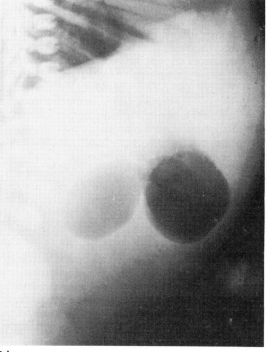

b)

g. 4.7   Duodenal atresia. (a) Posteroanterior and (b) lateral X-rays, showing the classic 'double bubble'.

Associated anomalies

About 70 per cent of cases have one or more associated congenital anomalies. One third have Down's syndrome, often itself associated with congenital heart disease; 15 per cent have cystic fibrosis. Other intestinal anomalies, such as malrotation, oesophageal atresia, imperforate anus and Meckel's diverticulum,. are fairly common, as are renal anomalies. Fifty per cent of these neonates weigh less than 2.5 kg at birth and 20 per cent less than 2 kg.

Anaesthetic problems

Since these neonates are generally operated upon within three days of birth, their general condition is usually quite good. They may, however, have evidence of pneumonitis or atelectasis from pulmonary aspiration. Gastric distension may be splinting the diaphragm and should be relieved with a nasogastric tube. The surgical procedure, usually duodenoduodenostomy, requires full muscle relaxation but otherwise presents few problems to the anaesthetist. Blood loss is usually slight and transfusion seldom required.

Late cases may present with dehydration, hypothermia, shock and severe metabolic and electrolyte disturbances.

Other atresias

With an incidence of between 1 in 1500 and 1 in 3000 live births, other atresias are usually jejunal or ileal and occasionally colonic. Multiple atresias occur in about 10 per cent of cases. In some the intestine is arranged in a spiral around a central mesenteric vessel and is known as apple peel' or 'maypole' atresia. These cases tend to have a familial incidence.

Whatever the cause, the proximal intestine dilates enormously and this may interfere with venous return from the bowel, causing bowel wall congestion or necrosis. Bile-stained vomiting occurs earlier with high lesions. Meconium peritonitis is present in approximately 30 per cent of cases, probably secondary to bowel infarction.

Associated anomalies

These are mainly other intestinal abnormalities such as volvulus. Birthweights are often within the normal range.

Anaesthetic problems

The main anaesthetic problems are respiratory embarrassment or aspiration from the gross distension that sometimes occurs, particularly with atresias low in the intestinal tract. The distension may be so gross as to impair respiratory function severely. The volume and complexity of the composition of fluid lost are also greater with low atresias. Intestinal losses should be replaced with physiological saline, although bicarbonate may also be needed to correct any metabolic acidosis. Increased capillary permeability causes loss of crystalloid and colloid from vessels in the bowel wall; if shock is present, colloid up to 20 ml.kg^{-1} should be infused rapidly. This is more likely to occur with low obstructions where the diagnosis may have been delayed and bowel infarction, meconium peritonitis or bacterial peritonitis may be present. Gaseous distension may be made worse by the use of nitrous oxide and severe metabolic derangement may potentiate the action of the muscle relaxants.

Malrotation and volvulus

Considering how complicated the process of rotation of the intestine is in the normal fetus, it is perhaps not surprising that things may go wrong and the gut may take up a number of abnormal positions. The commonest one is for the duodenum to lie behind or to the right of the superior mesenteric artery with the caecum in front of it. Folds of peritoneum, known as Ladd' bands, attach the caecum to the posterior abdominal wall, in the right hypochondrium, and these tend to obstruct the second part of the duodenum (Fig.4.8) Malrotations are, however, surprisingly rare.

If intestinal strangulation occurs due to volvulus blood may be passed per rectum and abdominal distension will ensue as with other causes of intestinal obstruction.

Associated anomalies

Exomphalos and duodenal atresia are sometimes associated with malrotation, as is diaphragmatic hernia.

Meconium ileus

Between 10 and 15 per cent of patients with cystic fibrosis (mucoviscidosis) present with meconium ileus, which has an incidence of about 1 in 20 000 live births. In this condition, the distal ileum is obstructed by inspissated meconium with a consistency similar to chewing gum. Atresias, volvulus, perforation, gangrene and meconium peritonitis are common complications (Fig.4.9).

A Gastrografin enema, containing the wetting agent polysorbate 80, may relieve obstruction in selected uncomplicated cases but since complications are sometimes hard to detect surgery is usually preferred in all cases. At laparotomy, the distal ileum is often found to be distended and surgery may involve resection of non-viable segments of bowel and the creation of an ileostomy. In addition, polysorbate 80 injected into the bowel lumen may enable some of the sticky meconium to be milked out of the cut end of the bowel, but too much handling of the bowel may make the situation worse.

Anaesthetic problems

These are related to the degree of obstruction and the presence of the complications mentioned above. The use of atropine is controversial, as it may increase the viscid nature of tracheal secretions. In addition, the respiratory problems of cystic fibrosis mean that careful attention must be given to humidifying the respired gases, especially in the postoperative period.

Meconium perforation

Intestinal obstruction may occur in the neonatal period following an intrauterine bowel perforation, with leakage of meconium causing an intense peritoneal reaction. The bowel is usually bound in extremely dense adhesions and specks of calcification may be visible radiologically. The perforation usually occurs proximal to an obstruction (e.g. from volvulus).

Anaesthetic problems

Intraoperative blood loss may be very heavy, equal to or even exceeding the entire blood volume in rare cases.

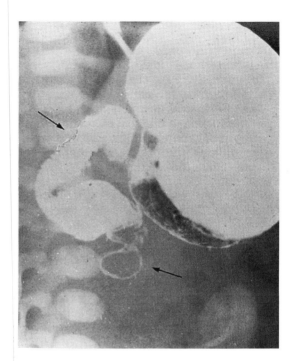

Fig. 4.8 Volvulus. Barium X-ray showing obstruction to the second part of the duodenum and the classic twisted ribbon sign.

Anaesthetic problems

The problems are either those of partial duodenal obstruction or of volvulus, where distension and fluid and electrolyte losses secondary to vomiting occur early. The situation may be complicated by pyrexia, bowel infarction or septicaemia. Surgery usually only involves division of Ladd's bands, derotation and fixation of the bowel, but occasionally resection of non-viable bowel and creation of a double-barrelled enterostomy is required. In the worst cases the amount of viable bowel left may be incompatible with life.

It has been claimed that the incidence of bowel necrosis can be reduced by the use of low molecular weight dextran. Similar claims have been made in animals for the use of hyperbaric oxygen, but these have not been substantiated in man.

embryology of the two systems. Vertebral and skeletal anomalies and congenital heart defects are also common, as are alimentary tract anomalies, particularly oesophageal atresia and Hirschsprung's disease.

Anaesthetic problems

Most of the anaesthetic problems are related to the associated anomalies. The surgical management of the covered anus is by the relatively simple procedure of anal 'cut-back' performed in the lithotomy position, whilst high rectal agenesis is usually treated by colostomy at birth followed by a definitive 'pull–through' procedure 6–9 months later.

Caudal analgesia with or without general anaesthesia is ideal for the anoplasty procedure, using bupivacaine 0.25 per cent 0.5 ml.kg^{-1}. Onset of analgesia takes approximately 15 minutes, but is more rapid if 1 per cent lignocaine is added. The infant usually goes to sleep during the procedure, presumably from the central effects of absorbed local anaesthetic agent.

Congenital pyloric stenosis

This is one of the commonest malformations of the digestive tract, its incidence having been estimated at between 1 in 300 and 1 in 400 live births. It is also one of the commonest of conditions in the first few weeks of life to be treated outside specialist neonatal surgical centres.

Approximately 85 per cent of affected infants are male and between 40 and 60 per cent are firstborns. The pathological abnormality is a gross thickening of the circular muscle of the pylorus, which forms a hard tumour and causes an increasing degree of obstruction to the passage of food from the stomach. The presenting symptom is vomiting, which does not usually start before the tenth day but increases in severity and generally becomes projectile. The infant loses weight and becomes dehydrated, and loss of chloride from the stomach may produce hypochloraemic alkalosis and even tetany. The physical signs which confirm the presence of pyloric stenosis are visible gastric peristalsis, especially after feeds (although this is an unreliable physical sign) and the presence of a palpable tumour usually felt just to the right of the umbilicus. The absence of a palpable tumour does not, however, exclude the diagnosis, and radiological examination can also be misleading.

Whilst medical treatment has been advocated in this condition, it is now standard practice to recommend surgical correction by pyloromyotomy in virtually every case. This operation is not an emergency procedure and must be preceded by complete correction of fluid and electrolyte abnormalities. Sodium, potassium and chloride ions are lost in the acid vomitus and the renal response to this is twofold. First, bicarbonate is excreted (combined with sodium) in an attempt to restore the pH and secondly, potassium is excreted and sodium retained in order to minimize the reduction in extracellular fluid. The first of these renal responses tends to produce an alkaline urine and the second an acid one.

The extent of the K$^+$ loss is not usually well reflected in serum levels. A compensatory respiratory acidosis is also seen with hypoventilation, possibly to the point of apnoea. Extremes of dehydration are rare nowadays, but would be seen with prolonged vomiting when pH falls with ketoacidosis and when a vicious circle develops with falling cardiac output, increasing acidosis and hypoxia.

No surgery should be undertaken until the chloride is at least 90 mmol.l^{-1}, the bicarbonate 24 mmol.l^{-1} and the sodium 135 mmol.l^{-1}; 0.9 per cent sodium chloride may be given and up to 400 ml may be necessary. (Giving 0.9 per cent NaCl 2 ml.kg^{-1} will raise the chloride by 1 mmol.l^{-1}.) Although surgery is not urgently required, correction of any degree of shock definitely is and a urine flow of 1–2 ml.kg^{-1}.h^{-1} should be established as soon as possible.

Most cases are diagnosed early nowadays, however, and little fluid or electrolyte replacement therapy is required.

Maintenance fluids should be 2 ml.kg^{-1}.h of 4 per cent dextrose in 0.18 per cent saline. Mild cases do not need potassium supplements, but in others it should be given at a rate not exceeding 3 mmol.kg^{-1}.24h. A large gastric residue is drained off and 4-hourly washouts of the stomach with physiological saline are carried out until the aspirate is clear and odourless (a secondary gastritis is often present).

Atropine premedication is usually given and the nasogastric tube aspirated before induction of anaesthesia. The tube is left in place because it does not reduce the effectiveness of cricoid pressure and will act as a 'blow-off' valve if the intragastric pressure should rise. There is a risk of reflux of stomach contents and subsequent aspiration during the induction of anaesthesia, though this is unlikely if the nasogastric tube is left open after aspiration. Induction of anaesthesia is by either inhalation or an intravenous method. Cricoid pressure is as effective in babies as it is in adults and may be applied after suxamethonium has been given for relaxation as part of a rapid sequence induction technique. Intubation and subsequent relaxation is also easily achieved by either atracurium or vecuronium.

The surgical procedure involves delivering the pylorus, splitting the muscle and then closing the abdomen. It is important that the child does not cough or strain at the time of muscle splitting, as the surgeon is attempting to cut down to, but not through, the mucosa. Postoperative morbidity increases if the mucosal layer is incised. The baby should be extubated awake in the lateral position. Excellent initial postoperative analgesia can be achieved by surgical infiltration of the wound with 0.25 per cent bupivacaine 0.25 ml.kg^{-1}.

Postoperative care

Oral feeding with clear fluids can usually be started 4–6 hours after the operation, but an intravenous infusion of 4 per cent dextrose in 0.18 per cent saline (3 ml.kg^{-1}.h) should be maintained for the first 12–24 hours until a normal oral intake has been re-established.

Necrotizing enterocolitis (NEC)

NEC is the most common gastrointestinal disorder affecting premature and SGA infants in the NICU; it is emerging as a major cause of mortality in very low birthweight infants, particularly as acute mortality from respiratory disorders decreases in infants in this weight group.[6] The incidence varies from 3.9–22.4 per cent of infants < 1500 gm; this variability is thought to reflect differences in the nature of the population served by individual NICUs, as well as by different NICU practices in early fluid and feeding regimens and PDA management.[7] The mortality rate is 10–30 per cent and directly correlated with the staging of the disease and the presence of perforation or peritonitis.[7–9] Morbidity is related to sepsis, the short bowel syndrome and malabsorption, cholestasis, recurrence of NEC, stricture formation and prolonged hospitalization; morbidity is also strongly correlated with the staging of the disease.[10]

Pathogenesis

Although numerous disorders have been associated with NEC, epidemiologic studies have emphasized three major pathogenic factors.

Vascular Compromise of the GI Tract

Factors which produce hypoxia and/or ischaemia with reduction in the splanchnic blood flow include fetal distress, RDS, shock, asphyxia, PDA, polycythaemia, dehydration, cyanotic CHD, use of umbilical catheters and the maternal use of cocaine (a powerful α-adrenergic vasoconstrictor).[11]

Enteral feeding

Ninety five per cent of infants affected with NEC have been enterally fed prior to the onset of the disease. Onset appears to be inversely related to gestational age, i.e. in larger term infants NEC tends to occur within the first few days of birth, whereas the more premature the infant the longer the duration of the risk period, such that NEC may be seen late in infants in whom enteral feeds are only initiated after two to three weeks of life.[7,12]

The type of feed, i.e. formula or breast, may be critically linked to the incidence of NEC; in Lucas' study formula fed babies had a higher incidence of NEC than those fed breast milk; those receiving combinations of formula and breast milk had an incidence between these two extremes.[8] Not only

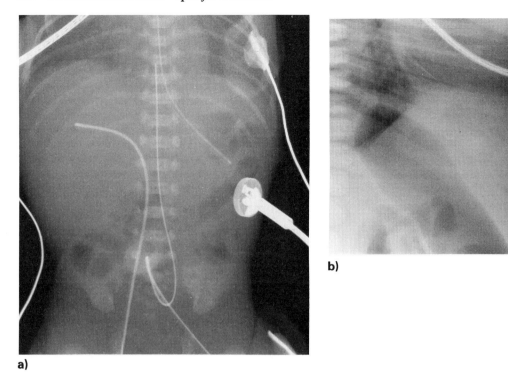

Fig. 4.11 Catheter placement. (a) Supine abdominal radiograph shows a normal bowel gas pattern. The nasogastric tube passes into the stomach. An umbilical arterial catheter passes up the left umbilical artery and the tip lies in the lower thoracic aorta. An umbilical venous catheter has inadvertently passed into the right branch of the portal vein. (b) Lateral view of the upper abdomen shows the tip of an umbilical venous catheter lying in the umbilical vein. Branching radiolucencies above the catheter tip represent air in the portal venous system. This can occur with difficult catheter placements or with necrotizing enterocolitis. The presence of portal venous gas is often well seen in the lateral view but might be more difficult to project in a supine AP view.

the nature of the feed, but also the rate of increasing feeds, total enteral intake and total fluid intake all appear to affect the incidence of NEC.[8,13–15]

Infection

Infection is thought to be operative in both epidemic and endemic cases of NEC. Epidemic NEC is more common in term infants where numerous pathogens have been incriminated, e.g. *Clostridia difficile* and klebsiella. In endemic NEC an infectious aetiology is suggested by the association with prolonged rupture of maternal membranes and chorioamnionitis,[7] the direct effect of bacterial toxins on the mucosa[16] and the effect of microbiologic agents in altering bowel flora and allowing bacteria to multiply to critical levels. In one multicentre study more than 40 per cent of infants with stage II and III disease had evidence of systemic infection; infants in stage I and II tended to

have positive blood cultures for S. epidermidis while enteric bacteria were more frequently cultured in infants with stage III disease.[7]

Attempts at unifying hypotheses propose that an interaction occurs between the vulnerable immature intestine and one or more of the above stimuli[12,17]; this facilitates the invasion of enteric microorganisms and may cause increased permeability of inflammatory mediators, endotoxin or hydrogen gas. Serious vascular compromise may then result from the increased intraluminal pressure leading to haemorrhagic necrosis of the bowel with gas filled cysts along subserosal and submucosal layers.

Despite many proposals the pathogenesis of NEC remains uncertain as it is seen in infants who have never been fed, infants who have been solely breastfed and in infants without other precipitating events.

Doppler flow studies may identify infants at risk for the development of NEC; absent or reversed end–diastolic flow velocities of the umbilical artery in high risk pregnancies have shown a correlation with the subsequent development of NEC.[18] Doppler ultrasound studies of the superior mesenteric artery flow velocity in preterm infants postnatally have documented a consistent intestinal blood flow response to feeding in some reports,[19] but not others.[20] The effects of postnatal age, quantity of milk fed and the presence of a PDA on the Doppler pattern limit its clinical usefulness.

Clinical Signs

The signs of NEC are both systemic and specific to the gastrointestinal tract. Systemic signs include: shock, temperature instability, apnoea, lethargy, acidosis and DIC. GI signs suggestive of NEC include: abdominal distension, intolerance of feeds or presence of aspirates, ileus, abdominal tender-ness, blood in the stool, bilious vomiting, perfora-tion and peritonitis.

Radiographic Signs

Non–specific generalized or focal bowel dilatation is an important radiographic sign in early diagnosis. The degree of dilatation usually correlates with the severity of the disease clinically and the progress of the distribution of dilated loops is important in evaluating the progress of the disease. (Persistent dilated loops often correlate with focal areas of necrosis.) Intramural gas and portal venous gas are more specific signs of NEC but may not be seen in all patients. (Intramural air is unusual in infants who have not been fed.) Pneumatosis is best seen in the colon and may be either curvilinear or bubbly in appearance. In most instances of perforation free air is readily seen on plain radiographs of the abdomen; occasionally this is absent and only ascites is noted.

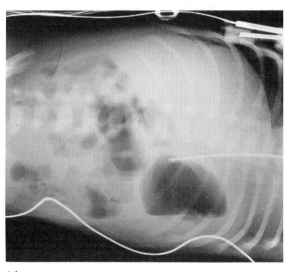

b)

a)

Fig. 4.12 (a) Necrotizing enterocolitis. Erect X-ray showing distended loops of bowel with fluid levels, intramural gas, and gas in the portal venous system. (b) Free air outlines the lateral surface of the right lobe of the liver. This emphasizes the importance of horizontal beam films to document the present of small amounts of free air which may not be seen in the supine film taken at the same time.

Table 4.2   Modified Bell staging criteria for NEC[7,21]

Stage	Classification	Systemic signs	Intestinal signs	Radiological signs
IA	Suspected NEC	Temperature instability, apnoea, bradycardia, lethargy	Elevated pregavage residuals, mild abdominal distension, positive stool	Normal or intestinal dilation, mild ileus
IB	Suspected NEC	Same as above	Bright red blood from rectum	Same as above
IIA	Proven NEC–mildly ill	Same as above	Same as above, plus absent bowel sounds, with or without abdominal tenderness	Intestinal dilation, ileus, pneumatosis intestinalis
IIB	Proven NEC– moderately ill	Same as above, plus mild metabolic acidosis and mild thrombocytopaenia	Same as above, plus absent bowel sounds, definite abdominal tenderness, with or without abdominal cellulitis or right lower quadrant mass	Same as IIA, plus portal vein gas, with or without ascites
IIIA	Advanced NEC– severely ill, bowel intact	Same as IIB, plus hypotension, bradycardia, severe apnoea, combined respiratory and metabolic acidosis, disseminated intravascular coagulation and neutropaenia	Same as above, plus signs of generalized peritonitis, marked tenderness and distension of abdomen	Same as IIB, plus definite ascites
IIIB	Advanced NEC– severely ill, bowel perforated	Same as IIIA	Same as IIIA	Same as IIB, plus pneumoperitoneum

Management of NEC

This includes:

1. Discontinuation of enteral feeds and decompression of the GI tract.
2. Septic work–up and administration of IV antibiotics.
3. Fluid and electrolyte management plus provision of parenteral nutrition.
4. Frequent clinical monitoring of systemic and abdominal signs plus laboratory assessment of CBC (particularly WBC and platelet responses) and acid–base status.
5. Frequent radiographic examination as perfo-

ration may occur without an overt change in clinical signs.

The indication for surgical intervention is generally documentation of a pneumoperitoneum. Other indications may include paracentesis evidence of intestinal gangrene or portal venous gas.[9,22] At operation there is often difficulty in differentiating potentially viable bowel from areas of necrosis; resection of necrotic bowel with an enterostomy is usually performed, provided that at least 30 cm of viable intestine remains.

Resumption of feeds depends upon the stage of NEC and the necessity for surgical treatment; parenteral nutrition is maintained until feeds are fully resumed.

Biliary atresia

Biliary atresia may be extrahepatic or, more commonly, intrahepatic and other major anomalies such as congenital heart disease may be associated. The differential diagnosis is with neonatal hepatitis. Surgical exploration of the bile ducts and intraoperative cholangiography are usually required to confirm the exact nature of the anomaly and to assess the feasibility of surgical correction by some form of anastomosis between the porta hepatis or biliary passages and the intestinal tract – the Kasai operation. The operation is most likely to be successful if it is performed early, before the liver is too damaged. The postoperative course may be complicated by ascending cholangitis.

Anaesthetic management

Because of reduced hepatic function these babies may have coagulation abnormalities and haematological studies should be carried out before surgery. It is probably wise to administer vitamin K_1 intramuscularly prior to surgery, as hypoprothrombinaemia is common. The operation may be prolonged, so maintenance of normothermia is important. Also, blood loss may be heavy so a reliable intravenous line must be inserted and adequate supplies of blood must be available for transfusion, if required. Hepatorenal failure does not seem to be a problem in infancy, so the administration of mannitol is probably unnecessary. Halothane is not contraindicated in anaesthesia for biliary atresia and increasingly regional anaesthesia, such as epidural techniques, is performed for this as well as other major abdominal procedures in small babies. Epidural analgesia is contraindicated in any baby with a coagulopathy.

Inguinal hernia

Inguinal hernias may present towards the end of the neonatal period; because these may become incarcerated, repair should not be delayed. The hernia is usually the result of a patent processus vaginalis and repair is by simple herniotomy. Most hernias can be reduced easily at this age and it is unusual for the patient to develop significant intestinal obstruction, provided diagnosis and treatment are carried out without delay. Inguinal hernia is especially common in low birthweight babies and is found in up to 15 per cent of such patients.

Anaesthetic management

Very many babies with inguinal hernia are ex-premature babies. Some are still oxygen dependent or have very poor respiratory reserve with residual bronchopulmonary dysplasia or are at risk from postoperative apnoea.

If strangulation has occurred, the baby may be shocked and dehydrated with loss of water and electrolytes by vomiting. Such babies are treated by nasogastric suction and intravenous therapy before surgery. For babies below 5 kg intubation with a relaxant technique using atracurium or vecuronium is very satisfactory, together with regional anaesthesia such as ilioinguinal/iliohypogastric block or caudal block. Spinal and caudal analgesia have been advocated for ex-premature babies without general anaesthesia.[23,24] Without a block, traction on the peritoneum is extremely stimulating and could cause laryngeal spasm if tracheal intubation has not been performed.

Postoperative care

If the child's general condition is satisfactory, a graduated feeding regimen can be started as soon as he is fully awake, as for pyloric stenosis.

Postoperative analgesia is seldom required at this age but intramuscular codeine phosphate in a single dose of 1 mg.kg^{-1} can be safely used, or paracetamol orally 15 mg.kg^{-1}. Patients below 44 weeks postconception should not be treated on a day-stay basis as there is significant risk of apnoeic problems postoperatively. They should be admitted to a high dependency unit for apnoea monitoring. The technique of anaesthesia appears to have no influence on the incidence of postoperative apnoea.[25] Intravenous theophylline (8 mg.kg^{-1}) is recommended by some to decrease the incidence of damaging apnoea.[26]

Urogenital abnormalities

Renal agenesis may occur, for example as part of Potter's syndrome, characterized by oligohydramnios, pulmonary hypoplasia, talipes and characteristic facies. The commonest lesions causing urinary tract obstruction in the newborn are pelvic hydro-nephrosis and posterior urethral valves.

Hydronephrosis

The cause of hydronephrosis is not fully understood but occurs by obstruction at the pelviureteric junction; considerable damage to the renal parenchyma may result, to a degree proportional to the length of time of obstruction. The condition is commonly diagnosed by prenatal ultrasound and some centres have undertaken surgery to the fetus. However, an isotope scan often shows good renal function and not all patients with hydronephrosis have an obstructed ureter so that fewer than half require surgery early in life. There seems to be no difference in the results between patients operated on before birth and those whose surgery is delayed until after birth – especially as some may need no urgent surgery at all. The commonest presenting postnatal symptoms are a palpable abdominal mass and non-specific symptoms such as failure to thrive associated with urinary tract infections. Investigations include ultrasound and isotope scan procedures and a Whitaker test performed under general anaesthesia consisting of determining rates of flow from the renal pelvis into the ureter by direct percutaneous puncture. Surgery consists of pyeloureteroplasty or bilateral nephrostomies if drainage is urgent. The babies occasionally have severe electrolyte and fluid disturbances which need to be corrected preoperatively.

Urethral valves

Posterior urethral valves which cause obstruction in the neonate usually present because of uraemia, acidaemia and the toxic effects of severe urinary tract infection. The diagnosis is often made by antenatal ultrasound and in some centres bladder drainage tubes are inserted by fetal surgeons. After birth the diagnosis is usually made because of a persistently palpable bladder, but should also be suspected when there is vomiting and failure to thrive as these are common presenting symptoms; in a severe case, cardiorespiratory collapse may occur following a vicious circle of vomiting, dehydration, reduced renal function, acidosis and, eventually, a fall in cardiac output. Abnormalities of micturition may go unnoticed.

The valves, which may be thick and rigid, tend to pass downwards and laterally, extending around the lumen of the urethra, and fuse together at a lower level. Catheterization and instrumentation are easily carried out, but the valve cusps obstruct the flow of urine. The obstruction to urine flow can have a very severe effect on the developing urinary tract, often before birth. The long-term prognosis must depend on the degree of renal damage; in one older series, 22 of 54 boys presenting within three months of age died. Now, no patients die in the early stages, but many develop chronic renal failure with the growth spurt of adolescence and eventually only 20 per cent have completely normal kidneys. The amount of irreversible kidney damage cannot be assessed from the initial degree of uraemia, which is caused also by dehydration, obstruction to urine flow and infection in a very sick baby.

Initial treatment must include intravenous fluids for dehydration, sodium bicarbonate to correct acidosis, antibiotics and urinary catheterization. Surgery is performed only when metabolic correction has taken place. Definitive diagnosis requires imaging (retrograde cystogram) and also urodynamic studies.

The great majority of urethral valves are destroyed by fulguration throughout their length using a hooked ball or a Whitaker hook electrode. When the instrument cannot be passed through a small anterior urethra, a urethrostomy in the perineum is created to enable the resectoscope to pass into the posterior urethra.

Anaesthesia should follow the basic principles for neonatal patients; if adequate medical treatment has been carried out initially, then no additional problems should ensue. After relief of the obstruction, a large fluid intake may be required, depending on the urine output and its osmolality. Up to 1 litre of fluid may be required over the first 12 hours postoperatively in severe cases. Potassium supplements are often necessary for these cases, although serum electrolyte values are unhelpful as a guide for intravenous doses of potassium.

Prune belly syndrome

The prune belly syndrome (Fig. 4.13), which involves defective muscularization of the anterior abdominal wall and the urinary tract, is only seen in its full extent in males. The full syndrome is a complex with several developmental errors. The severity of the muscular defect varies and may involve one or both sides of the abdominal wall. The skin over the abdomen is classically wrinkled like a prune, although it may merely have abnormal transverse creases. The costal margin is flared and the sternum is usually prominent. The upper parts of the recti and the oblique muscles of the abdomen are usually present.

Abnormalities of the gastrointestinal tract may include volvulus and intestinal obstruction, but changes in the genitourinary system are commonly seen and their severity is proportional to the deficiency of the abdominal musculature. The bladder is large and the urachus patent as far as the umbilicus. The ureters are dilated and the pelvices of the kidneys may be similarly affected: the degree of dysfunction depends on the back-pressure effect of the urine and subsequent urinary tract infection. The testes are always undescended.

These babies may have renal failure, acidosis and dehydration and may also be septicaemic. Because of the absent abdominal musculature, they may have reduced pulmonary function, with an inability to cough and clear the chest of secretions.

Surgery is designed to restore function of the urinary tract, to improve emptying of the bladder and to preserve or improve renal function.

The anaesthetist must take into account the possibility that renal function may be impaired, so care must be taken with those drugs known to

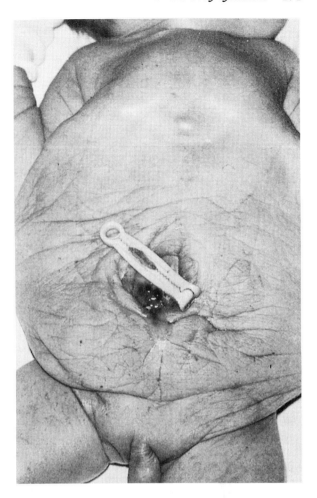

Fig. 4.13 The prune belly syndrome.

be excreted in the urine. There is usually a history of repeated chest infections, and any infection of the chest or urinary tract should be vigorously treated preoperatively. The babies should be managed during induction as if the stomach were full, because of the danger of regurgitation of gastric contents.

The neonate is intubated in the normal way, but eventually controlled ventilation may be maintained without the use of relaxants because the abdomen is very lax anyway. Postoperatively, hypoventilation and a reduced coughing mechanism may cause sputum retention and respiratory failure. Extubation takes place only when the baby is fully awake and moving vigorously. The condition is associated with perioperative morbidity and mortality, usually from respiratory causes such as secretion retention and hypoxia. Nasal CPAP, which allows lung volumes to be maintained, may be a very useful form of respiratory support postoperatively.

Bladder exstrophy

This serious congenital malformation affects approximately 1 in 20 000 babies: three times as many males as females. The mucosa of the bladder is laid open and the ureteric orifices are visible. The size of the exstrophy varies and sometimes the surface area of the mucosa is the same as that of a normal bladder. There is complete epispadias. As the mucosa of the bladder continues to be exposed, it becomes hyperaemic, friable and infected. Hydroureteronephrosis may develop because of oedema and, later, fibrosis which affect the ureteric orifices, causing obstruction to urine outflow.

Definitive surgical treatment is usually undertaken in the neonate before infection and secondary ureteric problems arise and while the bladder is still thinwalled and flexible. The open bladder exstrophy, if left, may predispose to carcinoma. The results of closure do not necessarily indicate that full continence and a normal upper urinary tract can be expected. Surgery usually takes place within the first 36–48 hours of life while the pelvis can be moulded. After 48 hours a pelvic osteotomy is necessary.

The operation involves very major surgery, starting with the baby prone if bilateral iliac osteotomies are to be performed, after which the baby is positioned supine for the formal mobilization and closure of the bladder. The pelvic osteotomies enable the pubes to be apposed and closure of the urethra to be attempted. Heavy blood loss may be expected and two good intravenous lines should be established, one of which should be central in the internal jugular vein. Hypotensive anaesthesia, so useful for this operation in older children, is rarely necessary in the neonate. Full monitoring should include oesophageal stethoscope and blood pressure cuff. Care should be taken to prevent heat loss during the long operation, particularly at the stage of turning from the prone to supine positions. The tracheal tube and intravenous lines should be very well secured to prevent accidental dislodgement during turning of the baby. While the baby is prone, pads under the pelvis and chest prevent pressure on the inferior vena cava which would increase bleeding and also decrease cardiac output.

Caudal analgesia may be used as an adjunct to anaesthesia for bladder exstrophy.

Anaesthesia for neuroradiology and neurosurgery

The principles of anaesthesia for neuroradiological investigation and neurosurgery in neonates do not differ greatly from those in adults. All patients need very careful neurological assessment preoperatively.

Cerebral blood flow

Cerebral blood flow is normally regulated automatically to match cerebral metabolism. Decreased oxygenation of arterial blood results in an increased rate of blood flow to the brain so that tissue oxygen tension is maintained at near-normal levels. This autoregulation operates throughout a wide range of systemic blood pressure (60–180 mmHg in the adult) and even as low as 45–50 mmHg in the newborn infant. Regulation of cerebral blood flow in the preterm baby is less precise and may not function after a period of hypoxia (p. 39). Cerebral blood flow increases with increasing $PaCO_2$ between 2.7 and 10.7 kPa (20 and 80 mm Hg): hypocapnia tends to modify the effects of agents which increase cerebral blood flow. Damaged areas of brain, such as occur with trauma, infarction or in the region of arteriovenous malformations and tumours, lose their autoregulation so the circulation in these areas varies passively with blood pressure. If the $PaCO_2$ rises and normal cerebral vessels dilate, blood is diverted from abnormal to healthy areas (intracerebral steal syndrome). The inverse intracerebral steal syndrome is seen when normally reactive cerebral vessels constrict.

The total volume of the intracranial contents cannot alter within the rigid skull of the adult, although compensatory decreases (or increases) may take place within the three constituents: brain, blood and cerebrospinal fluid (CSF). A slowly expanding space- occupying lesion will displace CSF and venous blood, so intracranial pressure (ICP) rises very slowly until no more compensation is possible. Any small increase in volume above this will cause a very large increase in ICP with severe symptoms. A neonatal skull has a capacity to expand not seen with the rigid adult skull and increasing head circumference is the main sign of hydrocephalus, preceding symptoms of raised ICP (vomiting, irritability, seizures or severe lethargy).

All inhalation anaesthetic agents increase cerebral blood flow, as does ketamine, although intravenous induction agents, barbiturates and drugs which depress neuronal activity tend to decrease it. Halothane, like all inhalation anaesthetic agents, increases cerebral blood flow and thus intracranial pressure. The effect is minimal if low doses of halothane are used and is not seen if hyperventilation is employed. This makes halothane combined with mild hyperventilation a very useful technique for neonatal neurosurgical anaesthesia. Isoflurane probably allows more cerebral depression than halothane without such marked increases in cerebral blood flow and nowadays is the maintenance agent of choice. However, as a smooth induction of anaesthesia is paramount for neurosurgery, halothane may be the preferred agent for an inhalational induction.

Anaesthesia for neuroradiology

General anaesthesia is invariably required for major neuroradiological investigations because of the need for immobility and the prolonged discomfort involved. In addition to the problems of anaesthetizing a neonate, there are those associated with working in the X-ray department. The commonest problems are a lack of facilities for keeping the baby warm (although this can be overcome with warm coverings and a draught-free environment), lack of easy access to the patient and, often, poor lighting. Because of the risk from radiation, protective aprons must be worn by the staff. Far fewer invasive investigations have been necessary since the advent of bedside ultrasound investigations, computerized axial tomography (CT) scanning and magnetic resonance imaging (MRI). Ultrasound is useful for primary diagnosis of haemorrhage ventricular size and cerebral shifts, and also for serial imaging as, for example, a guide to progressive ventricular tapping for hydrocephalus (see p. 49, 176).

CT and MRI scans

Neonates may not need anaesthesia for CT scanning as restraint with a blanket will immobilize the infant for a head scan. A fit child may be sedated with chloral hydrate 30 mg.kg^{-1} orally one hour beforehand. For high-speed body and head scans, periods of apnoea with anaesthesia may be required; occasionally, intubation is also necessary for airway security in patients who are having fits or who are comatose or in respiratory failure. Contrast CT scans to show configuration of the ventricles are commonly performed using iohexol which has very few side-effects, notably low allergenicity.

Investigations using MRI also require total immobility and no metallic objects must be in the field. A relaxant technique using one of the shorter-acting drugs such as atracurium or vecuronium is ideal and intubation should be with a preformed PVC tube which is not markedly radio-opaque. Tele-monitoring consists of precordial or oesophageal stethoscope, ECG, BP cuff, respiratory impedance and pulse oximetry.

Myelography

Myelography is nowadays rarely performed in newborns, but still does have a place for further investigations of spinal cord injuries at birth, for cord compressions and for dysraphic lesions of the cord.

Diastematomyelia is a fissure or cleft of the spinal cord in the lumbar region, caused by transfixion of the neural tissue by a bony septum. This prevents normal ascent of the cord in the vertebral canal as the child grows and, because the cord is tethered in the lumbar region, there will be progressive neurological damage. Cutaneous haemangiomata, a lipoma or a tuft of hair may overlie the site of the spinal defect.

During the X-ray examination there is a need for many changes in position of the patient, including marked flexion of the head, and a flexible reinforced tracheal tube is therefore recommended. If the investigation includes the cervical spine, a radio-lucent tube must be used; a plain Portex tube is suitable.

Premedication is with atropine and awake intubation is carried out after preoxygenation. Intubation difficulties are occasionally encountered, as lesions of the cervical spine which need investigation may be associated with conditions such as the Klippel–Feil syndrome (p. 129).

After intubation bilateral air entry should be sought for all positions of the head as flexion of the head may cause an overlong tube to slip into the right main bronchus.

Vital signs should be monitored using an oesophageal stethoscope, ECG and blood pressure cuff. The most satisfactory anaesthetic technique involves a relaxant, controlled ventilation with oxygen, nitrous oxide and halothane (0.25–0.5 per cent). Hypotension may occur during tilting of the patient.

Great care should be taken to prevent contrast medium from draining into the head, so a head-up posture is necessary postoperatively. It is perhaps wisest to give phenobarbitone 2 mg.kg^{-1} i.m. after the investigation, as a precaution against seizures.

Angiography

Carotid angiograms are performed for suspected vascular malformations and arteriovenous malformations and tumours (rare in the neonatal period). Arteriovenous malformations may present with severe cardiac failure and a bruit over the head will be audible. Fits will need to be controlled with specific agents such as phenobarbitone, diazepam or phenytoin.

Premedication is with atropine and awake intubation is carried out after preoxygenation. Ventilation, which needs to be controlled for neonatal anaesthesia, is also an advantage for cerebral arteriography. A flexible reinforced tracheal tube is used. If the patient is ventilated to a PaCO$_2$ of 4 kPa (30 mmHg normal vessels are constricted, which improves the definition of abnormal vessels. The dose of contrast medium must not exceed 4 ml.kg^{-1} body weight. Allergic reactions to contrast medium are relatively common and cause death in 1 in 40 000 cases. The contrast is hypertonic and causes a biphasic problem for the circulation; initial volume overload, followed by dehydration after an osmotic diuresis. Contrast media may also interfere with the clotting mechanism in which platelets are consumed. It is possible for a body to lose 10 per cent of the circulating blood volume during a carotid angiogram and fluid overload is possible as the result of excessive flushing of the artery with saline. Digital angiography with subtraction may require prolonged apnoea during the exposure.

Some arteriovenous malformations such as aneurysm of the vein of Galen may be controlled by an embolization procedure. Emboli of various substances including histoacrylic are flushed into a feeding artery if this can be localized. Success depends on the number of feeding vessels and several sessions may be necessary for very difficult situations. The prognosis is not good for those newborns that present in severe uncontrollable cardiac failure, but up to 50 per cent of patients may benefit from the procedure. Each session is likely to be more prolonged than an investigation, so extra care must be taken with heat maintenance and monitoring of vital signs. Great haemodynamic disturbances with hypertension, bradycardia and dysrrhythmias may occur during the embolization.

Anaesthesia for neurosurgery

Neurosurgery in the neonatal period usually involves operations for developmental anomalies in the spine and cranium, for hydrocephalus, extradural and subdural haematomas, or for elevating skull depressions from birth injury. Most operations for tumours, craniosynostosis or vascular lesions tend not to fall into this age group.

Myelomeningocele

Myelomeningocele occurs in 1–4 infants per 1000 live births, although encephalocele is much less common (1 in 5000). The measurement of α-fetoprotein (AFP) concentrations in the amniotic fluid has made possible the antenatal recognition of severe open neural tube anomalies and possible termination of the pregnancy. The maternal serum AFP may also be elevated in pregnancy when the fetus has an open neural tube anomaly (see p 77).

After 1952, when it became possible to relieve hydrocephalus by shunt operations, a period of aggresive surgery for myelomeningocele followed in which closure of the back lesion was one of the most common emergency neonatal operations. Because of the very large numbers of badly deformed children who survived as a result of this policy, many centres now try to restrict surgical treatment at birth to those babies whose handicap later in life will be minimal. Back closure is carried out in these babies within 24–36 hours of life because to delay increases the chances of wound infection and meningitis. Some untreated babies survive, however, and in these, back closure must be considered at some stage on humanitarian grounds.

Of babies with myelomeningocele or encephalocele, 80 per cent develop hydrocephalus with the Arnold–Chiari malformation (downward displacement of the pons and medulla and protrusion of the cerebellar vermis through the foramen magnum) and aqueduct stenosis. Occasionally, patients with the Arnold–Chiari malformation develop stridor as hydrocephalus progresses. This is possibly caused by traction on the vagus nerve in the posterior cranial fossa. Usually the stridor disappears after insertion of a shunt or following occipital craniectomy.

Occipital encephalocele is very commonly associated with other abnormalities such as Klippel–Feil syndrome (webbing of the neck and cervical vertebral synostosis), micrognathia and cleft palate. Such patients may be very difficult to intubate. If the neural damage is very extensive and possibly involving autonomic functions in the midbrain, surgery is usually withheld.

Surgery involves excision of the sac and preservation of the neural elements, then closure of the defect with fascial flaps and skin coverage. In the past, a very large defect needed a rotation flap of skin for cover.

Preoperatively the lesion is covered with sterile gauze, blood is cross-matched and atropine and vitamin K (1 mg) are given as premedication. Intubation is performed using a reinforced tube with the patient on his side to minimize damage

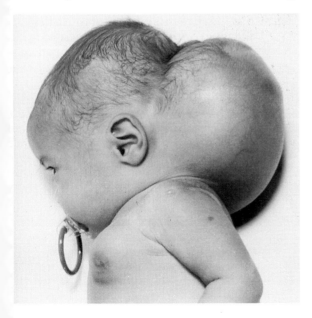

Fig. 4.14 A newborn baby with a large encephalocele.

to the myelomeningocele or encephalocele. An assistant presses the shoulders back and supports the head in an optimum position for laryngoscopy. An alternative is to support the baby's back on a 'head ring' to protect the lesion from pressure while the baby is intubated in the usual supine position. It is wise not to lubricate the outside of the tracheal tube because fixation becomes insecure as no tape will stick to it. It should be checked that air entry is bilateral with any position of the head.

For surgery, the infant is positioned prone, usually with pads supporting the chest and pelvis so that the abdomen remains free from external pressure and inferior vena caval obstruction is avoided. Any venous obstruction will greatly increase bleeding from the wound. When the patient is in the prone position, care must be taken to protect the eyes, which should be taped shut after chloramphenicol eye ointment has been inserted. In certain conditions such as gross hydrocephalus or hypertelorism, the eyes may be very difficult to close and tarsorrhaphy is occasionally necessary.

Anaesthesia is usually maintained with oxygen, nitrous oxide and isoflurane up to 0.5 per cent with relaxants and controlled ventilation. Controlled ventilation is especially necessary for neonates operated on in the prone position with pressure on the chest. The vital signs are monitored using an oesophageal stethoscope, ECG, blood pressure cuff and rectal temperature probe.

Maintenance of body temperature, which is so important in paediatric anaesthesia, is very difficult indeed in neurosurgery. Surgeons should be discouraged from using cold, wet drapes. The limbs and trunk must be wrapped in foil and as much contact as possible obtained between the baby and the heating pad. It is possible to put the support pads beneath the heating pad rather than between it and the baby. With most cases of occipital encephalocele some temperature fall during surgery is inevitable.

A further difficulty is encountered over the measurement of blood loss, as this is mixed with unknown quantities of CSF and saline used for irrigation. The need for transfusion is assessed not only by estimation of blood loss but also by changes in the patient's vital signs, including the state of the peripheral circulation, pulse rate and blood pressure. As a rule, blood is needed for encephalocele but not for myelomeningocele. In infants the suboccipital bone is very vascular. Surgery for occipital encephalocele involves a risk of air embolism because the suboccipital bones are exposed. Careful monitoring with an oesophageal stethoscope and ECG should give warning of this potentially disastrous complication. The surgeons may also be in a position to warn the anaesthetist. Venous distension, to discourage the passage of the air into the heart, is then possible by applying pressure to the reservoir bag of the anaesthetic T-piece. Early warning of air embolism using a capnometer is now feasible in the newborn, using a neonatal cuvette (Hewlett-Packard).

For spinal surgery in cases of diastematomyelia the general anaesthesia principles described for excision of myelomeningocele also apply. Blood loss may be expected to exceed 10 per cent of the blood volume and this must be replaced. Careful positioning of the chest and pelvis on pads will minimize venous bleeding from the edges of vertebrae. Occasionally lesions of the skin or subcutaneous tissues are haemangiomatous, so an increased blood loss is to be expected. If the lesion is greater than 4 cm in diameter, the need for transfusion is inevitable.

Hydrocephalus

A large proportion of neurosurgery in the neonate is carried out for hydrocephalus. The abnormal accumulation of CSF within the head is usually obstructive due to blockage of the fluid pathway. Communicating hydrocephalus with an open CSF pathway into the subarachnoid space may occur after meningitis. Non-communicating hydrocephalus is due to obstruction of the fluid pathway proximal to the subarachnoid space, such as aqueduct stenosis, or Arnold–Chiari syndrome.

Hydrocephalus is very commonly associated with myelomeningocele. The combined defect is present in 3 per 1000 live births. The excess CSF causes rapid dilatation of the ventricles, destroying the brain and producing enlargement of the cranium. The earliest sign is one of increasing head circumference, which is routinely measured in all babies following operation for myelomeningocele. Bulging fontanelle, the 'setting-sun' sign of the eyes and increased spasticity of the limbs are all later signs. Papilloedema is rare because of the capacity for the infant skull to enlarge. About 10 per cent of these children will grow up to be very retarded, both physically and mentally.

Surgical treatment involves the use of a low-pressure valve draining CSF from the ventricle to the right atrium, to the pleural cavity or to the peritoneum for cases of non-commnunicating hydrocephalus. For communicating hydrocephalus a shunt is inserted from the lumbar subarachnoid space to the peritoneum. If the CSF is infected, surgery must be delayed because the valve will become colonized.

The most important neonatal sign of raised intracranial pressure is the tendency to apnoeic attacks; patients may need to be intubated, ventilated and a ventricular tap performed. Cardiovascular signs such as bradycardia are also indicative of raised ICP.

Preterm babies frequently develop hydrocephalus following intraventricular cerebral haemorrhage in the early days of life. Because the CSF protein is high a ventriculoperitoneal shunt may not work well, frequently becoming blocked. These small babies are better managed with intermittent tapping of the ventricle or insertion of a percutaneous Teflon cannula until the CSF protein, and thus the viscosity, is back to normal. Many of these patients are a poor risk, having residual respiratory problems such as apnoeic attacks or residual oxygen dependency and reduced lung compliance from bronchopulmonary dysplasia. Occasionally a baby may be recovering from necrotizing enterocolitis in which case a Rickham cap is inserted for ease of tapping the ventricles when required or a ventriculoatrial shunt is inserted. The risk of infection increases enormously if tapping is performed too often.

Premedication is with atropine and, after preoxygenation, intubation is performed with a flexible tube. Difficulties with intubation associated with a very large head may be avoided if the patient's

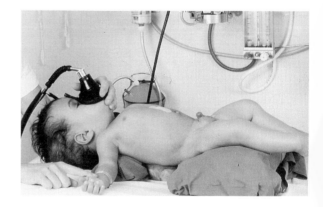

Fig. 4.15 Intubating position for a baby with severe hydrocephalus. (Reproduced with permission from [27].)

trunk is placed on a pillow so that the head is in neutral position. Controlled ventilation is established, preferably using a relaxant/nitrous oxide/oxygen technique and the baby is monitored with oesophageal stethoscope, ECG and blood pressure cuff. Because of the relatively very large head with its disproportionate radiating surface, temperature maintenance may be difficult.

Cardiovascular instability may occur at any time and is related to changes in ICP, especially hypotension at the time of CSF tap if the ICP and systemic blood pressure were previously raised. It is necessary to ventilate the patient with 100 per cent oxygen at this stage. The shunt most commonly used nowadays is the ventriculoperitoneal shunt. If ventriculoatrial shunts are employed, they are usually inserted under screening X-ray control so that the distal catheter is seen to lie in the right atrium.

At the moment that the internal jugular vein is opened for insertion of the catheter, positive pressure on the reservoir bag of the T-piece will raise the venous pressure and prevent air embolism. Many neurosurgeons infiltrate the surgical field with local anaesthetic and the maximum dose of 3 mg.kg^{-1} of lignocaine should not be exceeded. The patient should be wide awake before extubation and be returned to the intensive care unit for neurological assessment postoperatively. Although blood is always cross-matched for this operation, it is very rarely used.

Postoperatively phenobarbitone 1 mg.kg^{-1} 6-hourly i.m. can be given to babies irritable from cerebral causes such as residual intracranial blood.

For newborns simple analgesics such as paracetamol 10–15 mg.kg^{-1} orally or rectally are usually sufficient since very often the surgical field may lie in an insensitive area. For very vigorous babies codeine phosphate 1 mg.kg^{-1} i.m. can be given.

Other conditions

Other neurosurgical conditions in the neonate include intracranial haematomas and craniosynostosis (premature fusion of the cranial sutures, leading to deformities and mental retardation). Massive blood loss may be a feature of these operations, although anaesthesia follows the general pattern of that for neurosurgery in the neonate. Blood loss may be particularly large with craniectomy for craniosynostosis, and direct measurement of arterial pressure is useful so that the systolic blood pressure can be reduced to the range 50–60 mmHg using an increased isoflurane concentration and controlled ventilation. Induced hypotension with, for example, labetalol and/or sodium nitroprusside is not necessary in the neonate. After craniectomy, babies may lose at least 10 per cent of the blood volume into a drain or into the head bandages.

Surgery in the sitting position is very rare indeed in the neonatal period, although it is widely used for posterior fossa exploration and cervical surgery in the older child. However, the neonatal anaesthetist must be aware of the dangers of air embolism in any neurosurgical procedure where the head may be higher than the trunk.

Congenital lobar emphysema

Although rare, this condition may present as a cause of serious respiratory distress in the newborn period. The emphysematous lobe, which is commonly the left upper, right upper or right middle lobe, compresses the normal lung tissue and may displace the mediastinum (Fig. 4.16).

The aetiology was unknown in over half the cases reported in the literature. The condition can be caused by extrinsic bronchial obstruction from lymph nodes or abnormal vessels as in the absent pulmonary valve syndrome, or intrinsic obstruction associated with bronchial stenosis or cartilaginous

deficiency. It can present from birth to six months or so of age and the differential diagnosis includes congenital lung cyst, pneumothorax, diaphragmatic hernia and bronchial obstruction with compensatory emphysema as with inhaled foreign body. The presence of bronchial and vascular markings should help to differentiate the first two of these conditions from lobar emphysema. Chest radiographs show overdistension of one lobe which often herniates across the midline. The diaphragm on the affected side is flattened and the adjacent lobes may be compressed. As with congenital cystic adenomatous

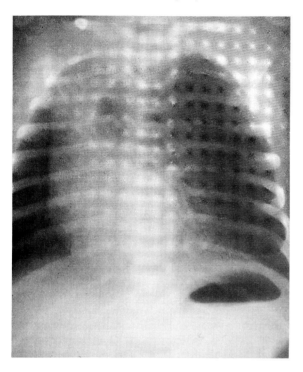

Fig. 4.16 Congenital lobar emphysema. X-ray showing mediastinal displacement to the right.

malformation, initial films may show a more solid homogeneous pattern associated with retained lung fluid. Serial radiographs show clearing of the fluid and reveal the radiolucent lobes. Prior to considering surgery, acquired lobar emphysema secondary to mucous plugs and mechanical ventilation must be excluded, if necessary by bronchoscopy. Lung cysts occasionally occur in isolation (Fig. 4:17)

Associated anomalies

The condition is frequently associated with congenital heart disease, particularly ventricular septal defect or patent ductus arteriosus. The relationship to absent pulmonary valve syndrome has been mentioned above.

Anaesthetic management

These children may present either for bronchoscopy or for lobectomy, although bronchoscopy is not usually indicated and is dangerous in the presence of intrapleural tension problems. The only safe way of performing bronchoscopy is with spontaneous ventilation and the bronchoscope should be passed under fairly deep anaesthesia, usually with halothane. The laryngeal inlet and upper trachea can be sprayed with lignocaine to a maximum dose of 4 mg.kg^{-1}. If the surgeon decides to proceed to lobectomy, the bronchoscope should be removed and a tracheal tube inserted.

The air in the emphysematous lobe may be under tension, and the presence of nitrous oxide can increase its volume significantly. Care should be taken with controlled ventilation because of the risk of making the emphysematous lobe even more distended or producing pneumothorax; only gentle ventilation is applied. However, once the chest is opened it is essential that controlled ventilation be performed and this is best carried out with full muscle relaxation. Cullum *et al.*[28] (1973) have described a technique for bronchial intubation in this condition but this is not usually required. It may be necessary to leave the tracheal tube in

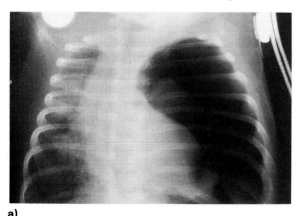

a)

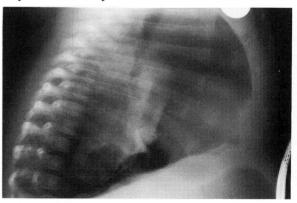

b)

Fig. 4.17 Lung cyst. (a) AP. (b) Lateral X-ray of the chest showing a left tension pneumothorax and collapse of the left lung.

place postoperatively, but if it is to be removed, this should not be done until the patient is fully awake.

Postoperative care

Usually these babies have a dramatic improvement in respiratory function postoperatively and respiratory support is not usually necessary. The infant should be nursed in an oxygen enriched environment using a head box and a postoperative chest X-ray should be taken to confirm adequate expansion of the remaining areas of lung.

Since this condition is sometimes associated with generalized chondromalacia of the bronchial walls, it is not unusual for further lobes to become emphysematous fairly soon after the operation. New alveoli continue to develop until about seven years of age, so the long-term outlook in terms of respiratory function may not be as poor as it first appears.

Congenital diaphragmatic hernia

Congenital diaphragmatic hernia (CDH) is a rare but serious emergency in the newborn period, with an incidence of approximately 1 in 4000 live births, although in terms of perinatal mortality this may be closer to 1 in 2000 as some continue to occur as stillbirths.

The condition is readily diagnosed by antenatal ultrasonography early in pregnancy which could allow the possibility of open fetal surgery,[29] but also may account for the dramatic fall in numbers of these cases seen in some centres if early termination of pregnancy is offered to the parents.

There are several types of anomaly, the commonest (about 80 per cent) occurring through a posterolateral defect in the left side of the diaphragm at the foramen of Bochdalek. Failure of fusion of the pleuroperitoneal folds and septum transversum by the 12th week of fetal life or premature return of the intestines from their extracoelomic position to the abdominal cavity allows the posterior portion of the dividing membrane to stay open. Closing of the right side is usually completed before the left, which may explain the greater incidence of left-sided hernia. The hernia usually consists of the whole of the midgut and may include the stomach, part of the descending colon, the left kidney, the spleen and the left lobe of the liver. The midgut fills with air soon after birth – usually at the time of the first feed – causing further displacement of the mediastinum to the right and compression of the right lung (Fig. 4.18).

The onset of respiratory distress depends largely on the degree of pulmonary hypoplasia present, which is usually bilateral, since the development of the contralateral lung is hindered by shift of the mediastinum in fetal life.[30] Mortality of up to 50 per cent is confined to that group of babies who develop severe respiratory distress within the first four hours of life. At postmortem the lung

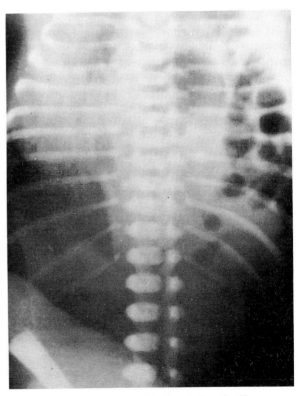

Fig. 4.18 Left-sided diaphragmatic hernia. X-ray showing gross mediastinal displacement caused by gas-filled intestine in the left hemithorax.

weights on the affected side may be found to be as low as 2 gm compared with a normal individual lung weight of from 17–35 gm in term babies. Survival is unlikely if the combined lung weights are less than 50 per cent of normal. Babies dying of CDH do have hypoplastic lungs in terms of weight and branching of bronchial generations, the distal airways being the greatest affected. The cell types, however, are normal for the gestation of the fetus. Together with this is a decreased pulmonary vascular bed causing an increased pulmonary vascular resistance. Increase in the muscular content of the media of the arterioles predisposes to the development of transitional circulation (persistent pulmonary hypertension of the newborn) in these patients. In some babies, congenital diaphragmatic hernia causes little respiratory embarrassment and occasionally the diagnosis is not made until early childhood or even later. These children presumably have little or no pulmonary hypoplasia.

The reason why some cases of diaphragmatic hernia have severe pulmonary hypoplasia and others apparently very little is not clear. Work in animals suggests that it depends upon the gestational age at which herniation of the intestinal contents into the chest actually occurs (Fig. 4.19). If lung maturation is arrested by the herniation, it is clear that when this occurs early in intrauterine life there is a greater chance of pulmonary hypoplasia than when it occurs later. Another point of view suggests that the failure of lung development is the primary defect and that

subsequent space in the chest is filled by abdominal contents before the diaphragm fuses.

Associated anomalies

The problem of associated pulmonary hypoplasia is discussed above. Other lung anomalies such as sequestrated pulmonary lobes may also occur. The commonest anomalies associated with diaphragmatic hernia are intestinal, and malrotation of the gut is almost a universal finding. Congenital heart disease and renal anomalies are less common, as are chromosomal anomalies.

Diagnosis

Increasingly, CDH is diagnosed in fetal life by ultrasound, although the condition should be suspected in any case of respiratory distress occurring soon after birth. Examination of the chest may reveal reduced movement and reduced breath sounds on the affected side, dullness to percussion, mediastinal displacement and a scaphoid abdomen (Fig. 4.20).

A straight X-ray will usually confirm the diagnosis, although this can occasionally be confused with congenital pulmonary lobar emphysema. Passage of a nasogastric tube will usually resolve any diagnostic uncertainty.

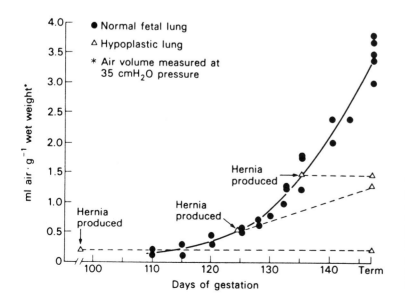

Fig. 4.19 Air capacity of lungs of lambs at gestational ages 100–147 days. The lungs of lambs with diaphragmatic hernia had air capacities equivalent to lungs at the gestational age at which the hernia was produced. (Reproduced with permission from [30].)

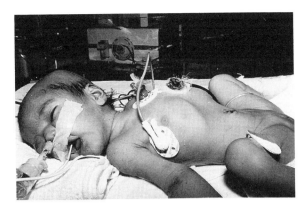

Fig. 4.20 Scaphoid abdomen typical of diaphragmatic hernia.

Management

The early onset of respiratory distress with severe hypoxia demands urgent treatment, usually by tracheal intubation and careful ventilation; deflation of the stomach via a large nasogastric tube keeps the stomach and intestines from distending in the chest. This, together with venous access should precede transfer of the infant to a regional centre for neonatal surgery. The lungs should not be inflated with a face mask because this will increase the amount of air passing into the stomach and intestines, increase mediastinal displacement and predispose to pneumothorax. The hypoplastic lungs always rupture before they are fully expanded, usually in areas of more normal lung development and frequently on the contralateral side.

Many centres have proposed that prolonged medical stabilization with delayed repair of the diaphragmatic hernia may improve survival.[31] Lung compliance is not only worsened by immediate surgery, it is very slow to improve postoperatively.[32]

The overriding aim of treatment for those presenting early with symptoms is the achievement and then maintenance of cardiopulmonary stability with direct monitoring of arterial pressure, preferably from the right radial artery (preductal blood) and right atrial pressure via right internal jugular vein. Mechanical ventilation with 100 per cent oxygen and moderately high inspiratory pressures (up to 40 cmH$_2$O) are employed using pancuronium 0.1 mg.kg^{-1} intravenously or vecuronium infusion 1–2 μg.kg^{-1}.min with fentanyl 2–5 μg.kg^{-1}.hr or morphine 20 μg.kg^{-1}.hr. Postductal PO$_2$ can be

estimated using a transcutaneous electrode over the lower half of the body. If surgery is to be delayed the gut is kept deflated via a large nasogastric tube and a stable cardiopulmonary state is of the greatest importance.

Bohn [33] has been able to predict outcome with conventional treatment accurately by using ventilatory parameters and plotting PaCO$_2$ against ventilation index (= ventilatory rate × mean airway pressure) based on a single measurement taken two hours postoperatively. A further predictor which is commonly used is the best postductal PO$_2$ and survival seems to be unlikely if this is much below 100 mmHg.[34] Certainly, the prognosis is poor if the A–aDO$_2$ exceeds 70 kPa (500 mmHg), if the arterial pH is less than 7.0 and if it is not possible to achieve a PaCO$_2$ below 5.5 kPa (40 mmHg) even with maximal ventilation. Many of the patients in the early presenting group will remain hypoxic postoperatively despite mechanical ventilation with high FiO$_2$ because of the degree of pulmonary hypoplasia. Other discouraging signs are the need for high inflation pressure (greater than 40 cm H$_2$O), CO$_2$ retention and progressive metabolic acidosis. The mortality in this group is as high as 50 per cent because the degree of pulmonary hypoplasia may be incompatible with life, so that no amount of intensive care will save the child. In addition to these patients, approximately 15 per cent develop signs of transitional circulation within 48 hours, usually with evidence of right-to-left shunting through the ductus (difference between pre- and postductal PaO$_2$) but also at atrial level which may be demonstrated by contrast echocardiography. Echocardiography can be used to monitor the pulmonary artery pressure and determine whether ductal flow changes from R-L to L-R, at which time the surgical repair could take place.

Transitional circulation is so common an event in CDH because the pulmonary vascular bed is reduced and the small pulmonary vessels remain unusually active because of failure of the smooth muscle of the media to regress in the normal way after birth and thus vasoconstrict readily in response to acidosis, hypercarbia and hypoxaemia or to a sympathetic stimulus. Most patients who develop transitional circulation will die with critical hypoxaemia unless attempts are made to reduce the reversible component of the pulmonary vascular resistance. The pH should be normal or greater than 7.4 and hyperventilation is usually impossible in these patients because of low lung compliance.

Many drugs have been used to reverse this situation – chlorpromazine, nitroprusside, phentolamine and phenoxybenzamine – but until recently tolazoline was undoubtedly the most specific agent for this purpose. Animal work has shown that this drug, although an α-adrenergic blocking agent, has its main action as a histaminergic agonist acting at H_2 receptors. This is the main action also in man as shown by the extraordinary 'lobster' red colour of the peripheries, by lack of response if histamine stores are already depleted by drugs such as morphine or curare, and by the effect on the secretion of gastric acid to cause mucosal erosions or hypochloraemic alkalosis. Tolazoline should be given to those patients with evidence of transitional circulation, but in practice it is also given to those patients who arrive deeply cyanosed and continue to be so in spite of normal resuscitative measures. Tolazoline may be given, cautiously, as a bolus of 1–2 mg.kg^{-1} followed by an infusion of 1–2 mg.kg^{-1}.h, with close monitoring of central venous pressure, as volume (blood or plasma) may be needed. The arterial pressure should also be closely watched, as these patients may need inotropic support, either dopamine 5–10 μg.kg^{-1}.min or a similar dose of dobutamine, as dopamine is thought to have a pulmonary vasoconstrictive action in infants.

If cardiac output and thus renal blood flow are maintained, renal failure is avoided. Gastric bleeding is avoided by instillation of antacid, such as magnesium trisilicate mixture, down the nasogastric tube. As with inotropes, weaning from tolazoline should be done very slowly, and only after the circulation has been stable for at least 24 hours (Fig. 4.21).

Tolazoline will act as a predictor of outcome because if there is no response then the mortality is 100 per cent whereas the mortality in the group that does respond is approximately 25 per cent.

Many centres are now using concentrations of up to 40 ppm of nitric oxide (NO) in the inspired gases to reverse the pulmonary hypertension seen with this condition.[35] NO, which has been identified as the endothelium-derived relaxing factor,[36] is the locally active principle of the nitrovasodilators, nitroprusside and nitroglycerine. NO is a selective pulmonary vasodilator because its half-life is extremely short, being immediately inactivated by haemoglobin.[37] The dramatic effect of NO on pulmonary vascular resistance was first seen in experimental animals and is now in use clinically in many centres (see p. 23). Attempts should be made to keep PaO_2 between 8 and 10.7 kPa (60–80 mmHg) and $PaCO_2$ as near to 5.3 kPa (40 mmHg) without excessive inflation pressure as hypoplastic lungs are especially prone to developing bronchopulmonary dysplasia. Weaning from the ventilator may be prolonged in severe cases and tachypnoea may persist for several weeks.

Extracorporeal membrane oxygenation (ECMO) is now widely practised in centres around the world for newborns with severe respiratory failure. Whether ECMO will make a great difference to the survival in babies with CDH is controversial and difficult to determine.[38,39] If available it should probably be reserved for those babies with initially good gas exchange with a 'honeymoon' period, but who later lapse and become unresponsive to pulmonary vasodilators. Even with the most advanced treatments, short of lung transplantation up to 50 per cent of those babies presenting immediately at birth die from pulmonary hypoplasia with or without persistent pulmonary hypertension.

Surgery

The surgical correction is via a laparotomy because of the associated malrotation of the bowel and

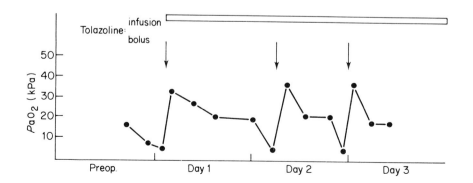

Fig. 4.21 Changes in PaO_2 as tolazoline reverses rises in pulmonary vascular resistance.

anaesthesia may comprise relaxant, high FiO_2 if necessary and supplementation with fentanyl. Because of the pulmonary hypoplasia, great care should be taken not to use excessive pressures when ventilating the lungs as these may cause pneumothorax. If possible, inflating pressures should be kept below 25–30 cmH_2O, using hand ventilation. The possibility of a pneumothorax on the contralateral side should always be borne in mind and drainage of the pleural cavity should always be considered if the baby's condition suddenly deteriorates. No attempt should be made to expand the ipsilateral lung at the end of the procedure, as this will invariably cause a pneumothorax. The monitoring of ECG, arterial pressure, nasopharyngeal temperature and $TcPO_2$ should be continued throughout the operation. The use of a precordial stethoscope may be impracticable if there is severe mediastinal shift and may interfere with the surgical field.

There is no agreement on the best arrangement for the chest drain. Some surgeons do not put one in but balance the mediastinum by putting a scalp vein needle into the left chest and allowing air to escape underwater – the needle is then removed. Another possibility is to put a chest drain into the left side but to clamp it and unclamp every eight hours to maintain stability of the mediastinum. Whatever the arrangement, the possibility of pneumothorax must always be borne in mind.

For babies not in the early presenting group, postoperative respiratory support should be given to those with symptoms within 24 hours of birth. Older babies who have not required preoperative respiratory support and who are breathing satisfactorily at the end of surgery may be extubated, but it is wise to return all babies to the ward breathing an oxygen-enriched mixture.

Pancreatectomy

Hyperinsulinism in the newborn causes increased glucose utilization and persistent hypoglycaemia extending beyond the first few days of life. Even moderate hypoglycaemia may result in neurological damage (less than 2.6 mmol.l^{-1})[40] and profound, prolonged hypoglycaemia will cause severe brain damage. A rise in plasma dextrose levels exceeding 1.6 mmol.l^{-1} (30 mg.dl^{-1}) following injection of glucagon (30 μg.kg^{-1}) is diagnostic of hyperinsulinism, as is the requirement for at least 10 mg.kg^{-1}.min dextrose infusion to maintain a normal blood sugar. Until surgery is performed treatment is with hypertonic dextrose infusions and diazoxide to a maximum of 20 mg.kg^{-1} per day. Concentrated dextrose must be given via a central vein. Hyperinsulinism may come from a functional defect in insulin secretion or from a diffuse pattern of β-cell hyperplasia known as 'nesidioblastosis' or

a focal adenoma.[41,42]

Surgical treatment for babies with refractory hypoglycaemia consists of subtotal pancreatectomy. The babies are often obese and have poor peripheral venous access. At least one central venous line is necessary, one for continuous infusion of hypertonic dextrose solutions and the other for very frequent sampling for estimation of blood sugar. Acute hypoglycaemia followed by hyperglycaemia may occur intraoperatively.

Epidural analgesia as an adjunct to general anaesthesia is very satisfactory. This can be as a 'one shot' technique or a catheter can be inserted and local anaesthetic agent infused to provide prolonged postoperative analgesia as well.

The postoperative course is often complicated with instability of blood sugar levels which requires very close monitoring.

Anaesthesia in patients with cardiac disease

The history, presentation and pathophysiology of congenital cardiac disease are discussed in Chapter 1. Anaesthesia and intensive care for infants with cardiac disease, whether for palliative or corrective cardiac surgery or for intercurrent disease, require a sound knowledge of the particular pathophysical process. The worldwide incidence of major congenital heart disease is estimated at 8 per 1000 live births. Without treatment, approximately 50 per cent of these children will die in the first year of life, one third of the deaths occurring in the first three months of life. Neonates with congenital heart disease may present as emergencies because of the effects of the cardiac anomaly itself, because of the effects of prematurity or because of the presence of other major congenital abnormalities. Of the coincident defects, renal abnormalities are the most common, although cleft palate, tracheo-oesophageal fistula, abdominal malformations and other defects also occur. In most cases no specific cause for congeni-

tal heart disease can be identified, but congenital rubella infection and fetal alcohol syndrome are known to be causative agents. 30–40 per cent of children with Down's syndrome (trisomy 21) have heart disease, mainly endocardial cushions defects (AVSD) and other chromosomal defects are also associated with different cardiac lesions.[43]

Ventricular septal defect is the commonest congenital cardiac anomaly, with an incidence of 2 per 1000 live births, although at least three-quarters of these defects will close spontaneously. Patent ductus arteriosus, pulmonary stenosis and atrial septal defect have incidences of 0.5–0.7 per 1000 live births. Transposition of the great arteries (TGA), although the commonest cardiac anomaly

Table 4.3 The incidence of treatment of congenital heart disease

Disease	Incidence	Treatment
Patent ductus arteriosus (PDA)	10–15%	Newborn – trial of indomethacin ligation or clipping Older – ligation
Ventricular septal defect (VSD)	10–20%	Closure on bypass
Atrial septal defect (ASD) (secundum)	5–15%	Closure on bypass
Atrial septal defect (ASD) (primum)	1–3%	Closure on bypass
Atrioventricular septal defect (AVSD)		Closure on bypass
Total anomalous pulmonary venous drainage (TAPVD)	1–2%	Immediate repair on bypass
Pulmonary stenosis (PS) (valvular)	5–10%	Newborn – valvotomy; inflow occlusion Older – valvotomy on bypass
Coarctation of aorta	2–5%	Subclavian angioplasty or resection
Aortic arch anomalies	0.5–1%	
Persistent truncus arteriosus	1–2%	Correction with conduit right ventricle to pulmonary artery (RV–PA)
Aortic stenosis (all types)	3–5%	Newborn – valvotomy; inflow occlusion Older – Konno on bypass
Tetralogy of Fallot	5–10%	Correction on bypass Blalock shunt; correction later
Pulmonary atresia + VSD	1%	Blalock shunt
Tricuspid atresia (TA)	1–3%	Blalock shunt; Fontan later
Transposition of great ateries (TGA)	5–15%	Rashkind septostomy Arterial switch on bypass Older – Senning on bypass
Corrected TGA (CTGA)	below 1%	
Univentricular heart (UVH)	1–2%	Banding of pulmonary artery
Ebstein's anomaly	below 1%	Tricuspid valve replacement ASD closure on bypass
Hypoplastic left heart syndrome	1–2%	Norwood on bypass

to cause cyanosis in the newborn, is an even rarer lesion, having a similar incidence to aortic stenosis, coarctation of the aorta and Fallot's tetralogy (0.3 per 1000 live births). Total anomalous pulmonary venous drainage, although having an incidence of only 0.1 per 1000 live births, is an extremely serious lesion in the newborn, often requiring emergency surgery because of severe hypoxia and congestive cardiac failure.

Although open heart operations in the first month of life are still associated with a higher overall mortality than in older infants and children, two points must be borne in mind. First, these operations are carried out on sick babies who would all certainly die without treatment. Secondly, many of the babies have complex, multiple lesions. If these are excluded, the mortality of the remainder is seen to be considerably lower. The exception to this is the 'arterial switch' operation performed for TGA in the first days of life where there is a very low operative mortality.

Congenital cardiac anomalies in the newborn can be classified into four basic functional categories, each of which poses distinct problems for anaesthesia:

1. Patients with *increased pulmonary blood flow*, including PDA, VSD, aortopulmonary window, truncus arteriosus and total anomalous pulmonary venous corrections (TAPVD). Respiratory failure is common because of pulmonary oedema, reduced pulmonary compliance and increased work of breathing. Untreated babies will fail to thrive and may die in cardiac failure or at a later stage develop pulmonary vascular disease. A fall in peripheral resistance, as may occur with induction of anaesthesia is not well tolerated when the pulmonary vascular resistance is high. Prolonged diuretic therapy may make this situation more likely as the blood volume may be depleted and hypotension occurs more easily.

2. Patients with *low pulmonary blood flow* causing cyanosis including Fallot's tetralogy, pulmonary stenosis, pulmonary atresia or tricuspid atresia. Cyanotic patients make a number of adaptations to compensate for reduced oxygen delivery to the tissues. The oxygen dissociation curve is shifted to the right to allow improved unloading of oxygen to the tissues, a shift caused by a mild persistent metabolic acidosis and a rise in level of 2,3-diphosphoglycerate

in red cells. There is a gradual enlargement of the systemic venous bed and increased blood volume with collateral formation, eventually causing clubbing. The oxygen carrying capacity of the blood is increased by a rising Hb and these babies do not usually display the physiological anaemia of infancy. As the haematocrit rises, there is an increase in viscosity of the blood and impairment of perfusion of organs such as the kidneys. Cerebral thromboembolism is not uncommon especially if the infant becomes suddenly dehydrated for example with preoperative starvation, diuretic therapy or sudden diarrhoea. A further compensatory mechanism is a coagulopathy with reduced prothrombin and poor platelet function which often causes bleeding problems after bypass surgery. Blood products such as platelet-rich plasma, fresh frozen plasma and cryoprecipitate should be available for any surgical procedure.

Babies with Fallot's tetralogy may not be cyanosed immediately after birth, but may later develop cyanotic attacks which are sometimes very severe (hypercyanotic) if systemic resistance is reduced or right ventricular outflow tract resistance rises.

Attacks can occur during crying or feeding but are commonly associated with cardiac catheterization or the pre-bypass phase of surgery, particularly induction of anaesthesia. The squatting which is so characteristic of the Fallot is an attempt to minimize right-to-left shunting by increasing peripheral resistance. Attacks can be controlled with β-blockade (e.g. propranolol) which is usually discontinued before surgery because of its myocardial depressant effect after bypass. Hypercyanotic attacks require urgent treatment, including sedation with morphine (0.2 mg.kg^{-1}), oxygen, sodium bicarbonate (1 mmol.kg^{-1}), propranolol (0.2 mg.kg^{-1}) and an infusion of noradrenaline. Noradrenaline (dose range $0.01–0.5 \ \mu\text{g.kg.}^{-1}\text{min}$, $30 \ \mu\text{g.kg}^{-1}$ in 50 ml 5 per cent dextrose at 5 ml.h^{-1} intravenously equals $0.05 \ \mu\text{g.kg.}^{-1}\text{min}$) is the drug of first choice for attacks occurring during surgery. Surgery becomes more urgent as the combination of systemic hypotension, hypoxaemia and acidosis may be rapidly fatal. Mechanical ventilation may further decrease pulmonary blood flow especially if more than minimal distending pressure is used.

Patients with *cardiac failure* may have large L–R shunts, valve atresias, mitral or aortic valve disease such as hypoplastic left heart syndrome or obstructed TAPVD. Babies with left ventricular tract obstruction, for example with preductal coarctation of the aorta, have a low cardiac output with myocardial ischaemia.

3. Patients presenting with symptoms early in life often have very poor cardiac function and may require considerable preoperative support – mechanical ventilation, prostaglandins, inotropes, vasodilators, renal dialysis, etc.; however, surgery should not be delayed too long.

4. Transposition of the great vessels, which may be complicated by PDA and ventricular septal defect (VSD) produces a combination of cyanosis and increased pulmonary blood flow. An arterial 'switch' operation is performed in the early days of life for 'simple' transposition before the pulmonary vascular resistance falls and the left ventricle can no longer support the systemic vascular resistance. If there is a VSD as well, the operation can be delayed, for example for the baby to gain weight, but not so long that increases in pulmonary vascular resistance occur. The combination of cyanosis and high pulmonary blood flow causes early onset of irreversible pulmonary vascular changes. If the anatomy of the coronary arteries is unsuitable for a 'switch' operation, the alternative is to perform an atrial direction of flow during the first year of life (Senning operation).[44] A Rashkinds balloon septostomy is always required soon after diagnosis to increase mixing of blood at atrial level, but even with good mixing the mortality without correction by two years of age approaches 50 per cent.

Preoperative management

Babies in cardiac failure usually develop severe hypoxaemia and acidosis, often complicated by hypoglycaemia or hypocalcaemia. Immediate assessment should include measurement of blood sugar, calcium and electrolyte levels, and arterial blood gas and acid-base analysis. Dextrose 50 per cent should be given intravenously: (0.2 ml.kg^{-1}) if the blood sugar falls below 2 mmol.l^{-1} in a term neonate or 1.5 mmol.l^{-1} in a premature neonate. If the serum calcium is less than 2.0 mmol.l^{-1}, intravenous 20 per cent calcium gluconate should be given (1 ml.kg^{-1}). ECG and body temperature should be monitored and the baby nursed in a suitably warm environment.

Details of initial management are discussed in Chapter 5 but treatment very often depends on respiratory support, prostaglandin and inotropic therapy. Intensive support may be beneficial before cardiopulmonary bypass and could include total parenteral nutrition to improve myocardial glycogen stores.

Diagnostic procedures

Detailed investigations are required to make the diagnosis in most neonates with suspected congenital heart disease. Modern echocardiography has revolutionized cardiac diagnosis and often information gained from a non-invasive technique is of superior quality. Doppler echocardiography detects changes in the velocity of blood flow so that shunts and obstructions as well as cardiac output can be measured.

Cardiac catheterization is required less often, but is necessary to obtain pressures, quantitative flows and for the calculation of systemic and pulmonary resistances. Many therapeutic manoeuvres are now performed – balloon atrial septostomy; transluminal angioplasty of aortic coarctation; balloon valvuloplasty of aortic and pulmonary valves; angioplasty of stenotic pulmonary arteries, occlusion of collaterals, PDA, ASD and some small, muscular VSDs.

Simple catheter investigations in relatively fit newborns are often performed using sedation and local anaesthesia (lignocaine up to 3 mg.kg^{-1}). In centres around the UK, one third of newborns have no sedation or anaesthesia, one third have sedation and one third general anaesthesia (Table 4.4). In addition, diazepam 0.1 mg.kg^{-1} may be injected

Table 4.4 Sedation for cardiac catheters in newborns

These investigations may be performed under basal sedation supplemented, if required, by i.v. diazepam (0.1–0.2 mg.kg^{-1}). *No atropine.*

Newborns	May have pethidine compound injection up to 0.05 ml.kg^{-1} i.m. 30 mins pre-catheter.
Over 5 kg	Trimeprajine orally 2 mg.kg^{-1} 2–3 hours pre-catheter Pethidine compound injection 0.1 ml.kg^{-1} i.m. 30 mins pre-catheter

through the cardiac catheter if increased sedation is required. Full monitoring includes ECG, blood pressure, often by direct femoral artery puncture and pulse oximetry.

Anaesthesia is required increasingly for sick babies with severe lesions, with rhythm problems and for the large number of patients undergoing therapeutic catheterization. If general anaesthesia is considered essential, tracheal intubation should be performed and a nitrous oxide/oxygen mixture administered using full muscle relaxation and controlled ventilation of the lungs. It is essential to monitor inspired oxygen concentration, as it is impossible to calculate shunts if the oxygen saturation of the venous blood is too high.

The newborn baby, if premature, is especially susceptible to heat loss and steps should be taken to prevent hypothermia. The temperature of the room should not be less than 24°C, the baby should be swathed in warm clothing and, if possible, be placed on a radiolucent heating pad. Wrapping the head and limbs in aluminium foil also helps to reduce heat loss.

In small infants, excessive amounts of blood can be removed during diagnostic sampling unless oximetry is carried out in a sterilized cuvette from which the sample can be returned to the patient. The blood volume in the neonate is approximately 85 ml.kg^{-1} body weight and loss of more than 10 per cent of this usually requires replacement. Blood should be cross-matched at the start of the procedure.

Other hazards of cardiac catheterization are rare. They include dysrhythmias from manipulation of the catheter, hypotension and occasional perforation of the heart or intramyocardial injection of contrast. Systemic hypotension may lead to increase in any right-to-left shunting and to intense hypoxia. Hypoxaemia itself may increase pulmonary vascular resistance and thus create a vicious circle of events.

The injection of contrast medium may lead to transient flushing of the skin from histamine release and, more importantly, may cause an increase in pulmonary vascular resistance with a fall in cardiac output. Angiography with its contrast load may be poorly tolerated in sick infants as the circulation has to cope with a biphasic insult – first a hyperosmolar load, then an osmotic diuresis – and isotonic fluid should be given to help offset the effect of the contrast medium.

Open heart procedures

General principles

The general principles of cardiac anaesthesia and conduct of the 'bypass' in newborns do not greatly differ from those used for older children or adults. Specific differences relate to the immaturity of all organ systems and a smaller blood volume may mean that sudden, major haemorrhage is more disastrous. Full doses of analgesia are required to reduce where possible stress responses to surgery and profound hypothermia. Systemic embolism in patients with R-L shunts such as transposition of the great arteries and ASD is a potential danger. Great care must be taken to avoid injection of air or particulate matter and cerebral, coronary and renal arteries are at particular risk from embolization.

The prevention of bacterial endocarditis is a major concern in children; antibiotic prophylaxis is routine to cover all heart surgery because transient bacteraemia asociated with intubation and vascular access is common. Routine cover is gentamicin 2 mg.kg^{-1} and flucloxacillin 25 mg.kg^{-1} i.v. at induction of anaesthesia, and again after bypass; then gentamicin 2 mg.kg^{-1} 8–hourly i.v. and flucloxacillin 12.5 mg.kg^{-1} i.v. 6-hourly for 24 hours postoperatively. For those allergic to penicillins vancomycin 20 mg.kg^{-1} is substituted – this requires infusion over one hour.

Open heart surgery in infancy has developed enormously in the last 20 years with a falling mortality. This is due to advances in equipment and techniques as well as to improved preoperative diagnosis. Better membrane oxygenators with increasingly low priming volumes are available, better intracardiac cannulae and suckers cause less red cell damage and the use of filters reduces platelet-fibrin aggregation with its embolization.

The use of deep hypothermia to 18°C with or without periods of circulatory arrest (DHCA) dramatically improved mortality and morbidity in newborns.[45] The technique allows the surgeon to carry out the intracardiac repair as a bloodless, motionless heart during periods of up to 60 minutes circulatory arrest, thus reducing time on bypass. Some surgeons prefer to keep a low flow where possible, reasoning that postoperative neuropsychological dysfunction may be lessened, but there is very little evidence for this.[46] In some centres bypass is started with very cold perfusate, disregarding the conventionally accepted maximum temperature gradients between patient and perfusate of 15°C. The use of this rapid cooling technique may improve myocardial function. The technique of surface cooling to 26–28°C prior to sternotomy is not now used by most major centres except in certain cases such as newborns with interrupted aortic arch where core cooling may be uneven. The technique is very time-consuming and allows very little control over haemodynamics at a critical period of the operation. Very little, if any, advantage can be demonstrated for surface cooling over core cooling on bypass.[47]

If surface cooling is used, icebags are packed around the baby over the major arteries after anaesthesia and insertion of all monitoring lines. Care is taken to avoid the precordium, kidneys or extremities of the limbs. Peripheral vasodilatation is promoted by adequate anaesthesia and analgesia and supplements of isoflurane are useful. As the temperature falls, CO_2 production is diminished so 2.5–5 per cent CO_2 is added to the inspired gases to maintain $PaCO_2$ over 6 kPa (45 mmHg) to improve cerebral perfusion, though cerebral blood flow and cerebral CO_2 reactivity are retained down to low levels of cerebral perfusion pressure.[48] Frequent temperature corrected blood gas analyses are essential and any severe acidosis is corrected. Cardiac stability is easily achieved during cooling if K^+ supplements are given (0.5–1 mmol) as K^+ levels fall with K^+ shifts into the cells. Crystalloid 10–20 ml.kg^{-1} i.v. helps to maintain peripheral blood flow. When the core temperature reaches 26°C active cooling is discontinued and surgery proceeds. A 2°C after drop is to be expected.

Perfusion techniques

Until recently, fresh heparinized blood was chosen to prime the bypass for neonatal surgery because of the risk of coagulation disorders following the use of stored blood and because of the metabolic alkalosis which follows the transfusion of citrated blood. Fresh blood may be difficult to obtain, especially in an emergency, but the freshest stored blood obtainable should be used. Blood which is more than four days old should not be accepted unless undue delay in obtaining fresher blood threatens the patient's life.

Haemodilution should not lower the haematocrit below 30 per cent because the neonate has difficulty in excreting a large fluid load. Haemodilution does, however, improve the flow characteristics of the perfusate, especially at low temperatures, and improves postperfusion urine flow; 20 mg heparin, 3 ml of 20 per cent calcium chloride and 80 mmol sodium bicarbonate are added to each unit of blood used in the prime. Mannitol (0.5 gm.kg^{-1}) may be added to improve urine output, and methylprednisolone sodium succinate (Solu-Medrone) (30 mg.kg^{-1}) to stabilise membranes. Some also add albumin to increase the oncotic pressure of the prime. Bypass flow rate is calculated at 2.4 l.m^{-2}·min^{-1}, although lower flows are often used during hypothermia.

Blood sugar levels are always well maintained on bypass, but require close monitoring afterwards. Up to 1 mmol.kg^{-1} of potassium is required and this may be given into the pump after cross-clamping of the aorta, to maintain a serum K^+ of at least 4.5 mmol.l^{-1}.

Anaesthetic management

Premedication

Neonates are given atropine 0.02 mg.kg^{-1} either orally or intramuscularly either alone or with an oral agent such as chloral hydrate 30 mg.kg^{-1} one hour preoperatively. EMLA cream applied over a suitable vein, e.g. on the dorsum of the hand, allows a cannula to be inserted painlessly before induction of anaesthesia. This cannula is vital for administration of fluids and any drugs required during the induction.

Before bypass

During induction of anaesthesia full indirect monitoring of ECG, BP and SaO_2 should be established. All newborns should be adequately anaesthetized for intubation of the trachea and insertion of arterial and venous lines.

It is known that halothane produces at least 50 per cent greater depression of contraction in neonatal cardiac muscle than in adult muscle so that 50 per cent of all *normal* infants develop sustained hypotension and bradycardia with halothane, partly reversed by atropine.[49] Halothane also causes loss of sinus rhythm in some children and this may be critical in infants with right–sided cardiac problems. In addition, there are potential changes in both systemic and pulmonary vascular resistances with all potent inhalational agents. Hensley *et al.*[50] found that induction with halothane, nitrous oxide and oxygen actually increased oxygen saturation in children with cyanotic congenital heart disease, particularly in those with the potential for variable pulmonary outflow tract obstruction, e.g. Fallot's tetralogy. The cause of the increased oxygen saturation is probably complex, but may relate to increasing pulmonary blood flow, increased inspired O_2 concentration in patients with R-L shunts of less than 40 per cent, a decrease in dynamic infundibular pulmonary stenosis in Fallot's tetralogy by a direct effect or a decrease in cardiac output with maintenance of pulmonary blood flow.

Murray *et al.*[51] found in children that halothane and isoflurane both decrease mean blood pressure from an awake level; both decrease cardiac index at 1.25 MAC (minimum alveolar concentration) with a significant decrease in ejection fractions. After a fluid load the ejection fraction decreased significantly with halothane but increased with isoflurane. This response to fluid may show that a greater cardiovascular reserve exists during isoflurane anaesthesia than with halothane. However, isoflurane is more irritant to the infant airway and may cause undesirable changes in myocardial blood flow.

Theoretically R-L shunts affect the speed of inhalation induction and Tanner *et al.* showed that with a 50 per cent shunt the induction was slowed only with insoluble agents such as nitrous oxide and not with a relatively soluble agent such as halothane. Where pulmonary blood flow is very limited inhalation induction may be so slow as to make its use impractical.

Intravenous induction agents are increasingly used as a venous line can be painlessly established if EMLA cream has been used. Injection should be slow in the presence of a R-L shunt as transfer to the arterial circulation is very rapid indeed affecting the brain and myocardium immediately. Thiopentone ($2–4$ mg.kg^{-1}) significantly decreases cardiac output by at least 30 per cent by reducing the availability of calcium to the muscle fibres and decreasing sympathetic output. It also causes an increased heart rate and does not attenuate the stress response to intubation. These effects are dose related and related to fast injection, but are much greater in patients with heart disease, patients who are hypovolaemic, or other poor risk infants. This is a useful agent, but must be given with great caution.

The benzodiazepines, diazepam or midazolam, are amnesic which is an advantage in older babies. They cause mild to moderate reduction in cardiac output and other unpredictable effects such as tachycardia in some, but bradycardia in others. Fentanyl with midazolam may exert a slightly more depressant effect together than when given alone, probably by reducing the normal sympathetic tone and by direct negative inotropism. Fentanyl may be used for induction by itself or together with, for example, midazolam or even thiopentone. Its tendency to cause bradycardia is offset by pancuronium so that excellent cardiovascular stability can be achieved even in sick small babies. Doses of as little as 10 μg.kg^{-1} have been shown to obtund undesirable stress responses in newborns and sick infants, particularly in the pulmonary vasculature which is so reactive at this age.

Ketamine ($1–2$ mg.kg^{-1} intravenously) may be the drug of choice for induction of small babies. It produces a non-dose-related increase in heart rate, cardiac index and in systemic and pulmonary artery pressure, increasing myocardial oxygen consumption. There are no changes in the direction of balanced shunts and oxygen saturation increases during ketamine induction in infants with cyanotic disease. Ketamine actually has a direct negative inotropic effect on the myocardium, but a centrally mediated sympathetic response overcomes this, unless noradrenaline stores have been recently depleted. There is potential for a rise in pulmonary vascular resistance, but this effect is trivial if the airway has been secured and mechanical ventilation started. This drug which is now in routine use again seems to have the fewest unsuitable side effects. Halothane is potentially dangerous at this stage in small babies where hypotension and ventricular fibrillation occur very readily, especially in those with left ventricular outflow tract obstruction.

A tracheal tube of 3.0 or 3.5 mm internal diameter is passed and either the oral or the nasal route can be used. The former is usually easier and quicker and less likely to cause hypoxia, but a nasal tube can be secured more satisfactorily for intra- and postoperative care. It is important to make sure that there is air entry to both lungs after intubation, as it is quite easy to intubate either main bronchus because of the relatively short trachea.

Pancuronium 0.1–0.2 mg.kg^{-1} is used for relaxation routinely. Central venous and arterial lines are inserted percutaneously. Two 20G cannulae are placed in the right internal jugular vein by direct puncture, one for monitoring and the other for continuous infusion of drugs. Alternatively, a double or triple lumen catheter can be placed using the Seldinger technique. Other sites for central vein catheterization include the femoral and left internal jugular veins which should be used if there is a persistent left superior vena cava or if a Glenn anastomosis is planned. Three venous cannulae are a basic requirement for open heart surgery.

Central venous pressure readings in infancy may not be reliable because the venous system has a great capacity as the liver is so distensible. Considerable volumes of fluid may be given with no rise in central venous pressure at all, though the liver has enlarged enormously. Right atrial pressure does not necessarily correspond with severity of congestive cardiac failure in small infants.

Direct monitoring of arterial pressure is via a 22 or 24G Teflon cannula inserted into a radial artery. Alternative sites include the axillary and femoral arteries, both of which last longer in the postoperative period than the radial.

In infants the technique of transfixation is likely to be more successful than a direct puncture technique. The cannula is connected to a short extension with a three-way stopcock to allow frequent sampling and is continuously flushed with heparinized saline (1 μ.ml^{-1}) using an 'Intraflow' type of device (3 ml.h^{-1}) except in very small babies when a syringe pump set to 1 ml.h^{-1} is used.

Major complications of cannulation of the radial artery are rare in children, provided a fine (22–24 gauge for neonates) cannula is used, possibly because the arterial wall is healthier or because there is a better collateral blood supply. Internal jugular and subclavian vein cannulation are not free from hazard, particularly from puncture of the carotid artery with haematoma formation or from pneumothorax. The advantages outweigh the risks involved, which may be minimized if the tip of the needle is kept well above the thoracic inlet.[53]

In patients at risk from postoperative pulmonary hypertension a 20 or 22G catheter may be passed from the internal jugular vein and allowed to coil up in the right atrium to be passed on into the pulmonary artery (PA) by the surgeon before completing the operation. The alternative is for the surgeon to implant this line directly into the heart. A urinary catheter is inserted and urine output recorded regularly.

Maintenance of anaesthesia

Oesophageal and nasopharyngeal or rectal temperatures should also be monitored, the former reflecting blood temperature and the latter core temperature. Intermittent positive pressure ventilation (IPPV) is continued with nitrous oxide/oxygen as the basic anaesthetic and pancuronium 0.1–0.15 mg.kg^{-1} for muscle relaxation. Inspired oxygen concentration should be adjusted according to the arterial oxygen tension and inspired gas should be warmed and humidified, at least in the post bypass period. Opioid supplements such as fentanyl are given, usually after a test dose, after which generous doses may be given (up to 50 μg.kg^{-1}). These fentanyl doses provide unique cardiovascular stability. Heparin 3 mg.kg^{-1} is given prior to insertion of the aortic cannula and it is wise to check the level of heparinization by ensuring that the activated coagulation time (ACT) is greater than 350 seconds. A baseline ACT is also useful information.

FiO_2 is adjusted to give a reasonable PaO_2, depending on the lesion, but 100 per cent oxygen should be used if cardiac output falls and the balance can be made up with air or nitrous oxide. Additional full doses of relaxant and opioid should be given a few minutes before the start of bypass.

Serial blood gas analyses should be made as a tendency to an increase in acidosis is common and should be corrected if the base excess is greater than 5 mmol.l^{-1} (weight/5 × ½ base deficit = ml 8.4 per cent HCO_3).

Metabolic alkalosis is associated with a low total body potassium and increments of 0.5–1 mmol K$^+$ diluted are given slowly to keep serum levels over 4 mmol.l^{-1}.

Rapid transfusion may be necessary at any time, e.g. during aortic cannulation, so equipment to pressurize the infusion should be available. Surgical manipulation always interferes with cardiac output, especially when putting in venous pursestrings and 'snuggers' for the venous tourniquets. It is now usual to begin bypass with only the superior vena cava cannula and to put the second in as soon as bypass is established. A bolus injection of $CaCl_2$ is a powerful inotropic stimulus but it should be remembered that severe bradycardia and even asystole may occur if K$^+$ is low or if myocardial oxygenation is very borderline. It is probably better to administer a small dose of 1 in 100 000 adrenaline to improve cardiac output if it does not return after surgical manipulations have ceased.

Bypass

Ventilation of the lungs continues until full flow from the bypass pump has been achieved, after which the lungs may be allowed to collapse or may be maintained slightly distended to a pressure of 3–5 cms H_2O with oxygen or air/O_2 mixture. Damage to the lungs is more likely to occur from the vascular side and blood from the left side of the heart must be vented continuously. Left to right shunts through a PDA or Blalock shunt are controlled as soon as bypass is started. Heparinization should be checked every 30 minutes using the ACT, but since relatively large amounts of heparin are added to the perfusate during priming, incremental doses of heparin are seldom required.

Myocardial function is preserved during bypass by the use of ice-cold cardioplegic solution injected into the aortic root and hence to the coronary arteries during aortic cross-clamping. The composition of the cardioplegic solution varies from centre to centre, but the common constituents are potassium, magnesium and procaine. 20–30 ml.kg^{-1} of solution are infused until the myocardial temperature has dropped to 10°C. Because the aorta is clamped and the solution is aspirated to waste via the coronary sinus, little of it enters the perfusate. Half doses of cardioplegic infusion are repeated every 30 minutes to ensure that the myocardial temperature remains below 20°C and that the heart does not commence beating. The presence of procaine may increase the incidence of atrio ventricular block in the immediate post-bypass period, but this does not seem to be of any great clinical significance.

Perfusion pressures on bypass are kept between 40 and 70 mmHg. Higher pressures are caused by peripheral vasoconstriction from either light anaesthesia or deep hypothermia. Patients at risk from postoperative pulmonary hypertensive crisis are routinely given the long-acting α-adrenergic blocking agent phenoxybenzamine 1 mg.kg^{-1}. This agent attenuates the responses of the muscularized pulmonary arterioles to stimuli such as a rising $PaCO_2$ and is given prior to bypass without serious cardiovascular effects. It may also be necessary to infuse sodium nitroprusside (5–20 $\mu g.kg^{-1}.min$) and this agent is routinely used during rewarming, but the rate of infusion must be carefully controlled, especially during periods of reduced flow in order to avoid the risk of cyanide toxicity.

At low temperatures cerebral oxygen requirements are reduced to 17 per cent of basal requirements at 18–20°C so periods of circulatory arrest of up to 60 minutes may be used as required to perform complex intracardiac procedures.

Catecholamine levels are enormously elevated after DHCA[54] but lactate and pyruvate levels are surprisingly low even after long periods of arrest. Myocardial protection is maximized by covering the heart with ice-slush and thus preventing the heart from being rewarmed by the surrounding tissues. Alternatively low flow can be maintained where possible (venous cannulae left in situ) at flow levels as low as 0.5 l.m^2.min. Uniform cooling before arrest is very important and requires all temperatures to read 17–18°C with at least 12 min of bypass. Methylprednisolone 30 mg.kg^{-1} to stabilize membranes is given before arrest and moderate haemodilution to a haematocrit of 20 is used to promote peripheral blood flow. Newborns who have difficulty in excreting a large fluid load may require ultrafiltration towards the end of or after bypass or peritoneal dialysis in the early postoperative period.[55]

Potassium levels are checked during perfusion, but 1 mmol.kg^{-1} supplement is always necessary and may be safely given into the pump after the aorta has been clamped.

Rewarming is commenced as the intracardiac repair is completed, but is started gradually with gradients not exceeding 15°C. After the aorta is unclamped a period of low flow should continue in order to minimize reperfusion injury. During rewarming heat is provided mainly by the heat exchanger, but in addition to this, heat also comes from the heating mattress which is now turned on and from heated humidified inspired gases. At this stage it is routine to infuse sodium nitroprusside to overcome the intense vasoconstriction which hypothermia induces and to allow rapid and even rewarming. Higher doses than those used postoperatively are required at this stage and a mean perfusion pressure of 35–45 mmHg is satisfactory. The infusion is stopped at 36°C. Suction is attached to the aortic needle vent as the cross-clamp is removed. Removal of every trace of air is crucial to avoid cerebral air embolism. The cardiac action should be vigorous and the lungs inflated to drive air out of the pulmonary veins; venous pressure is increased and the heart, especially the left atrial appendage is massaged. The heart begins to eject at this point and mechanical ventilation is recommended. It is also usual to position the patient in the head-down position so any ejected air bubbles do not go to the brain.

Intracardiac lines are placed in the left atrium and pulmonary artery if necessary. LA pressure readings are necessary when left ventricular or mitral valve function requires close monitoring, for example in the Fontan operation to monitor the transpulmonary gradient. These intracardiac lines have a low morbidity if placed with care.[56] It is wise to leave the chest drains in situ and to have a unit of blood cross-matched before these lines are removed in the postoperative period.

Post perfusion

When the heart ejects with increased venous pressure, bypass is withdrawn and the patient transfused via the aortic cannula to a systemic pressure of 60-80 mmHg, SVC 10-12 mmHg and LA no more than 12 mmHg. If arterial pressure remains low with high filling pressures then inotropic support is necessary, as it is essential that the heart is not left with poor myocardial perfusion pressures and poor myocardial oxygen delivery, causing increasing hypoxia and acidosis. It is acceptable to provide an intial inotropic 'kick' to the myocardium with a small bolus of 1 in 100 000 adrenaline or 10 per cent $CaCl_2$ and occasionally this is all that will be necessary. Should blood pressure be low despite adequate filling pressure, it may be necessary to commence inotropic support with dopamine, isoprenaline or, occasionally, adrenaline. Dopamine 5–10 μg.kg^{-1}.min is the drug of first choice, although isoprenaline may be added if the cardiac rate is below 100 as the cardiac output is rate-dependent in infants. Dobutamine is increasingly used as a first-line inotropic agent for neonates and infants because it has no effect on pulmonary vascular resistance. It is also logical to use both dopamine and dobutamine, the former in a low renal vasodilating dose (2–4 μg.kg^{-1}.min) and the latter in higher dosage for inotropic action without pulmonary vasoconstriction (up to 20 μg.kg^{-1}.min). The venous system is very compliant and it is dangerously easy to overload an infant with colloid without any change in CVP.

Recently ultrafiltration has been used after bypass to remove excess water and to achieve a final haematocrit of approximately 40 and incidentally greatly improved haemodynamics. The haematocrit is maintained at this level with judicious use of red cells and colloid, e.g. fresh frozen plasma, platelet rich plasma, which may also be required to achieve final haemostasis.

Protamine is given to reverse heparin in doses up to 6 mg.kg^{-1} with ACT control though very small patients may require greater doses. Heparin levels in the patient coming off bypass are often in excess of those before going on as a result of heparin added to the prime; although ACT is not specific for heparinization, it is useful to know whether the level has returned to the baseline. Protamine causes a degree of hypotension in most patients and this is occasionally profound, possibly coming from the release of histamine or other vasoactive substances by the heparin protamine moiety.[57] Vascular effects of protamine can be minimized by very slow infusion, possibly after a small test dose, into a peripheral rather than central vein or even into the left side of the heart via the LA line, although this should be done with meticulous care to avoid air embolism.

Towards the end of bypass and afterwards, urine flow should be at least 1 ml.kg^{-1}.h. Because the incidence of renal failure associated with cardiopulmonary bypass is high in the very young, attempts to minimise this should include mannitol 0.5 gm.kg^{-1} to the pump prime, low renal vasodilating doses of dopamine (3–4 μg.kg^{-1}.min) and low doses of frusemide (0.25 mg.kg^{-1}). If renal failure exists preoperatively and with major lesions a peritoneal catheter is inserted after bypass to allow either drainage of peritoneal transudate or dialysis if necessary. Failure to respond to diuretics is an indication for early dialysis.

Routine placement of temporary pacemaker wires allows either direct ventricular pacing or atrioventricular sequential pacing. Troublesome dysrhythmias are not uncommon and occur when the myocardium is under stress. Slow dysrhythmias are often easily corrected by small doses of isoprenaline. Fast dysrhythmias with an acute fall in cardiac output may be treated by DC shock or adenosine. If the change in rhythm is less catastrophic it can be treated by digoxin, β-adrenergic blockade or amiodarone 5 mg.kg^{-1} by slow i.v. infusion.[58]

Direct measurements of cardiac output are not performed as thermodilution techniques have many limitations in the infant. Indirect methods may be more useful.[59]

Many patients benefit from reduction in the left ventricular afterload, particularly in infants where vasoconstrictive compensatory mechanisms are very active. Sodium nitroprusside $1–2$ $\mu g.kg^{-1}$.min is the first choice, but nitroglycerine, which in low doses may specifically dilate venous capacitance vessels, is particularly valuable in patients with mitral valve lesions and possible coronary artery dysfunction, e.g. after the arterial 'switch' operation for transposition of the great arteries.

The arterial switch

The arterial switch operation for transposition of the great arteries is the most physiological of the surgical procedures for this congenital defect, but must be performed in the first few days of life for 'simple' TGA, before the left ventricle can no longer pump to a systemic resistance. If there is a large PDA or VSD, there is less urgency.

Pulmonary hypertension is an advantage as it allows left ventricular normality to persist which is essential for the success of the operation, but a disadvantage as a reactive pulmonary vasculature is a potential problem intra- and postoperatively.

All induction agents change cardiac output, but ketamine $1–2$ $mg.kg^{-1}$ intravenously has many favourable characteristics and is widely used, one major advantage being profound analgesia for the intubation and insertion of venous and arterial lines. The α-adrenergic blocking agent phenoxybenzamine 1 $mg.kg^{-1}$ is given before the start of bypass. This partly offsets the profound catecholamine–induced vasoconstriction with profound hypothermia, but also partially obtunds the responses of the pulmonary vasoactivity to stimuli such as a rising $PaCO_2$.

Nitroglycerine is used during rewarming on bypass as it is a more potent venodilator, promotes coronary perfusion and has some specificity for the pulmonary circulation. Dopamine is used only in doses for renal vasodilation and dobutamine is the first choice for positive inotropism. Weaning from bypass is undertaken very slowly indeed with minimal L and R filling pressures as the ventricles are already functioning at the top of the Starling curve. Ultrafiltration to a haematocrit of 40 is routine after bypass.

Aprotinin (Trasylol, Bayer), the proteinase inhibitor has a beneficial effect on the bleeding tendency after cardiac bypass, by inhibiting the contact phase of coagulation.[60] The agent is used routinely in some centres but in others is reserved for major cases or re-operations. No firm dose regimen has evolved, but 1 $ml.kg^{-1}$ as a bolus to the patient and also to the pump prime followed by 1 $ml.kg^{-1}$ per hour continuing into the postoperative period until bleeding stops has proved satisfactory.

Norwood procedure

Hypoplastic left heart syndrome (HLHS) affects up to 7 per cent of babies with congenital heart disease and is a complex of anomalies of the aorta, left ventricle and mitral valve. The condition is very frequently diagnosed antenatally and many parents are advised that termination should take place. The condition carries 100 per cent mortality without palliative treatment by heart transplantation[61] or the Norwood procedure.[62] This is a staged procedure of firstly the reconstruction of the aortic arch and a central shunt performed before three weeks of age, secondly when the baby is a few months old a bidirectional Glenn shunt (SVC to PA) and later a Fontan-type procedure with an overall survival in the very best centres of 75–80 per cent. During surgery and postoperatively for the first stage PVR must be maintained at a high level or myocardial blood flow becomes inadequate. Manoeuvres such as normo- or hypoventilation to give a $PaCO_2$ of at least 6 kPa (40 mmHg) or the addition of CO_2 to inspired gases, reduction of FiO_2, distending pressure or temporary occlusion of the right pulmonary artery may all be necessary. Drugs which increase SVR or decrease PVR should be avoided.

Closed heart procedures

Approximately one third of surgical procedures for congenital cardiac disease are performed without bypass often via a thoracotomy. The patients may be very sick and require intensive care pre- and postoperatively. Direct monitoring of arterial and central venous pressure is usual except for ligation of a PDA in an older child. Many PDAs and valve lesions can be dealt with during therapeutic catheterization, but the main procedures performed in the neonatal period are Blalock-type shunts, closure of PDA and resection of coarctation of the aorta. The Blalock–Hanlon procedure to increase interatrial mixing of blood has largely been replaced by the balloon atrial septostomy, but is still performed occasionally in some complex congenital lesions such as mitral atresia. Banding of the pulmonary artery to reduce pulmonary blood flow is nowadays performed only for very complex lesions such as multiple VSDs.

Blalock shunts

Anastomosis of a subclavian artery to the pulmonary artery of the same side is frequently required to improve pulmonary blood flow in babies with pulmonary or tricuspid atresia or severe Fallot's tetralogy if the diameter of the PA is less than 30 per cent of the aorta. Blood flowing through the shunt increases oxygen saturation and prevents dangerous hypercyanotic attacks, but also the increased flow will stimulate small PAs to grow. The most commonly performed shunt is with 4–6 mm Gore-Tex tubing usually on the side opposite the aortic arch.

The patients are usually cyanotic, often with a very high haematocrit and will be receiving prostaglandin infusion to maintain ductal patency. Excessive mechanical ventilation will further reduce pulmonary blood flow. Arterial monitoring should be on the side opposite to the thoracotomy.

An anaesthetic technique with relaxant, oxygen, nitrous oxide or oxygen, air and fentanyl is satisfactory and hand ventilation may help the surgeon during the delicate anastomoses in the mediastinum. Heparin 1 mg.kg^{-1} i.v. is given after the Gore-Tex has been sutured to the subclavian artery, before it is joined to the pulmonary artery. Increasing acidosis is a common finding and 1 mmol.kg^{-1}

sodium bicarbonate is invariably necessary during the procedure. Transfusion during the procedure is with plasma to replace the blood loss.

After the shunt is completed peripheral oxygenation and graft patency depend on a normal perfusion pressure and an infusion of, for example, dopamine 6 μg.kg.$^{-1}$.min may be necessary to achieve this. A short period of intubation postoperatively is invariably beneficial, particularly if the shunt is large and pulmonary compliance falls.

Patent Ductus Arteriosus (see also p. 37)

Any premature baby is at risk from PDA because the mechanisms which cause the duct to close are also immature; fluid overload in the neonatal period may also cause the ductus to remain open. PDA is also associated with many forms of congenital heart disease, but may be a single chance finding. It is estimated that 25 per cent of babies weighing below 1500 mg and recovering from hyaline membrane disease have a PDA. The greatly increased pulmonary blood flow contributes to persistent chest infections and failure to thrive in spite of diuretics and may allow the development of bronchopulmonary dysplasia. Echocardiographic investigation should be routine for any ventilator-dependent baby as there may be no murmur. Occasionally the operation to ligate the PDA is performed in the intensive care unit.

A relaxant technique with oxygen/nitrous oxide or air/oxygen mixtures with fentanyl 10 μg.kg^{-1} is a very satisfactory technique for a baby not expected to breathe spontaneously in the early postoperative period.[63,64] Otherwise, the fentanyl dose should not exceed 5 μg.kg^{-1}. To minimize the risk of retinopathy of prematurity oxygen saturation should be kept between 90–92 per cent. The surgical approach is via a left thoracotomy and the ductus is either clipped or ligated twice. Sudden ligation of the ductus may cause a surge in arterial pressure and increase the possibility of intraventricular cerebral haemorrhage in the preterm age group. Before the PDA is finally ligated, a trial clamping takes place to demonstrate any serious cardiovascular consequences and there should be two suckers, vascular clamps and blood ready to transfuse in the unlikely event that the ductus is torn during ligation. Transfusion of blood is otherwise rarely necessary.

Coarctation of the aorta

The infantile type of coarctation is preductal with much of the blood supply to the lower body coming via the PDA. Other anomalies such as TGA or VSD may be present. These babies are often in terminal left ventricular failure with a tight preductal stenosis or a hypoplastic aortic arch and little, if any, collateral flow. Clinical diagnosis is confirmed by echocardiography.   Preoperative care should include mechanical ventilation, prostaglandin and dopamine therapy and all vascular access should have been achieved in the intensive care unit before surgery is undertaken. The arterial line must be in the right arm as the left subclavian artery is often incorporated in the surgical repair which takes place via a left thoracotomy. The anaesthetic technique which provides the greatest stability for these very sick patients is relaxant, oxygen and fentanyl (10–25 μg.kg^{-1}); inhalation agents such as halothane are contraindicated. Total body potassium is frequently very low and contributes to cardiac instability.

The time of greatest risk is at unclamping of the aorta when hypotension reduces myocardial perfusion. The aorta can be repeatedly clamped to increase coronary perfusion pressure and with transfusion of 10-20 per cent blood volume, the clamp can eventually be completely removed. The peripheral vasculature is often reactive so an infusion of sodium nitroprusside may be necessary later to maintain the blood pressure between 80 and 100 mmHg in the postoperative period. Respiratory support should continue for up to 48 hours postoperatively, though recovery is usually rapid if the repair is satisfactory and other lesions, e.g. VSD, are not present.

Blalock-Hanlon procedure

This operation was designed to improve interatrial mixing of blood in TGA by the creation of an atrial septal defect. In neonates it is now performed only in cases of complicated TGA.

The common method is to expose the right pulmonary artery and veins via a right thoracotomy and place a clamp on the right and left atrial wall near the interatrial groove so as to include part of the septum in the clamp. The atrium is opened and a portion of septum excised. The clamp is then partially opened, allowing the septum to slip out of it, then quickly reapplied. The snares previously applied to the pulmonary vessels are then released and the atrial incision is closed. Alternatively, the operation can be performed after inflow occlusion.

Whichever technique is used, it is wise to ventilate the lungs with 100 per cent oxygen for three minutes before the clamps are applied , and during closure of the atrium. Major blood loss may occur and myocardial stimulant drugs should be available. Intra-arterial blood pressure monitoring is mandatory and blood gas and acid-base state should be checked immediately before and after the period of clamping. Controlled ventilation may be required for several days after this procedure.

Pulmonary artery banding

This procedure, which reduces pulmonary blood flow in patients with left-to-right shunts, is nowadays seldom performed in uncomplicated VSD because the risks of total correction have been reduced to a low level. It is, however, used in complex lesions which are not suitable for early correction, such as a univentricular heart with high pulmonary blood flow, multiple VSD and occasionally VSD with coarctation, to prevent the onset of pulmonary hypertension and to allow the baby to thrive.

The pulmonary artery is usually approached through a left thoracotomy although it may be reached from the right. A thick ligature is passed round the artery, and when this is tightened the systemic arterial pressure rises and the distal pulmonary artery pressure falls. If the band is applied too tightly, oxygen tension will fall dramatically because of inadequate pulmonary blood flow, so intra-arterial pressure monitoring and sampling facilities are mandatory. Pulse oximetry can be used as an early indicator of an excessively tight band and the final PaO_2 should be at least 7 kPa (80 per cent saturation).

Closed valvotomy

If balloon valvuloplasty fails in the small infant aortic and pulmonary valvotomy may be performed without bypass, using a very short period of inflow occlusion and circulatory arrest. This is simple, avoiding the use of cardiopulmonary bypass and is the technique of choice for sick newborns. The approach is a median sternotomy and monitoring is as for a bypass with reliable venous access for the rapid transfusion of warmed blood. For aortic valvotomy, the patient is ventilated with 100 per cent oxygen for a few minutes and 1 mmol.kg^{-1}

HCO_3 is given before the cavae are snared. The aorta is clamped and opened and the valvotomy performed under direct vision in a time not exceeding three minutes. After the cavae are unsnared, the heart ejects any air which escapes via the aortic suture line. Postoperative respiratory support may be required for several days if ventricular function is poor.

Phrenic nerve palsy

Infants rely solely on a functioning diaphragm to breathe and the phrenic nerves are vulnerable during cardiac and thoracic surgery. Damage may be caused by diathermy, traction or cold injury. A phrenic palsy should be suspected if a small baby fails to wean from the ventilator when cardiac output and pulmonary compliance are normal. The plain chest X-ray may show an elevated hemidiaphragm – two vertebral spaces above the contralateral side are diagnostic, but the

diagnosis should also be confirmed by fluoroscopy and occasionally both sides are affected. Often, recovery can be expected between theee and six weeks from the injury; however, the period of respiratory support will be greatly reduced if surgical plication of the diaphragm is undertaken to prevent the damaging respiratory effects of paradoxical movement. Plication will not prejudice normal diaphragmatic function if the nerve regenerates at a future time.[65]

Non cardiac surgery

Many patients with cardiac disease, uncorrected, corrected or only palliated, may require surgery for non-cardiac reasons. The patients may not be able to respond to stress with great increases in cardiac output or may poorly tolerate the change from spontaneous to controlled respiration or have balanced shunts depending on stability of SVR and PVR. Many conditions predispose to dysrhythmia and to other organ damage, e.g. liver and kidneys.

Exercise tolerance is a good guide to tolerance of anaesthesia and in newborns or infants this is assessed by the ability to feed and suck without breathlessness and whether the baby has developed and grown normally.

The choice of technique should allow cardiac output to be maintained and involves carefully

controlled ventilation with relaxants and small doses of opioid or inhalational agent or if possible together with a regional technique. Monitoring should be full and careful with direct arterial monitoring for major cases. The blood volume must be fully maintained with crystalloid and/or colloid to cover all losses and to maintain the peripheral temperature. A high FiO_2 allows a margin of safety if cardiac output falls or pulmonary blood flow decreases. The heart rate should be maintained, using atropine if necessary. Appropriate antibiotic prophylaxis is required. Postoperatively, respiratory support may be necessary, but all such babies should be nursed in a high-dependency area where close monitoring and oxygen therapy can be delivered if required.

Anaesthesia and respiratory obstruction

The anatomical differences between the upper airway of the neonate and that of the adult are

described on p. 9. The fact that neonates are obligatory nose breathers makes them particularly susceptible to respiratory distress should blockage of the nasal airway occur. This is probably more important for caucasian babies than for black infants, in whom nasal resistance is lower.[66] A nasogastric tube may also cause respiratory difficulty, particularly if too large or if placed in the larger nostril.

Obstruction of the upper airway in the newborn may lead to acute respiratory distress and/or stridor. Infants with nasal obstruction manifest severe distress with cyanosis and retractions; narrowing or partial collapse of the larynx and upper trachea produces prolongation of the inspiratory phase of breathing and the distinctive sound of stridor. As the site of obstruction moves towards the level of the cricoid, an expiratory component to the stridor may be noted. A high-pitched sound is usually indicative of a laryngeal abnormality, while a lower pitch tends to emanate from the trachea or pharynx. A normal cry generally rules out lesions affecting the vocal cords, while a weak, aphonic or hoarse cry suggests vocal cord paralysis or cord anomaly, e.g, laryngeal cyst, laryngeal cleft. It is important to determine whether any relationship exists between stridor and feeding.

'Fixed' lesions of the airway such as tracheal stenosis, where little change in diameter can occur with respiration, may produce a picture of combined inspiratory and expiratory stridor.

Immediate assessment of severity

The urgency for diagnostic investigation of stridor depends upon the severity of the respiratory distress. Upper airway obstruction, if severe and prolonged, may cause serious hypoxia which can easily be fatal or may lead to cerebral ischaemia and resultant mental retardation. The fact that a high proportion of infants with Pierre Robin syndrome are found later to have mental retardation may be due to hypoxia subsequent to severe and prolonged episodes of airway obstruction. The immediate assessment of the severity of the obstruction must be based on a rapid and thorough appraisal of the clinical signs and recent history. The amount of stridor is not on its own the most significant feature because stridor diminishes as the infant tires, so the moribund child may be almost silent.

Increase in respiratory frequency is a reliable sign of respiratory failure, rates over 60 per minute giving cause for concern. Any baby able to take a feed without undue distress is unlikely to require urgent treatment although other signs may show that immediate action is necessary to relieve the obstruction. These signs may include severe intercostal and subcostal recession, paradoxical movement of the chest and abdomen with abdominal protrusion on inspiration, tracheal tug, sweating cyanosis, peripheral hypoperfusion, head retraction and general restlessness. Because the compliance of the rib cage is high, intercostal recession is particularly marked. Arterial blood gases tend initially to be well maintained although hypercarbia, hypoxia and metabolic acidosis develop in sequence, as respiratory failure ensues

Cardiovascular deterioration occurs early in severe respiratory obstruction, with initial tachycardia, pallor or cyanosis progressing to bradycardia and cardiac arrest. Cardiac arrest is particularly likely to result in brain damage if it has been preceded by a period of severe hypoxaemia, which is usually the case in respiratory obstruction.

Clinical examination may give a clue to the site and possible cause of obstruction. There may be an obvious external abnormality such as malformation of the nares, micrognathia, cleft palate or swelling around the neck and face.[67] Diagnosis of upper airway obstruction may on occasion require plain soft tissue lateral and AP radiographs of the neck, ultrasound, CT, MR imaging, pulmonary angiography, or upper GI contrast studies.

Endoscopic examination is the mainstay of diagnosis; vocal cord function and overall general dynamic motion of the larynx can be evaluated, with identification of the nature and exact anatomic location of the airway obstruction. Gastrointestinal contrast studies allow the air column to be visualized when the oesophagus is contrast filled; with tracheomalacia the air column will show collapse with expiration; with vascular rings there will be a characteristic pattern of indentation on the trachea and oesophagus.

Causes of respiratory obstruction

The main causes of respiratory obstruction in the neonate are shown in Table 4.5. In many of these there is some underlying pathology – congenital or acquired – to which an acute or subacute obstructive episode may be added. In addition, however, obstructive apnoea may occur during sleep in the absence of apparent underlying disease, particularly in preterm infants.

Table 4.5　Causes of respiratory obstruction in the neonate

Site	No pre-existing anomaly	Pre-existing anomaly
Nose	Nasal congestion Nasogastric tube	Congenital absence Choanal atresia
Pharynx	Sleep apnoea Burns	Macroglossia (e.g. Beckwith syndrome) Cretinism Pierre Robin syndrome Treacher Collins syndrome Cystic hygroma
Larynx	Acute laryngospasm Acquired vocal cord palsy Acquired subglottic stenosis	Atresia Laryngomalacia Congenital webs, cysts, Haemangiomata Secondary to raised intracranial pressure Congenital vocal cord palsy Congenital subglottic stenosis
Trachea	Foreign body Acquired tracheal stenosis	Tracheomalacia, often associated with oesophageal atresia Congenital tracheal stenosis Extrinsic pressure: cyst, tumour, vascular ring

Although obstructive apnoeic episodes are usually shorter in duration than central apnoeas, they are frequently associated with hypoxia. Several theories have been put forward to explain the mechanism behind these episodes, including laryngeal hyperexcitability and pharyngeal inco–ordination. Neck flexion appears to make the airways more susceptible to collapse.

Nasal

Nasal obstruction may be fatal, as the neonate is an obligatory nose breather. Extreme respiratory distress with cyanosis is characteristically relieved when the infant cries, thus using its mouth for breathing.

Choanal atresia

Choanal atresia/stenosis is a rare condition (1 in 60 000) which, if bilateral, causes severe respiratory symptoms in the first minutes to hours of life. The infant is characteristically pink while crying but cyanotic when quiet and with the mouth closed. Unilateral obstruction may lead to poor feeding and/or disturbed sleep. Choanal atresia is readily diagnosed by the inability to pass a catheter through the nares into the pharynx. The placement of an oral airway will relieve the obstruction until further diagnostic work-up can be performed. Transnasal puncture and dilatation is usually performed at the age of 1–2 days.

Premedication is with atropine and intubation is performed after preoxygenation through the oral airway. Ventilation is controlled with all the precautions necessary for neonatal anaesthesia and surgery. Care must be taken to avoid compression of the tracheal tube by the mouth gag. After the nasal punctures are completed the surgeon inserts short plastic tubes which are fixed in place in the nose for six weeks. The operation usually takes 20–30 minutes. The patient is extubated fully awake after careful suctioning of the pharynx. Pulmonary aspiration of regurgitated stomach contents is very likely to occur after this operation: careful nursing observation must start at once in the postoperative ward.

Atresia may be unilateral or bilateral and may also be associated with other congenital abnormalities such as CHARGE association, Apert's or Treacher Collins syndrome (Fig. 4.22).

Nasal obstruction may also be due to dermoids, gliomas and encephaloceles. Nasal stuffiness may be seen with reserpine given to the mother, or in infants with congenital syphilis and a profuse rhinitis ('snuffles').

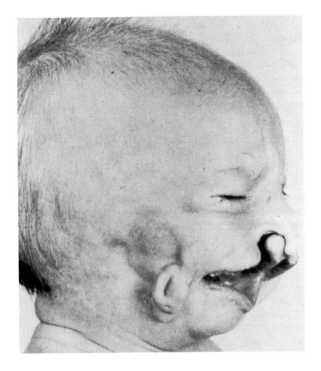

Fig. 4.22 The Treacher Collins syndrome.

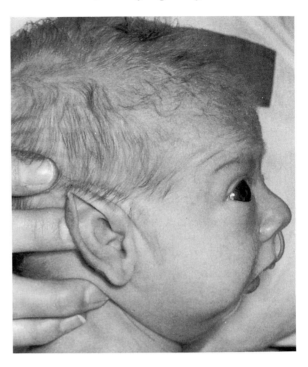

Fig. 4.23 The Pierre Robin syndrome.

Pharyngeal

Recent evidence has shown that pharyngeal obstruction may be an important cause of apnoea in some preterm infants, possibly due to pharyngeal or laryngeal dysfunction. It has been shown that transmural pressures greater than those normally seen during peak inspiratory flow are required to keep airways patent, suggesting that a neuromuscular mechanism is required to maintain airway patency in some infants. Neck flexion increases the opening pressure, making the airways more liable to collapse.

Pierre Robin syndrome (Fig. 4.23)

This syndrome consists of cleft palate, underdevelopment of the mandible (micrognathia) and a relatively large tongue (macroglossia) which may cause pharyngeal obstruction, particularly in the supine position. Severe cases provide a challenge to airway management in the first few months of life. Traditionally, the infant was nursed in the prone position, but even in this position fatalities do occur. A nasopharyngeal airway avoids the need for tracheal intubation and is commonly used, but the most severe cases may require tracheostomy.

Cystic hygroma

This cystic lymphangioma presents at birth as a multiloculated cystic swelling in the neck (Fig. 4.24) or, rarely, in the axilla. The swelling is soft and fluctuant and although it is benign it frequently invades neighbouring tissues and may recur. It may not be possible to perform complete surgical removal, especially if the tumour is large or extends around the trachea or brachial plexus. Involvement of the base of the tongue and oropharynx is common and may cause respiratory difficulties. Intrathoracic extension of this tumour is rare.

Anaesthetic management

The intraoral extension of this multilocular cystic tumour may make identification of the larynx difficult and, more importantly, may make inflation of the lungs impossible in the apnoeic patient. It is therefore essential to maintain spontaneous breathing until intubation has been performed. In the worst cases the only way to identify the larynx may be to observe the movement of air in and out of the lungs, which usually causes a number of frothy bubbles to appear between two lobules of the hygroma. Surgical removal of the tumour may be

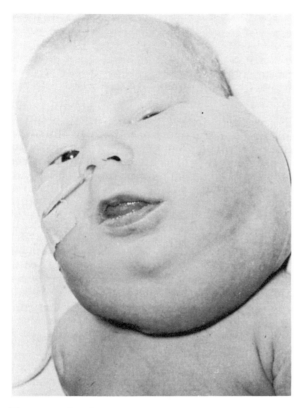

Fig. 4.24 Cystic hygroma.

difficult as it crosses tissue planes and blood should be available for transfusion. The child should not be extubated until fully awake and in the worst cases tracheostomy may be necessary.

Postoperative care
Because of the danger of bleeding into the operative site causing respiratory obstruction in the early postoperative period, these children must be observed very closely. Even the aperture of a tracheostomy tube may become obstructed by recurrent swelling in the neck.

Laryngeal

Congenital laryngeal stridor (laryngomalacia) is the commonest cause of stridor at birth and is probably due to immaturity of the laryngeal muscles and cartilages. It may be present at birth or more often develops within the first weeks after delivery. The highpitched stridor is worse with straining or crying and improves in the prone position or when the infant is relaxed or with the jaw thrust manoeuvre.

The voice and cry are usually normal. Stridor may disappear when the infant cries vigorously and increases the tidal volume.

Laryngomalacia may occur in association with other congenital defects such as subglottic stenosis. The laxity of the supraglottic larynx allows it to be drawn into the glottis during inspiration, causing the characteristic inspiratory stridor. The condition is seldom life–threatening although it may cause feeding problems, and repeated respiratory infections are common. The diagnosis is made by direct laryngoscopy and may require aryepiglottopexy. The long–term prognosis is usually good, although in some cases symptoms of persisting respiratory obstruction may remain into childhood.

Vocal cord palsy may be unilateral or bilateral and congenital or acquired. Congenital vocal cord paralysis may present with stridor at birth; it is associated with the Arnold–Chiari malformation, cardiovascular malformations or is often idiopathic. Acquired vocal cord paralysis has been associated with birth trauma, recurrent laryngeal nerve injury, dislocation of the arytenoid cartilage during traumatic intubation or secondary to raised intracranial pressure, and rarely from tumours in the neck or thorax. Partial paralysis may leave the adductors relatively unopposed, creating severe stridor. In some but not all cases the stridor gradually resolves over a period of several months, during which time intubation or even tracheostomy may be required. Diagnosis is made at direct laryngoscopy, with spontaneous breathing to allow vocal cord movement to be properly assessed.

Other laryngeal abnormalities include congenital webs, cysts, stenosis (very rare), clefts, haemangiomas and lymphangiomas. Stridor has also been associated with hypocalcaemia without anatomic abnormality of the upper airway. Hyperexcitability of the laryngeal adductors has also been demonstrated in prematures, aggravated by hyperthermia.

Congenital webs and cysts may arise anywhere in the larynx. The most common are situated in the glottic or subglottic area and lateral X-ray of the neck or xerogram usually demonstrates the lesion clearly. Laryngeal haemangiomata should be suspected in any child with significant cutaneous haemangiomata, especially over the neck or anterior chest wall. They seldom give rise to airway problems at birth; stridor tends to develop within the first three months of life. Crying, struggling or partial airway obstruction

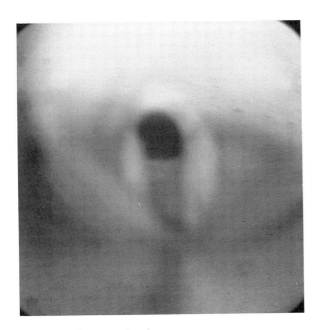

Fig. 4.25 Laryngeal web.

will increase the size of the tumour by venous engorgement. Direct laryngoscopy confirms the diagnosis and treatment is by steroid injection or laser resection. Tracheostomy is often required.

Congenital subglottic stenosis is a relatively rare cause of airway obstruction, found more frequently in association with tracheo–oesophageal fistula or Down's syndrome. Acquired stenosis, on the other hand, still occurs more frequently than it should and is due either to the pressure of too large a tracheal tube or to trauma from the shoulder of a tapered tube such as the Cole pattern.

Since the subglottic area, which is the narrowest part of the neonate's upper airway, is the site of the complete cartilaginous cricoid ring, there is no room for expansion and 1 mm of oedema or fibrosis will narrow the airway by as much as 65 per cent. Stridor usually occurs within a few hours of extubation and mild cases may respond to humidity, oxygen, intravenous dexamethasone (0.25 mg.kg^{-1} followed by 0.1 mg.kg^{-1} 6-hourly for 24 hours) and possibly nebulized racemic adrenaline. More severe cases require a cricoid split operation or period of reintubation with a small tube and the worst cases may require tracheostomy and eventual laryngotracheoplasty.

Tracheal

Congenital lesions

Congenital tracheal lesions include stenosis, subglottic haemangiomas (silent at birth but symptomatic within a few months), cysts, vascular rings or tracheomalacia. Tracheomalacia may be a primary malformation of the cartilaginous rings of the trachea; it is associated with oesophageal atresia, particularly with a concomitant tracheo-oesophageal fistula (TOF) located in the proximal trachea above T3. Infants with TOF and tracheomalacia or with vascular compression of the trachea may develop sudden cyanotic episodes with the rapid development of apnoea and bradycardia, particularly during or immediately after feeding. Extrinsic tracheal compression may also be due to congenital goitre, cystic hygromas or other mediastinal masses.

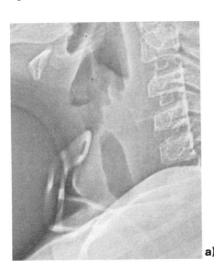

a)

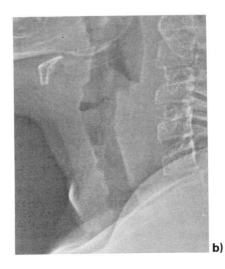

b)

Fig. 4.26 Xerograms showing (a) complete respiratory obstruction due to subglottic stenosis, and (b) the same child after relief of the obstruction by laryngotracheoplasty (courtesy of J.N.G Evans).

Vascular anomalies of the aortic arch may cause compression of the trachea and oesophagus. A vascular ring is most commonly due to persistent right and left aortic arches, but can also be caused by a right–sided aortic arch and left patent ductus arteriosus, or by aberrant right subclavian, innominate or left common carotid arteries (Fig. 4.27).

The trachea and oesophagus are enclosed within the vascular ring and pressure on the trachea causes the main clinical problem, airway obstruction. This obstruction usually develops within the first few weeks after birth, is exacerbated by feeding and may become very severe. The clinical picture is that of intrathoracic respiratory obstruction, with a croaking cry, brassy cough, signs of hyperinflation of the chest, expiratory wheezes and rhonchi.

Respiratory infections are common and the diagnosis should be considered in cases of repeated chest infection. In severe cases the infant may adopt the hyperextended posture of opisthotonus and sudden death from respiratory obstruction may occur. Associated cardiac anomalies may be present, particularly ventricular septal defect or bicuspid aortic valve.

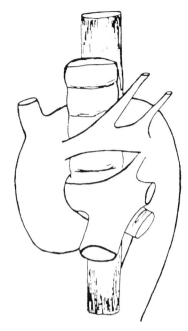

Fig. 4.27   Double aortic arch.

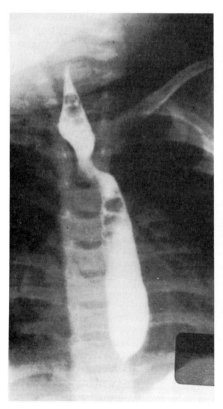
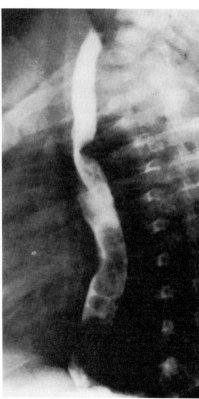

Fig. 4.28 Barium swallow, showing oesophageal compression caused by double aortic arch. (Reproduced with permission from [67].)

Diagnosis should be confirmed as soon as possible, either by endoscopy or by barium, propyliodone (Dionosil) or water–soluble non–ionic contrast medium swallow (Fig. 4.28).

These investigations should be carried out only when a skilled anaesthetist can be standing by with full resuscitation equipment. Laryngoscopy and tracheal intubation may be necessary in order to suck out any aspirated propyliodone and to relieve hypoxia.

Treatment is surgical and incomplete division of the ring has been reported. Because the airway obstruction is low in the trachea it may occasionally be necessary to use a long tracheal tube passed into the right main bronchus, with a side hole cut 1.5–2 cm from the tip to allow ventilation of the left lung. Care should be taken not to pass too large a tube through the obstructed area because of the risk of oedema causing postoperative stridor and it is better to keep the tube above the lesion if possible. Surgical manipulation may cause complete airway obstruction and severe haemorrhage may occur.

Symptoms of airway obstruction may be slow to improve postoperatively, as the trachea has often been severely distorted and some degree of tracheomalacia and tracheal stenosis is almost always present. The infant should be nursed in a humidified head box with some oxygen enrichment and may be helped by dexamethasone (0.25–0.5 mg.kg^{-1}). In severe cases, continuous positive airway pressure, using either a nasal prong or a small tracheal tube, may be necessary. Tracheostomy may have to be considered, although the low position of the obstruction often makes this unsatisfactory. The possibility of incomplete resection of the vascular ring should be considered if post-operative respiratory obstruction persists, as in some cases a ligamentum arteriosum may be responsible for continuing symptoms.

Acquired Lesions

Intraluminal pressure on the tracheal cartilage secondary to high pressure endotracheal ventilation, particularly chronically elevated intrathoracic airway pressures, may lead to secondary tracheomalacia with the development of widened, flaccid membranous portions of the trachea. Inhalation of a foreign body is unusual in the neonatal period.

Acquired subglottic stenosis is a relatively frequent upper airway obstructive lesion in premature infants. A number of factors have been incriminated in its pathogenesis. These include patient factors (gestational age, birthweight, severity of illness, physical activity) and tube related factors (tube size, method of intubation, method of fixation, physical and chemical properties of the tube, duration of ventilation and the number of intubations). The maximal tube contact is at the cricoid, the only complete ring of cartilage and the smallest diameter in the normal infant. Prolonged intubation leads to pressure necrosis, mucosal oedema and ulceration with scar tissue formation. Adherence to protocols avoiding tight fitting tubes, better stabilization of tubes, higher humidification of gases and minimizing intubation frequency have led to a lowering in the incidence of intubation injury.

Subglottic stenosis may present with raspy, stridorous breathing weeks after prolonged intubation. Symptoms may progress with increasing respiratory difficulty and cyanotic episodes. The voice and cry may be affected if the process has involved the true vocal cords.

Management of respiratory obstruction

Intubation, laryngoscopy, bronchoscopy or tracheostomy may be necessary for the management of these cases. Infants with subglottic oedema and stridor developing immediately after prolonged intubation may benefit from racemic adrenaline and/or corticosteroid therapy. Routine use of corticosteroids is not recommended but may be of benefit in very low birthweight infants[68] In those infants demonstrating postextubation stridor, reintubation of the trachea is often necessary to secure airway patency and re-establish effective ventilation. These patients may or may not go on to develop an organized stricture.

In infants with repeated failed extubations and demonstrated subglottic stenosis the anterior cricoid split operation (with the tracheal tube left in situ to act as a stent) has been utilized with good results; in the large majority of infants it has precluded the requirement for tracheostomy.

Bronchoscopy and laryngoscopy should never be undertaken lightly, especially in the neonate. Bronchoscopy is never indicated merely for removal of secretions. It should not be performed in the presence of tracheal infection or subglottic stenosis, as oedema and stridor will be intensified.

Laryngoscopy

Some of the conditions for which laryngoscopy is performed can progress to partial or complete respiratory obstruction under anaesthesia; this applies particularly to patients with micrognathia, large tongues, rigid jaws and pharyngeal or glottic cysts or tumours. A selection of laryngoscopes and tracheal tubes of various lengths must be on hand and a surgeon must be ready to perform a tracheostomy if that becomes urgently necessary. Great care must be taken to maintain the infant's body temperature during induction of anaesthesia and surgery; pulse oximetry and ECG and precordial stethoscope should be employed. Premedication consists only of atropine, and this should always be given because local topical analgesia is essential and only works well if adequate drying of secretions has been achieved. In spite of the advantages generally cited for controlled ventilation in neonatal anaesthesia, these are usually outweighed by the advantages of spontaneous ventilation in anaesthesia for laryngoscopy. Spontaneous ventilation is mandatory in respiratory obstruction unless the anaesthetist is certain he will be able to inflate the lungs of the paralysed patient. In children with laryngeal papillomata or cystic hygroma the movement which occurs around the glottis only during spontaneous breathing, with possible bubbles of saliva, may provide the only means of identification of the laryngeal inlet.

Induction of anaesthesia for laryngoscopy is usually performed with oxygen and halothane via a well-fitting face mask. The application of constant distending pressure by controlling the gas leak from the open-ended T-piece reservoir bag is sometimes extremely useful during induction in cases of respiratory obstruction and may even lead to the complete disappearance of stridor. It is essential, therefore, that the mask used is one which can make a good seal with the face: the Rendell–Baker mask is not ideal for the purpose and one with an inflatable rim is preferable despite its larger dead space. A vein should always be cannulated as soon as possible, though in the absence of severe obstruction it may be acceptable to leave this until after induction. Topical lignocaine ($3–5$ mg.kg^{-1}) is sprayed into the larynx and trachea when the patient is fairly deeply anaesthetized and at this time the anaesthetist can make a first assessment of the larynx. If microlaryngoscopy is to be performed it is wise to intubate the trachea first, in order to assess the diameter of the larynx and upper trachea, and

to provide a secure airway while the microscope is set up. A small nasotracheal tube is convenient for this purpose. This is usually withdrawn into the nasopharynx during the microlaryngoscopy and oxygen and halothane are insufflated through it. Spontaneous ventilation allows the surgeon to observe the movements of the larynx during the procedure and this is essential to the diagnosis of prolapsing larynx, laryngomalacia, cleft larynx and vocal cord palsy.

The Sanders injector[69] is often unsatisfactory for use during laryngoscopy in infants because it cannot be easily fitted to the microlaryngoscope blade and there is often difficulty in aiming the jet directly down the larynx. There is also a risk of seeding papillomata further down the airway. Intratracheal jets have been used in older children, but are dangerous if the cords close and probably should not be used in neonates.

Controlled ventilation through a small nasotracheal tube will be required for the occasional patient in respiratory failure.

Bronchoscopy

Anaesthetic techniques for bronchoscopy depend on the apparatus available.

Paediatric bronchoscope systems such as the Storz (Fig. 4.29) are designed as 'ventilating' bronchoscopes, but it is very unwise to give relaxants to the patient during such an endoscopy unless one is sure that it is possible to inflate the lungs adequately through the bronchoscope. Assisted or spontaneous ventilation is possible using the side arm of the bronchoscope. The smaller sized bronchoscopes originally had very little gap within the bronchoscope when the telescope was in place and ventilation was difficult in these circumstances.

The latest models have a finer telescope and significantly lower resistance to ventilation. Manual ventilation is not possible during suction and insertion of the telescope, during which time a paralysed patient will become increasingly hypoxic. Bronchoscopy is performed under general anaesthesia with full local anaesthesia to the respiratory tract as described above, with oxygen and halothane delivered to the side arm of the bronchoscope, ventilation being spontaneous or gently controlled.

Monitoring should include pulse oximetry, ECG and precordial stethoscope; if a hand is placed over

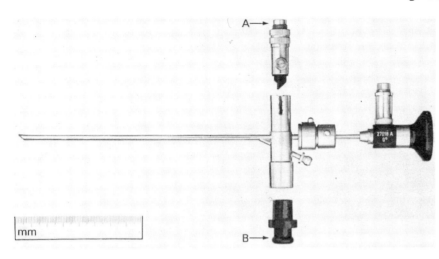

Fig. 4.29 The Storz bronchoscope showing (a) the light carrier, and (b) the attachment for the anaesthetic T-piece.

the epigastrium, each breath can be felt and the thumb on the apex can feel each heart beat. It is useful to attach two precordial stethoscopes; one on the left for breath and heart sounds and the right only for breath sounds. This allows monitoring of respiration to both lungs independently and is especially useful when the bronchoscope is down one or other main bronchus.

Most laryngotracheal lesions are diagnosed by laryngoscopy or bronchoscopy. The characteristic small, floppy glottis and epiglottis of laryngomalacia and vocal cord palsies will be observed. Tracheomalacia is seen during spontaneous respiration. Pulsatile swellings may be vascular in origin, although such pulsation may be transmitted and is not therefore diagnostic of a vascular origin. If the compression is caused by an aberrant subclavian artery making a vascular ring, the pressure of the tip of the bronchoscope may produce changes in the character of the radial pulses. This condition usually requires a cine swallow with contrast medium, using the image intensifier to visualize the obstruction and so make for a definitive diagnosis.

After the examination, the patient should be placed in the lateral position, the lower side being the side of any bleeding from trauma or biopsies. The patient must be observed until he is fully awake, as stridor and respiratory distress may not reappear until then.

Bronchoscopy may precipitate complete respiratory obstruction in very marginal cases by minimal oedema caused by the instrumentation. Bronchoscopy is not necessary and may be dangerous in the diagnosis of subglottic stenosis. Postoperatively the baby is nursed using a head box

with humidified air or air and oxygen mixture and should have nothing by mouth until three hours after the lignocaine spray to the glottis. Oxygen saturation, if available, can be extremely helpful. Dexamethasone should be given (p. 201) for laryngeal oedema if stridor reappears.

Tracheostomy (see also p. 218)

This is very rarely an emergency procedure. With the advent of long-term nasotracheal intubation, tracheostomy is never required nowadays merely for respiratory support in the neonatal period. The indications for tracheostomy vary from centre to centre, but it is generally accepted that for ventilator-dependent patients tracheostomy may be delayed for many weeks and then performed, not for airway reasons but because handling, nursing and stimulating a growing baby are easier with a tracheostomy. Tracheostomy is most commonly performed for conditions of the upper airway for which tracheal intubation is unsuitable, such as subglottic stenosis, severe tracheomalacia or vocal cord palsy.

Many patients who require tracheostomy already have a tracheal tube in place. Premedication is with atropine and preoxygenation is followed by intubation if a tube is not already in place. A very small tube may be necessary in cases of subglottic stenosis. A relaxant technique with controlled ventilation may be used. The patient is positioned with a sandbag behind the neck to extend the head maximally and to throw the trachea into prominence. Monitoring must include pulse oximetry, ECG and oesophageal stethoscope.

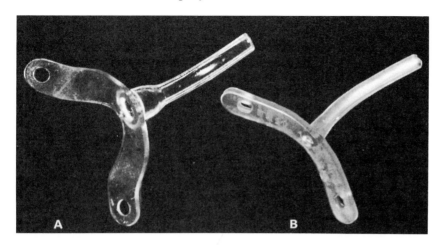

Fig. 4.30 Neonatal tracheostomy tubes. (a) Great Ormond Street; (b) Portex.

Infant tracheostomy is a specialized and difficult operation. Cartilage must never be excised because of the risk of subsequent tracheal collapse and stenosis, nor must the incision be too high in the trachea because of the risk of subglottic stenosis. The surgeon usually makes a vertical incision through the second and third tracheal rings. If it is made lower than this, there is a risk of bronchial intubation or tube dislodgement. Some surgeons insert two stay sutures which remain in place for seven days until the tube is changed for the first time. The uncuffed tracheostomy tube is chosen, usually one size larger than the tracheal tube in place, and then a check is made that all connections are available and that they fit (Fig. 4.30).

The patient is ventilated with 100 per cent oxygen before the tracheal incision is made and the tracheal tube withdrawn only enough for the tracheostomy tube to be inserted. Anaesthesia is continued through the tracheostomy with a sterile connector. The tube must fit with a small air leak around it and be fixed tightly round the neck with tapes after removal of the sandbag and flexion of the neck. Unless this step is taken the tapes will be too loose and accidental decannulation may occur. Postoperatively a chest X-ray is taken to check the position of the tip of the tube.

The complications of tracheostomy are more severe than those of tracheal intubation. Accidental dislodgement in the first week before a track is established can be disastrous, although less so if stay sutures are employed. Severe infection, tracheal granuloma and vascular erosion are reported complications.

A tracheostomy mask with humidified air is used to prevent crusting of secretions in the tube. Eventually the epithelium in the trachea becomes stratified and humidification is usually discontinued after about three weeks.

References

1. Pollack MM, Alexander SR, Clarke N, Ruttimann UE, Tesselaar HM, Bachulis AC. Improved outcomes from tertiary center pediatric intensive care: a statewide comparison of tertiary and non-tertiary care facilities. *Critical Care Medicine*. 1991; **19**, 150–9.
2. Waterston DJ, Bonham-Carter RE, Aberdeen E. Congenital tracheo-oesophageal fistula with oesophageal atresia. *Lancet*. 1963; **2**, 55-7.
3. Spitz L, Kiely E, Brereton RJ. Esophageal atresia: five year experience with 148 cases. *Journal of Pediatric Surgery*. 1987; **22**, 103-8.
4. Chamberlain PF, Manning FA, Morrison I, Harman CR, Lange IR. Ultrasound evaluation of amniotic fluid volume. II. The relationship of increased amniotic fluid volume to perinatal outcome. *American Journal of Obstetrics and Gynecology*. 1984; **150**, 250–4.
5. Reyes HM, Meller JL, Loeff D. Neonatal intestinal obstruction. *Clinics in Perinatology*. 1989; **16**, 85–96.
6. Kliegman RM. Neonatal necrotizing enterocolitis:

Bridging the basic science with the clinical disease. *Journal of Pediatrics*. 1990; **117**, 833–5.

7. Uauy RD, Fanaroff AA, Korones SB, Phillips EA, Philips JB, Wright LL. Necrotizing enterocolitis in very low birth weight infants: Biodemographic and clinical correlates. *Journal of Pediatrics*. 1991; **119**, 630–8.
8. Lucas A, Cole TJ. Breast milk and neonatal necrotising enterocolitis. *Lancet*. 1990; **336**, 1519–23.
9. Grosfeld JL, Cheu H, Schlatter M, West KW, Rescorla FJ. Changing trends in necrotizing enterocolitis: Experience with 302 cases in two decades. *Annals of Surgery*. 1991; **214**, 300–6.
10. Walsh MC, Kliegman RM, Hack M. Severity of necrotizing enterocolitis: influence on outcome at 2 years of age. *Pediatrics*. 1989; **84**, 808–14.
11. Czyrko C, Del Pin CA, O'Neill JA, Peckham GJ, Ross AJ. Maternal cocaine abuse and necrotizing enterocolitis: outcome and survival. *Journal of Pediatric Surgery*. 1991; **26**, 414–21.
12. Kliegman RM. Models of the pathogenesis of necrotizing enterocolitis. *Journal of Pediatrics*. 1990; **117**, S2–5.
13. Anderson DM, Kliegman RM. The relationship of neonatal alimentation practices to the occurrence of endemic necrotizing enterocolitis. *American Journal of Perinatology*. 1991; **8**, 62–7.
14. Goldman HI. Feeding and necrotizing enterocolitis. *American Journal of Diseases of Children*. 1980; **134**, 553–5.
15. Bell EF, Warburton D, Stonestreet BS, Oh W. High volume fluid intake predisposes premature infants to necrotizing enterocolitis. *Lancet*. 1979; **2**, 90.
16. Scheifele DW, Bjornson GL, Dyer RA, Fussell S, Olsen E. Delta-like toxin produced by coagulase-negative staphylococci is associated with neonatal necrotizing enterocolitis. *Infections in Immunology*. 1987; **55**, 2268–73.
17. Kosloske AM. A unifying hypothesis for pathogenesis and prevention of necrotizing enterocolitis. *Journal of Pediatrics*. 1990; **117**, S68–74.
18. Malcolm G, Ellwood D, Devonald K, Beilby R, Henderson-Smart D. Absent or reversed end diastolic flow velocity in the umbilical artery and necrotising enterocolitis. *Archives of Disease in Childhood*. 1991; **66**, 805–7.
19. Leidig E. Doppler analysis of superior mesenteric artery blood flow in preterm infants. *Archives of Disease in Childhood*. 1989; **64**, 476–80.
20. Daneman A, Baby P, Garcia P, Stringer DA, Hellmann J. Doppler sonography of intra-abdominal vessels in premature infants. *Pediatric Radiology*. 1987; **17**, 342(A).
21. Bell MJ, Ternberg JL, Feigin RD, Keating JP, Marshall R, Barton L, Brotherton T. Neonatal necrotizing enterocolitis: Therapeutic decisions based upon clinical staging. *Annals of Surgery*. 1978; **187**, 1–7.
22. Kosloske AM, Musemeche CA. Necrotizing enterocolitis of the neonate. *Clinics in Perinatology*. 1989; **16**, 97–111.
23. Abajian JC, Mellish RWP, Browne AF, Perkins FM, Lambert DH, Mazuzan JE. Spinal anesthesia for surgery in the high risk infant. *Anesthesia and Analgesia*. 1984; **63**, 359-62.
24. Spear RM. Anesthesia for premature and term infants: Perioperative implications. *Journal of Pediatrics*. 1992; **120**, 165-76.
25. Liu LMP, Cote CJ, Goudsouzian NG, Ryan JF, Firestone S, Dedrick DF, Liu PL, Todres ID. Life-threatening apnea in infants recovering from anesthesia. *Anesthesiology*. 1983; **59**, 506-10.
26. Welborn LG, Hannallah RS, Fink R, Ruttiman UE, Hicks JM. High dose caffeine suppresses postoperative apnea in former preterm infants. *Anesthesiology*. 1989; **71**, 347-9.
27. Mackersie AM. Anaesthesia for neurosurgery in paediatrics. In: Sumner E, Hatch DJ (eds) *Textbook of Paediatric Anaesthetic Practice*. London: Baillire Tindall, 1989; p. 387.
28. Cullum AR, English ICW, Branthwaite MA. Endobronchial intubation in infancy. *Anaesthesia*. 1973; **28**, 66-9.
29. Longaker MT, Golbus MS, Filly RA, Rosen MA, Chang SW, Harrison MR. Maternal outcome after open fetal surgery; a review of the first 17 human cases. *Journal of the American Medical Association*. 1991; **265**, 737-41.
30. de Lorimer AA, Tierney DF, Parker HR. Hypoplastic lungs in fetal lambs with surgically produced congenital diaphragmatic hernia. *Surgery*. 1967; **62**, 12-17.
31. Cartlidge PHT, Mann NP, Kapila L. Preoperative stabilisation in congenital diaphragmatic hernia. *Archives of Disease in Childhood*. 1986; **61**, 1226-8.
32. Nakayama DK, Motoyama EK, Tagge EM. Effect of preoperative stabilization on respiratory system in newborn infants with congenital diaphragmatic hernia. *Journal of Pediatrics*. 1991; **118**, 793-9.
33. Bohn D. Ventilatory and blood gas parameters in predicting survival in congenital diaphragmatic hernia. *Pediatric Surgery International*. 1987; **2**, 336-40.
34. Wilson JM, Lund DP, Lillehei CW, Vacanti JP. Congenital diaphragmatic hernia: Predictors of severity in the ECMO era. *Journal of Pediatric Surgery*. 1991; **26**, 1028-34.
35. Frostell CG, Lonnqvist PA, Sonesson SE, Gustafsson LE, Lohr G, Noack G. Near fatal pulmonary hypertension after surgical repair of congenital diaphragmatic hernia. Successful use of inhaled nitric oxide. *Anaesthesia*. 1993; **48**, 679–83.
36. Johns RA. Endothelium-derived relaxing factor; Basic review and clinical complications. *Journal*

of Cardiothoracic and Vascular Anaesthesia. 1991; **5**, 69-79.

37. Frostell C, Fratacci M-D, Wain JC, Jones R, Zapol WM. Inhaled nitric oxide. A selective pulmonary vasodilator reversing hypoxic pulmonary vasoconstriction. *Circulation.* 1991; **83**, 2038-47.

38. Breaux CW, Rouse TM, Cain WS, Georgeson KE. Improvement in survival of patients with congenital diaphragmatic hernia utilizing a strategy of delayed repair after medical and/or extracorporeal membrane oxygenation stabilization. *Journal of Pediatric Surgery.* 1991; **26**, 333-8.

39. Charlton AJ, Bruce J, Davenport M. Timing of surgery in congenital diaphragmatic hernia. *Anaesthesia.* 1991; **46**, 820-3.

40. Lucas A, Morley R, Cole TJ. Adverse neurodevelopmental outcome of moderate neonatal hypoglycaemia. *British Medical Journal.* 1988; **297**, 1304-8.

41. Aynsley-Green A, Polak JM, Bloom SR, Cough MH, Keeling J, Ashcroft SJH, Turner RC, Baum JD. Nesidioblastosis of the pancreas: definition of the syndrome and the management of severe neonatal hyperinsulinaemic hypoglycaemia. *Archives of Disease in Childhood.* 1981; **56**, 496-508.

42. Goossens A, Gepts S, Saudubray JM, Bonnefont JP, Nihoul-Fekete, Heitz PU, Kloppel G. Diffuse and focal nesidioblastosis: A clinico-pathological study of 24 patients with persistent neonatal hyperinsulinemic hypoglycemia. *American Journal of Surgical Pathology.* 1989; **13**, 766-75.

43. Lenz W. Aetiology: incidence and genetics of congenital heart disease. In: Graham G, Rossi E (eds) *Heart Disease in Infants and Children.* London: Edward Arnold, 1985, pp. 27–35.

44. Stark J, de Leval MR (eds) *Surgery for Congenital Heart Defects.* Philadelphia: WB Saunders, 1993.

45. Hickey PR. Deep hypothermic circulatory arrest is preferable to low flow bypass. *Journal of Cardiothoracic and Vascular Anaesthesia.* 1991; **5**, 635-7.

46. Greeley WJ. Deep hypothermic circulatory arrest must be used selectively and discreetly. *Journal of Cardiothoracic & Vascular Anaesthesia.* 1991; **5**, 638-40.

47. Hickey PR, Anderson NP. Deep hypothermic circulatory arrest: A review of pathophysiology and clinical experience as a basis for anesthetic management. *Journal of Cardiothoracic Anaesthesia.* 1987; **1**, 137-55.

48. Prough DS, Stump DA, Roy RC, Gravlee GP, Williams T, Mills SA, Hinshelwood L, Howard G. Response of cerebral blood flow to changes in carbon dioxide tension during hypothermic cardiopulmonary bypass. *Anesthesiology.* 1986; **64**, 576-81.

49. Rao CC, Boyer M, Krishna G. Effects of halothane, isoflurane and enflurane on the isometric contrac-

tion of the neonatal isolated rat atria. *Anesthesiology.* 1984; **61**, A424.

50. Hensley FA, Larach DR, Martin DE, Stauffer R, Waldhausen JA. The effect of halothane/nitrous oxide/oxygen mask induction on arterial haemoglobin saturation in cyanotic heart disease. *Journal of Cardiothoracic Anaesthesia.* 1987; **1**, 289-96.

51. Murray D, Vadewalker G, Matherne P, Mahoney L. Pulsed Doppler and 2-dimensional echocardiography: comparison of halothane and isoflurane on cardiac function in infants and small children. *Anesthesiology.* 1987; **67**, 211-17.

52. Tanner GE, Angers DG, Barash PG, Mulla A, Miller PL, Rothstein P. Effect of left-to-right, mixed left-to-right and right-to-left shunts on inhalational anesthetic induction in children. *Anesthesia and Analgesia.* 1985; **64**, 101-7.

53. Forrest ETS, Silk JM, Mackersie A. An audit of percutaneous central venous catheters in paediatric practice. *Paediatric Anaesthesia.* 1993; **3**, 147–52.

54. Firmin RK, Bouloux P, Allen P, Lima RC, Lincoln JC. Sympathoadrenal function during cardiac operations in infants with the technique of surface cooling, limited cardiopulmonary bypass, and circulatory arrest. *Journal of Thoracic and Cardiovascular Surgery.* 1985; **90**, 729–35.

55. Naik SK, Knight A, Elliott M. A prospective randomised study of a modified technique of ultrafiltration during paediatric open-heart surgery. *Circulation.* 1991; **84**, 422-31.

56. Gold JP, Jonas RA, Lang P, Elixson EM, Mayer JE, Castaneda AR. Transthoracic intracardiac monitoring lines in pediatric surgical patients: a 10-year experience. *Annals of Thoracic Surgery.* 1986; **42**, 185-91.

57. Colman RW. Humoral mediators of catastrophic reactions associated with protamine neutralisation. *Anesthesiology.* 1987; **66**, 595-6.

58. Deanfield J. Arrhythmias: paediatrics. *Current Opinions in Cardiology.* 1987; **2**, 109-11.

59. Tibballs J, Osborne A, Hochman M. A comparative study of cardiac output by dye dilution and pulsed Doppler ultrasound. *Anaesthesia and Intensive Care.* 1988; **16**, 272–7.

60. Bidstrup BP, Royston D, Sapsford RN, Taylor KM. Reduction in blood loss and blood use after cardiopulmonary bypass with high dose aprotinin (Trasylol). *Journal of Thoracic and Cardiovascular Surgery.* 1989; **97**, 364-72.

61. Martin RD, Parisi F, Robinson TW, Bailey L. Anesthetic management of neonatal cardiac transplantation. *Journal of Cardiothoracic Anaesthesia.* 1989; **3**, 465-9.

62. Pigott JD, Murphy JD, Barber G, Norwood WI. Palliative reconstructive surgery for hypoplastic left heart syndrome. *Annals of Thoracic Surgery.* 1988; **45**, 122-8.

63. Robinson S, Gregory GA. Fentanyl-air-oxygen

anesthesia for ligation of patent ductus arteriosus in preterm infants. *Anesthesia and Analgesia*. 1981; **60**, 31–62.

64. Anand KJS, Sippell WG, Aynsley Green A. Randomised trial of fentanyl anaesthesia in preterm babies undergoing surgery: effect on the stress response. *Lancet*. 1987; **i**, 243-8.

65. Hamilton JRL, Elliott MJ, deLeval M, Stark J. Paralysed diaphragm after cardiac surgery in children: value of plication. *European Journal of Cardiothoracic Surgery*. 1990; **4**, 487–91.

66. Stocks J, Godfrey S. Nasal resistance during infancy. *Respiration Physiology*. 1978; **34**, 233–46.

67. Hatch DJ. Acute upper airway obstruction in children. In: Atkinson RS, Adams AP (eds) *Recent Advances in Anaesthesia and Analgesia 15*. Edinburgh: Churchill Livingstone, 1985, p. 133.

68. Couser RJ, Ferrara TB, Falde B, Johnson K, Schilling CG, Hoelstra RE. Effectiveness of dexamethasone in preventing extubation failure in preterm infants at increased risk for airway edema. *Journal of Pediatrics*. 1992; **121**, 591–6.

69. Miyasaka K, Sloan IA, Froese AB. Evaluation of jet injector Sanders' technique for bronchoscopy in paediatric patients. *Canadian Anaesthetists' Society Journal*. 1980; **27**, 117–24.

5 Neonatal intensive care

Scope and organization

The neonatal intensive care unit (NICU) of today is not merely a group of physicians and nurses working in an isolated area of the hospital trying to master technology and break new ground, but an open, analytic, changing and hopefully self–critical and responsive environment providing care to newborn infants, and support to their parents and to the individuals working within this milieu.

Neonatal units

Levels of care

A major factor contributing to the reduction in perinatal mortality over the past 20–25 years has been the development of neonatal intensive care units. The proliferation of these facilities has led to definitions and classifications of care based on the relationship to obstetric services (in-born versus out-born units) and the level of resources available (Levels I, II, and III).[1] Further distinctions are made between units that provide predominantly assisted respiratory and allied care and those providing surgery or extracorporeal membrane oxygenation (ECMO) – the latter sometimes referred to as Level IV units. Although these definitions may be indistinct and applied differently in many regions, a facility, for example, providing care for the newborn with a surgical disorder needs to reflect that emphasis in its organization, function, personnel and technical facilities. Care for newborn infants with surgical disorders should be provided in a Level III unit with the full range of surgical, anaesthetic and neonatal expertise for the management of any complication in the newborn, as well as skilled transportation and subspecialty services in areas such as genetics, cardiology, neurology and radiology that are often required in the management of these infants.

Regionalization

Intensive care units function within a network of perinatal care or regionalized programmes so that rational use is made of these expensive human and technical resources. Regionalization implies that patients receive the care appropriate to their needs as close to home as possible and that all infants have access to a higher level of care when required.[2]

Implications of regionalization also include the coordination of data collection and outcome evaluation and the provision of collaborative assistance in the introduction of new technologies and educational programmes for that region.

Although the primary objective of a Level III neonatal unit is to provide care to individual high risk newborns and their families at a tertiary level, triage and transport systems, the provision of educational programmes and leadership in areas of research and clinical care are also part of that regional centre's mandate. Efficient use of facilities and personnel is essential, particularly in current times of financial constraints; priorities have to be set and the suitability and appropriateness of every referral to a regional centre evaluated.

Provision of care

The multidisciplinary team:

Care within the NICU is provided by a multidisciplinary team of individuals with expertise in all areas of medicine, nursing, respiratory therapy, nutrition, pharmacology, psychosocial services, rehabilitation medicine and biomedical engineering. This is a reflection of the increasing complexity of clinical problems due to the increased survival of very sick, small babies, the increasing body of scientific knowledge, the feasibility of surgery for most congenital disorders and the increasingly sophisticated technological support available.

Medical staffing of NICUs via the traditional role of doctors in training programmes is no longer always feasible. The dependence of patient care on technical procedures and the need for continuous attention to sudden changes in management place great pressure on medical staff. Restrictions have been placed on working hours of doctors in training and service demands can no longer overshadow educational needs.[3,4] Also, the complexity of care and limited time constraints create the potential for producing procedure-orientated physicians who, though they may be very efficient, may not have the time, energy or enthusiasm to maintain other contact with patients and parents.[5] A number of tasks previously considered resident duties have been assumed by administrative personnel and staffing requirements of NICUs have had to be met by enhancing the roles of many other members of the clinical team.[6]

The increased expertise of neonatal nursing practice has led to a variety of expanded roles for nurses within the NICU: it has been well shown that clinical nurse specialists or neonatal practitioners with advanced training can undertake many direct aspects of patient care.[7] Neonatal transport can be performed almost exclusively by specially trained nurses certified in neonatal resuscitation, stabilization, assisted ventilation and transportation. Neonatal nursing management has also recognized the need and created a number of new directions in neonatal nursing practice including discharge planning, bereavement programmes, infection and quality control and nutritional and breastfeeding support.

In North America, the role of respiratory therapists has expanded from the utilization and maintenance of mechanical ventilators, to participation in resuscitation procedures, transportation, administration of surfactant and full involvement with the medical team in managing and monitoring ventilation and oxygen therapy for the sick newborn.

The progress made in nutritional research in the newborn and the constant introduction of new products make it important that individuals with nutritional expertise be a part of the multidisciplinary NICU team.[8]

The increasing complexity of clinical problems encountered in the NICU has also led to changes in the practice of other support services, e.g. physiotherapists and occupational therapists expert in neurodevelopmental assessment provide strategies for handling and stimulation of longer-term infants with asymmetry of movements, abnormal tone, cognitive delays or feeding difficulties. Furthermore, physiotherapists and occupational therapists are actively involved in designing and providing developmentally appropriate care of the premature infant whose behavioural responses are easily overwhelmed by the multitude of environmental stimuli in the NICU.

Numerous other support personnel are required to maintain the full function of an NICU. These include laboratory and blood bank services, social work services, pharmacists (see therapeutic drug monitoring), radiology and biomedical technicians and data managers.

Although care is provided by a large number of different individuals, designation of primary responsibility to a specific physician or team is extremely important. Management is coordinated and a coherent and consistent flow of information is provided to parents.

The quality of communication between physicians, nurses and other intensive care staff has a direct impact on the effectiveness of the unit, its responsiveness to clinical needs and the quality of care provided.[9] A sense of mutual interdependence must be attained such that every member of the team's observational, intellectual and technical skills collectively contribute to patient care. This will enhance job satisfaction and staff retention despite the stresses of the work environment.

Teaching in the NICU

The educational needs of all the health care professionals must be integrated into the functioning of the unit, while at the same time respecting patients' and parents' needs for privacy and family interaction. It is a great challenge in any busy department to accomplish this; but teaching within the unit must be maximized so that a daily schedule is developed to utilize teaching opportunities with specific time set aside for achieving educational objectives. It is essential that doctors in training take direct responsibility for patients, that they learn technical procedures under supervision, that they are encouraged to take care of critical situations and show leadership in management, triage systems and collaboration with the multidisciplinary team.

The challenge for senior staff is to create an atmosphere of academic discussion and debate and to critically examine accepted concepts rather than merely to follow protocolized management which can often become the routine in busy intensive care units. The atmosphere within a unit should also reflect a concern for psychosocial issues and the responsibilities toward the very ill and their parents, as a practical demonstration that technology and compassionate medicine are complementary and not contradictory to one another.

In addition, it is imperative not only to train the staff within the neonatal unit but also to develop programmes of continuing education in neonatal medicine for physicians, nurses and allied professionals in the larger regional area.

Parental support

An extremely important function of the medical, nursing and psychosocial team is to provide support for the parents of the infants in the unit. It is necessary to plan how, when and what information can be provided and the general manner in which parents' needs can be handled throughout their child's hospitalization. This has a major impact on parents' short-term adaptation to their child's illness and the NICU environment and also on their long-term relationship with their child.

Parents' reactions to the birth of infants with congenital defects or to any seriously ill infant requiring intensive care may range from initial shock, denial, anger, guilt or fear of their infant's impending death, through adaptation to the intensive care milieu and the development of coping strategies. Eventually most parents realize that their child will survive, possibly with special long-term needs. An awareness and understanding of the body of knowledge concerning parental reactions and parents' perspectives on the stresses of an ICU stay[10-12] should ideally enable the clinical staff to counsel parents and recognize their needs appropriately during the hospitalization.

Many obstacles have to be overcome by the medical team, including the lack of prior knowledge by the parents, the fast-paced environment and time limitations of intensive care, the degree of medical uncertainty about the child's condition and prognosis, as well as limitations in the physician's own psychological and communication skills. Furthermore, the multitude of care-givers and consultants in the NICU make the establishment of a doctor–patient/parent relationship extraordinarily complex. This certainly pertains to the care of the complex surgical newborn with multiorgan involvement. In these cases the designation of primary responsibility for the care of the child and communication with the parents is particularly important.

Communication

At the time of admission and with any unexpected deterioration or significant intervention communication must be initiated without delay such that parents are kept abreast of all significant events as they unfold. Communication whenever possible should be more formalized than chance encounters at the bedside but should occur at regular intervals unless unanticipated complications have arisen. Preferably meetings should be with both parents, together with other family members or support people where appropriate, and should be done in combination with members of the multidisciplinary team, such as the primary nurse for the child, while at the same time attempting to preserve privacy and confidentiality for parents.

The nature of the communication may be for providing information or it may be to derive a decision as to a particular course of management.

Providing information
Physicians should provide information about diagnosis, management and prognosis in an honest and open manner with an awareness of the impact of that information on the parents. The question often arises as to how much parents should be told and whether the whole truth, if that can be known, is a real concept. Parents often display a greater capacity to deal with bad news than physicians think. It is what patients [parents] do not know, but vaguely suspect, that causes them corrosive worry.[7,13] In many instances there is more dissatisfaction with the way information is given than with the content of the information itself. It is often difficult to know what the emphasis of medical information should be. In one study, parents thought that the initial information they received in relation to their child's management was inadequate, although physicians had given detailed information about diagnosis and prognosis.[14]

Dealing with medical uncertainty requires reflection not only on whether the uncertainty is the result of the physician's own knowledge base or the limitations of medical knowledge itself, but also on the potential impact of that uncertainty on parents. In general, openness and honesty about what is known will promote a relationship of trust with parents. Striking the right balance is difficult and of course must be tailored to the individual. Attempts to express this balance are encapsulated in the familiar but still valid axioms: 'be cautiously optimistic'; 'be honest but not cruel'[15]; 'never destroy hope whenever possible'.

The provision of clinical service by physicians who rotate on weekly, monthly or other bases may often lead to difficulties in consistency in both medical care of the infant and in the care of the parents. This requires recognition by the staff of the NICU and the development of appropriate strategies to deal with this issue. One such alternative is the designation of a physician, often the staff physician who first admitted the infant or the one who has developed a relationship with parents, to remain involved in the child's long-term care.

Decision making

Professional responsibility should ensure that a decision to pursue a particular course of management is made jointly between the physician and the parents. It is implicit that the physician has the necessary expertise and knowledge of all the available treatment options, that full input has been enlisted from all consultants and care-givers, and that parents are fully informed and encouraged to express their own values and beliefs.

Usually it is clear that a particular therapy or course of action is either beneficial or harmful and consensus is easily reached. However, if the course is not clear because of uncertainty, a decision to continue treatment should be made until more certainty is achievable. Occasionally conflict may arise between the parents and the medical team due to differences in perception as to the best course of action for the child. The physician should allow time for agreement to develop and for further appropriate information to be given to parents. Attempts must be made to identify the underlying reasons for parental insistence on a point of view contrary to what is perceived by the medical staff to be in the best interests of the child. All efforts are made to preserve family integrity and to harmonize family interests with those of the child.[16] In the rare situation where this cannot be achieved involvement of a bioethicist may help to clarify the ethical issues involved, to ensure that all legitimate interests are duly considered and to assist parents and the medical team in coming to conclusions that are mutually and socially acceptable (see p. 267).

Many of these issues arise in the NICU around decisions involving withdrawal of life-sustaining care. The quality of any preceding communication with parents, the physician's approach, the parents' understanding of the child's condition, their coping mechanisms and strength of their relationship will all have a bearing on this.

Monitoring of unit activity

Data Collection

Data collection in the NICU has evolved from laborious notes and card systems, through huge hospital mainframe computer systems to dedicated unit-based computers with appropriate data and management software systems.

The aim of a database is to provide the informational support for any or all of the activities of the NICU, e.g.:

Administration   Level of activity markers, utilization of resources, quality assurance and staffing requirements. (The concept of quality assurance, although in its early stages of development, is being increasingly applied within the NICU because of the frequency of adverse events.[17])

Clinical   Specific patient data, diagnostic categories, referral patterns, use of transport and regionalization systems, trends in disease patterns as well as major morbidity and mortality statistics.

Educational   Generation of research ideas, enhancing computer skills of staff, teaching of clinical epidemiology.

Research   Identification of patients for retrospective research studies, sample size estimation and selection of cases and controls for prospective projects, research in health care services, etc.

Economic evaluation

The ability to accurately monitor a unit's activity is essential if informed decisions about clinical care, the introduction of costly new technology or procedures and allocation of health care resources are to be made. As more infants survive after prolonged hospitalization, some of whom may endure life-long disability, the demand for economic evaluation and justification of neonatal intensive care has increased.[18–22] A framework for evaluation has been described both by Sinclair[23] and by Torrance[24] and involves an assessment of efficacy, effectiveness, efficiency and availability of NICU programmes. The type of evaluation depends on the question raised because third party payers are interested in cost-benefit analysis, whereas health care groups are more interested in the outcome of treatment or analysis of cost-effectiveness. Most outcome studies have not addressed these issues.[25] Costs are difficult to define and the rapidly changing nature of neonatal care, survival rates and morbidity statistics make frequent replication of studies imperative.

Despite these difficulties it is important that neonatal intensive care units develop the capability of monitoring their activity. This demands a greater consciousness of the costs of services, learning to prioritize finite resources and attempting to standardize outcome measures such that decisions regarding the provision of neonatal intensive care do not become random or politically determined but are based on as accurate and appropriate information as is possible.

Discharge planning

For parents, discharge from a supportive environment may be a very stressful time and this has led to the development of prospective discharge planning. It is extremely important that parents be provided with the knowledge and skills to care for their child, particularly those with residual problems. Standardized teaching for specific needs such as low flow oxygen, gastrostomy feeding, nasogastric tube feeding, or ventriculoperitoneal shunt care, etc. are provided for parents and other relevant health care workers. The time and energy spent in the detailed follow-up arrangements, identifying the needs of the individual child and their family, and communication with other hospital or community resources greatly improves parental confidence in caring for their special child and decreases inappropriate outpatient or emergency department visits.[26]

Follow-up

A follow-up programme is an integral part of any acute neonatal intensive care unit's activities. Outcome data provide important measures of the quality of acute care and may be used to modify practice.

The objectives of a follow-up programme usually include the following:

1. To evaluate the outcome of NICU patients in a comprehensive and systematic manner to determine the incidence and degree of disability in growth and neurodevelopment and specific morbidity such as bronchopulmonary dysplasia or retinopathy of prematurity.

2. To provide early identification of problems or special needs so that intervention and continuing care can be instituted.

3. To provide education, support and counselling for parents since their involvement in follow-up has a significant impact on the success of any treatment.[27] There is controversy over whether early intervention programmes or physiotherapy influence developmental outcome.[28] Parental encouragement and demonstration of simple measures, such as language and visual stimulation, handling techniques, positioning, etc., are appropriate[29] and may significantly affect outcome.

4. A further objective is the collection of longitudinal data and long-term outcome measures of specific research protocols, interventions or modes of therapy.

The focus of most follow-up programs is the 'high risk' infant, identified by birth weight < 1500 gm or medical complications such as intraventricular haemorrhage, meningitis, chronic lung disease, perinatal asphyxia, growth restriction or major social factors. Post surgical infants have not been generally regarded as high risk unless their hospital course has been complicated by one or more of these factors.

Assessments in follow-up include full general and neurological examination, measurement of growth parameters (weight, linear growth and head circumference) and developmental, hearing and speech evaluation.

Developmental disabilities are usually evident within the first two years and include fine and gross motor abnormalities, sensory and cognitive deficits including visual and hearing loss, receptive and expressive language delay, behavioural disorders, attention deficits and seizure disorders.

Any infant who displays evidence of one developmental disability should be globally evaluated, as brain damage is more likely to be diffuse than focal. Motor problems identified early may require intervention. However, delay in visual or mental development may only become evident later, but may be more handicapping in the long-term.[29]

While these major sequelae have been easiest to quantify, current longer–term studies are bringing to light a 'new morbidity', the neurodevelopmental and behavioural sequelae in very low birthweight infants as they enter the school system. This involves more subtle identification of average to borderline intelligence, school difficulties requiring the repeating of courses or special education, difficulty with visual–motor integration, fine and gross motor incoordination and behavioural problems.[28,30–32]

A wealth of literature over the past ten to 20 years has appeared on the outcome of very low birthweight infants. In infants 1000–1500 gm, where survival is currently 95 per cent, there is little debate regarding the provision of neonatal intensive care diminishing returns. However, the value of extending intensive care to progressively smaller infants has been questioned.[33,34]

Numerous factors make the interpretation of outcome data difficult, e.g. methodological problems, in-born versus out-born differences, population- or centre-based studies, eligibility criteria for studies, lack of control groups, lack of description of treatments provided, socioeconomic and demographic characteristics of the groups of infants being compared, as well as difficulties in the classification and standardization of morbidity.

Death in the NICU

The frequency with which death occurs in the NICU and the impact that it has on parents and staff make it imperative that each member of the medical and nursing team learns to face their own fears, anxieties and potential sense of failure. Every unit should develop its own philosophy for the management of this important issue. Death may come within hours of admission or may be months after a prolonged and difficult course; it may be totally unexpected or relatively easily predicted; it may occur as the result of the withdrawal of life-sustaining therapy or in spite of its continued use. Although every situation is different, it is essential that the NICU staff provide consistent and compassionate support to parents through the dying and death of their infant, as the nature of this support may have a major impact on the parents' grief and mourning process.[35,36]

Even though there is increasing sensitivity to the wishes of parents of dying infants and more open discussion about the entire subject, parents may still often perceive an unwillingness of medical staff to talk about the possibility of death, or parents themselves may be reluctant to discuss the topic. This makes it extremely difficult to determine the level of staff input that is appropriate in each situation and calls for a flexible and individual approach.

While an individual staff member's display of sensitivity and empathy will often be remembered by parents, it is important that they are supported by all staff in a systematic way. This entails formalizing, to a degree, a series of steps in support of the family. This will incorporate many of the following[37,38]:

1. Consideration of the possibility of the child being transferred to a hospital closer to home, the parents taking the child home to die or, as a minimum, providing a quiet room ensuring privacy within the NICU, so as to encourage parents to participate in a hospice-type care in the child's last days.[39]
2. Consideration of the use of narcotics to provide relief of pain and suffering.
3. The promotion of open expression of feelings and preparation for death by extended family members, and discussion about death with siblings.
4. Providing advice on the expected grieving process.
5. Providing written resource material on bereavement support groups.
6. Assembling a memory package including photographs.
7. Discussion about the potential usefulness of an autopsy examination as an aid to establishing the cause of death and discerning any other possible factors which may impact on future pregnancies.
8. Follow-up with parents via telephone or direct review or discussion of autopsy findings where an autopsy has been done.[40,41]

Support for the NICU staff includes participation in a coordinated bereavement programme and providing them with opportunities to express their own responses to death.

Respiratory support

Management of the airway

The technique for prolonged tracheal intubation as an alternative to tracheostomy in children quickly gained favour following Brandstater's[42] initial report in 1962 of its successful use in 12 children and the recommendations of several groups in 1965.[43–5] Although tracheostomy had previously been extensively used in infants by some groups with good results,[46] others had reported considerable morbidity.[43,47,48]

Intubation

If the infant is to be intubated postoperatively for IPPV or CPAP, it is better to change the tube from an orotracheal to a nasotracheal one for what may be prolonged respiratory support. Nasal tubes are preferred for long-term intubation because the fixation is more secure, there is greater comfort for the patient and ease of nursing, which includes improved mouth care, and also allows the infant to suck.

Although oral tracheal intubation is very widely practised by neonatologists and is satisfactory in the immediate newborn period, particularly in preterm infants, paediatric anaesthetists tend to favour the nasal route for the advantages of comfort and security. The oral fixation which may be associated with dental, palatal and tracheal damage, is certainly unsuitable for prolonged intubation after the immediate neonatal period. Prolonged nasotracheal intubation for respiratory support is now a well accepted technique for all age groups in paediatric practice. Ratner and Whitfield[49] report a significant incidence of acquired subglottic stenosis in infants below 1500 gm who were orally intubated.

Each neonatal centre tends to develop its favoured method of fixation, but that described by Reid and Tunstall[50] is particularly popular in the United Kingdom. The tube should be radio-opaque, have clear centimetre graduations and a Murphy 'eye' to overcome inadvertent obstruction of the bevel of the tube by the side wall of the trachea. Shouldered tubes of the Cole type are not used because they have significantly greater resistance to gas flow caused by turbulence at the shoulder and are associated with an incidence of laryngeal damage.[57]

With the oral tracheal tube still in place and an assistant ventilating the baby, an uncut 3 mm (or 2.5 mm) plain PVC (tissue tested) nasotracheal tube is lubricated and passed through the nares as far as the glottis. This is done using a laryngoscope. The tracheal tube is cut to the desired length so that its tip lies midway between the glottis and the carina – an extra 3 cm on the length of the tube. A Tunstall connection or similar device is fixed into the nasal tube and, as the oral tube is removed by the assistant, the nasal one is inserted through the glottis using intubating forceps and then secured. Auscultation should reveal bilateral air entry and a check chest X-ray should show the tip of the tracheal tube lying in the midpoint of the trachea, i.e. between the heads of the clavicles. The correct size of tracheal tube is that which allows normal controlled ventilation with the application of constant distending pressure if this is required, but which also allows a slight air leak at an airway pressure of 25–30 cmH$_2$O (Table 5.1).

Table 5.1 Nasal tracheal tube sizes for newborns

Patient's weight (kg)	Tube size (i.d.) (mm)	Tube length (cm)
0.7–1.0	2.5	8.5–9.0
1.0–1.5	2.5	9.0–9.5
1.5–2.0	3.0	9.5–10.0
2.0–2.5	3.0	10.0–10.5
2.5–3.0	3.0	10.5–11.0

The leak must be present at all times and checked daily. If the leak disappears (subglottic oedema), this is an indication for the tracheal tube to be changed to one a size smaller (not smaller than 2.5 mm internal diameter). It is common practice to change the tube from one nostril to the other every ten days to preserve the symmetry of the nostrils and to minimize pressure sores at the nares.

After this length of time, the plastic of the tube hardens as plasticizers are leached out. Small rings of 'Stomadhesive' or plastic foam around the tube also help to prevent pressure of the tube and connector on the nares. When the tube is changed the tip of the old tube should be sent to the laboratory for microbiology examination.

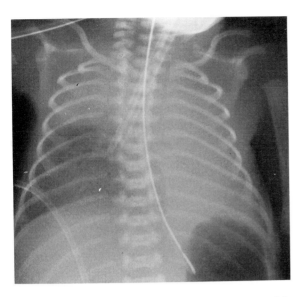

Fig. 5.1 Complication of ventilation. AP X-ray of the chest shows the tip of the tracheal tube in the bronchus intermedius. The right lower and middle lobes are aerated, but there is collapse of the right upper lobe and the entire left lung, with shift of the heart and nasogastric tube towards the left.

Earlier changing of the tube may be necessary in patients with low cardiac output or cyanotic congenital heart disease, as ulceration occurs more commonly in these patients.   With meticulous care it is possible to use tracheal tubes for respiratory support for prolonged periods with a very low complication rate.

All the complications of prolonged tracheal intubation are avoidable.[52,53]

1. Dislodgement by accident is prevented by firm fixation of the tube which is of the correct length. Secondary fixation of a short catheter-mount to the forehead prevents traction on the ventilator tubing being directly transmitted to the tracheal tube. Such an accident need not be a disaster in a good intensive care unit if the problem is recognized promptly. Dislodgement is less likely to occur if the patient is maintained in a lightly sedated state.

2. Blockage of the tube by inspissated secretions is prevented by humidification of the inspired gases to full saturation at a temperature approaching that of the body (35–44 mg of water vapour per litre gas flow at 37°C = 80–100 per cent relative humidity). When the trachea is intubated, together with increases in inspired oxygen concentrations, ciliary action is decreased and the cough mechanism ineffective and yet mucus production may be increased. Most commercial humidifiers do not come up to these standards and some of the water vapour condenses in the patient tubing. Good practice, therefore, is to instill 0.5 ml physiological saline down the tracheal tube every 2–3 hours or more often if necessary, followed by suction with a sterile soft catheter.

Tracheobronchial secretions must be suctioned frequently as retained secretions cause atelectasis, decreased pulmonary compliance and a predisposition to infection.

However, suctioning is potentially hazardous, as it may introduce infection; disposable gloves should be worn and a sterile technique used. It may also cause dangerous hypoxia because ventilation is discontinued and intrapulmonary oxygen concentration is reduced to a degree proportional to the length of time suctioning takes place. The application of negative pressure causes a greater degree of hypoxia than would an equal period of apnoea. Suction pressure should be limited to 100–150 mmHg and suction time to 15 seconds with suction taking place only on withdrawal of the catheter. Techniques do exist whereby suctioning can take place while IPPV continues. Negative pressure is minimized in the airways if the diameter of the suction catheter does not exceed 70 per cent of the tracheal tube diameter – this is difficult when small tubes are used. Suction can also cause traumatic lesions of the tracheal mucosa, but these are minimized if soft catheters with an end hole (not whistle-tip) are used. The nursing staff should always know the exact length of the tracheal tube and ensure that the suction catheter passed is longer than this, otherwise secretions at the tracheal end of the tube may not be reached.

3. Subglottic stenosis is potentially the most serious long-term complication. Stocks[54] demonstrated convincingly that subglottic stenosis could be avoided if the tube used was always small enough to allow a slight leak of air around it when positive pressure is applied, i.e. the tube is never too tight in the subglottic cricoid ring of cartilage. The effectiveness of this policy in avoiding subglottic stenosis has recently been confirmed in a large series including over 700 neonatal patients.[55]

Pressure on the mucosa causes necrosis and

ulceration which eventually heals with fibrous stricture. When the trachea is intubated for infective lesions in older infants, such as laryngotracheobronchitis or acute epiglottitis, exactly the same criteria are used for sizing the tracheal tube, although usually a tube considerably smaller than normal is needed to achieve the mandatory leak.

In a series of 5000 babies and children with prolonged intubation over the past ten years at Great Ormond Street there has been no case of subglottic stenosis.

4. Postextubation stridor occurs rarely and is most commonly seen after short intubations (24–36 hours) or in patients with Down's syndrome. Very rarely does the condition require reintubation, but usually responds to dexamethasone 0.25 mg.kg^{-1} i.v. followed by 0.1 mg.kg^{-1} i.m. 6-hourly for 12 hours, or nebulized adrenaline (0.5–1 ml of 1 : 10 000 plus 1 ml saline). If a baby does require to be reintubated because of laryngeal or subglottic oedema a tube 0.5 mm smaller should be used.

5. Nasal ulcers may occur even with careful techniques. These heal normally if the tube is changed to the other nostril.

Suctioning and instillations of saline take the place of natural expulsion of secretions by mucociliary activity and coughing. Intubated patients should also receive chest physiotherapy 2- to 4-hourly as a prophylactic measure and all the techniques of physiotherapy – vibration, percussion, manual lung expansion – are applicable to the neonate, although care must be taken in patients whose cardiac function is poor as a fall in PaO$_2$ may cause a further fall in cardiac output. An electric toothbrush may be used for vibration of consolidated lobes and manual ventilation with air or oxygen with a few sustained breaths of 25 cm H$_2$O pressure will expand alveoli collapsed by suction or atelectasis associated with secretions.

There is no place for bronchoscopy for removal of secretions or for treatment of lobar collapse. These conditions are more safely dealt with by intubation and physiotherapy.

Because of the very low morbidity of tracheal intubation in all sizes of neonates it is usual to institute mechanical ventilation only after the patient has been intubated. This is not universal practice, as in some centres babies are ventilated with tightly fitting face masks or through a nasal prong. This is possible only if pulmonary compliance is near normal and ventilating pressures are low.

Securing the airway with a tube has the additional advantage of allowing full tracheal toilet.

Tracheostomy

The indications for tracheostomy in neonates are now almost exclusively limited to those with upper airway abnormalities such as micrognathia, congenital subglottic stenosis, vocal cord paralysis, laryngomalacia and subglottic haemangioma. Neonates requiring very long-term ventilatory support may occasionally be better managed with tracheostomy, though long-term tracheal intubation can be performed with an acceptably low incidence of complications and tracheostomy has virtually no role in patients without pre-existing upper airway pathology for the first three to six weeks. However, at the end of this time, if there is no sign that full respiratory support can be discontinued in the foreseeable future, then tracheostomy may be a better alternative.

Tracheostomy is more convenient for the nursing staff and enables the patients to become more mobile and more easily stimulated. There is a lower resistance to gas flow and a small but often significant decrease in dead space and occasionally a patient previously dependent on mechanical ventilation will start to wean from full respiratory support.

Management of respiratory distress

Supportive measures and oxygen administration:

1. Skilled and effective resuscitation at the time of delivery and early recognition of distress may significantly reduce the severity of subsequent respiratory distress and the incidence of complications.

2. Thermal neutrality is necessary to maintain oxygen consumption at minimal levels. This is usually achieved via servo-controlled temperature monitoring of the infant.

3. The administration of oxygen to prevent and/or correct the effects of hypoxia requires careful monitoring; oxygen should be administered in the lowest concentration and for the briefest periods needed to achieve the desired therapeutic goal. The aim of oxygen therapy in the newborn with acute respiratory distress is to

maintain the PaO_2 in the range of 7–10 kPa (50–70 mmHg). In term or post-term infants the range may be somewhat higher, 7.5–12 kPa (60–80 mmHg) (Table 5.3).

Monitoring of oxygenation

When oxygen requirements exceed 40 per cent or where it is anticipated that accurate oxygen measurement will be required in a distressed infant for more than 24 hours, direct or invasive means of measurement of arterial oxygenation are usually undertaken.

Arterial PO_2 measured via umbilical artery catheterization (UAC) is the most common method of oxygen measurement, particularly in premature infants. Umbilical arterial catheters should be placed either 'high', T8 to T10 (above the origin of the coelic axis), or 'low', between L3 and L4 (below the renal arteries and above the bifurcation of the aorta). An abdominal radiograph must be taken to confirm the correct positioning of an umbilical catheter.

Umbilical artery catheters are occasionally complicated by vasospasm, thromboembolism, blood loss, infection or NEC. The most common of these is vasospasm, manifested by ischaemia to the ipsilateral leg or toes; if blue or pale discolouration persists after brief warming of the contralateral leg, the catheter should be removed. The UAC has been the easiest and most reliable means of monitoring O_2 therapy; however, in the light of the potential risks, greater use is being made of percutaneous arterial catheters placed in the radial, posterior tibial or dorsalis pedis arteries. These catheters have lower rates of complications.

Intermittent arterial sampling via percutaneous aspiration of the radial or brachial artery must be performed without unduly disturbing the infant for the sample to be an accurate reflection of the infant's oxygenation status. It is commonly used as an adjunct to continuous non–invasive monitoring.

Arterialized capillary PO_2 obtained by heel puncture after warming the infant's foot provides an accurate measurement of pH and PCO_2, but systematic underestimation of PO_2 measurements when compared to arterial values.

Intermittent sampling of arterial blood is not necessarily as accurate a reflection of the steady state of the infant as desired and it is therefore used in conjunction with non-invasive means of continuous oxygen monitoring.

Non-invasive monitoring

Transcutaneous ($TcPO_2$) monitors are an accurate reflection of arterial oxygen tension, provided that an appropriate electrode temperature is used for a given skin thickness and the circulatory status of the infant is adequate. The accuracy of $TcPO_2$ monitoring is affected by patient factors, e.g. decreased perfusion, the presence of oedema or an increase in the infant's temperature, as well as a decrease in skin permeability with increasing postnatal age. Equipment factors such as the calibration and clinical application of the electrodes also affect accuracy.

Skin surface carbon dioxide electrodes measure the concentration of CO_2 on the surface of the skin. The electrodes are less affected by skin thickness or membrane permeability.

Pulse oximetry is the estimation of oxygen saturation of arterial blood (SaO_2) using pulsatile changes in light transmission by comparing the absorbances of light during systole and diastole. It has become widely used in the NICU because of its accuracy and the fact that no calibration, heating or membrane changes are required.[56,57] The response time of the pulse oximeter to changes in SaO_2 is almost immediate; this fast response time, coupled with a high degree of sensitivity to interference with movement or even brief physiological changes in the infant, requires that appropriate clinical assessment be made prior to an immediate response to a low SaO_2 reading. The disadvantage of pulse oximetry is its potential inaccuracy in the detection of hyperoxaemia because of the non linear relationship between PO_2 and SaO_2. Minimal changes in haemoglobin oxygen saturation may occur in association with large changes in oxygen tension in the upper portion of the oxyhaemoglobin dissociation curve e.g. a small rise in SaO_2 from 90 to 98 may represent an increase in PO_2 of 5.5–7 kPa (40–50 mmHg). Therefore if pulse oximetry is used to monitor the oxygen status of the low birthweight neonate it is essential that a correlating PaO_2 sample be within acceptable range.

Patient factors which may prevent the valid application of pulse oximetry include hypotension, severe oedema or inadequate peripheral perfusion.

Venous obstruction does not reduce accuracy but delays detection time, as do vibration and movement of the probe. There is a greater incidence of artefact with small fingers, and probes perform well if movement between finger and probe can be minimized.[58]

Table 5.2 Comparison of transcutaneous and pulse oximetry

$TcPO_2$	Pulse oximeter
Requires heat, therefore potential for skin burns	Does not require heat
Not as rapid response and not as subject to wide swings with minor changes in infant	Very rapid response time (may be inaccurate and overly sensitive to small changes in oxygenation, movement artifacts, etc)
Affected by skin thickness and skin blood flow	Not affected by skin thickness
Affected by circulatory status and may be indicator of poor perfusion	Affected by circulatory status but not to same degree as $TcPO_2$
Protection from hypoxia and hyperoxia	Protection from hyperoxia not assured because of oxygen dissociation curve
Requires calibration and frequent site changes but requires infrequent correlation with arterial PO_2	No calibration or site changes but more frequent requirement for PaO_2 correlation
More applicable in acute care of premature infants	More applicable to older infant with chronic lung disease

Table 5.3 Guidelines for acceptable ranges of values

$TcPO_2$	SaO_2
Preterm 7–10 kPa (50–70 mmHg)	88–92
Term 7.5–11 kPa (60–80 mmHg)	90–95
PPHN>13 kPa (>90 mmHg)	>95
BPD >7 kPa (>50 mmHg)	90–94

Nowadays, pulse oximetry is a mandatory form of monitoring postoperatively and in the intensive care unit.

Arterial blood gas monitoring

The measurement of arterial blood gases is an indispensable component of the management of respiratory distress as they provide essential information regarding oxygenation, ventilation and acid-base status of the infant. Measurement of the partial pressure of oxygen, the partial pressure of carbon dioxide and the pH is performed from samples of whole blood collected anaerobically. Measurement of the PCO_2 and pH, according to the Henderson–Hasselbalch equation, is sufficient for calculation of $[HCO_3]$ in the same specimen. Analysis must be done within minutes to avoid changes in gas tension caused by RBC metabolism and gas diffusion across the walls of plastic syringes; air bubbles increase PO_2 and pH and decrease PCO_2; excess heparin also alters the results. If immediate analysis is not feasible the sample should be stored in ice and analysed as soon as possible. In the interpretation of blood gases it is essential to know the inspired oxygen concentration, the sampling site (pre or postductal) and the potential effect of the sampling itself, e.g. if the infant is crying. Although arterial blood is customarily used as it is essential for assessment of oxygenation, the arteriovenous differences in pH and PCO_2 are small and relatively constant and venous blood can occasionally be used if one is interested only in the assessment of acid-base balance. The venous pH is usually 0.03 to 0.04 units lower and venous PCO_2 approximately 1 kPa (7 mmHg) higher than arterial values.

Blood gases should be measured within 15 to 30 minutes of initiation of mechanical ventilation, changes in respiratory settings or changes in an infant's clinical condition. Alterations in respiratory settings are dictated by changes in PaO_2 and $PaCO_2$ and by the clinical situation.

Assessing the adequacy of oxygenation.

The PaO_2 is generally maintained between 7–10 kPa (50–70 mmHg). PaO_2 values less than 6–7 kPa (45–50 mmHg) are associated with vasoconstriction of the pulmonary vasculature, pulmonary hypertension, reduced pulmonary blood flow, right to left shunting and systemic hypoxia and acidosis. PaO_2 values greater than 14 kPa

(100 mmHg) have been associated with retinal vascular injury and other forms of oxygen toxicity.

In RDS the severity of the hypoxaemia is related to the severity of the hypoxia in the open underventilated lung units, the alveolar PAO_2. Calculation of the alveolar–arterial PO_2 difference therefore provides an indication of the severity of the respiratory distress. The alveolar oxygen tension (PAO_2) can be calculated with a simplified version of the alveolar–air equation: $PAO_2 = PIO_2 - PACO_2$, where PIO_2 is the partial pressure of oxygen in the inspired gas and $PACO_2$ is the partial pressure of CO_2 in the alveoli. PIO_2 is determined by multiplying FIO_2 by the barometric pressure minus water vapour pressure (at body temperature this has a constant value of 47 mmHg). $PACO_2$ approximates arterial PCO_2.

The difference between the alveolar and arterial O_2 (A–aDO_2) can therefore be calculated. The A–aDO_2 is normally < 3 kPa (< 25 mmHg) while the infant is breathing room air and may be as high as 85 kPa (600 mmHg) in an infant with RDS breathing 100 per cent oxygen.

The assessment of the oxygenation status provided by measurement of the PaO_2 must obviously be supplemented by assessment of other components of the oxygen delivery system, i.e. cardiovascular function, the amount and function of haemoglobin, the distribution of peripheral blood flow and the oxygen utilization by tissues. Assessment of the total oxygen delivery system is therefore via a combination of clinical signs, oxygen saturation monitoring, arterial PaO_2 and assessment of the acid-base status.

Assessment of ventilation

Adequacy of alveolar ventilation is assessed simply in terms of arterial PCO_2. The normal resting arterial PCO_2 in the newborn is ± 4.7–5.1 kPa (33–36 mmHg) in the first 12–48 hours. Whenever CO_2 production (derived from tissue respiration) is increased, if ventilation, either spontaneous or assisted, does not adjust to keep the PCO_2 within normal range it will increase, leading to a respiratory acidosis. A usually accepted goal of assisted ventilation is to maintain the $PaCO_2$ at 7 kPa (50 mmHg) or less and the pH 7.3 or greater. However, the upper limit for CO_2 must be individualized for each infant based on birthweight, gestational age, underlying disease process, stage and progression of the disease, chest radiograph, pH and degree of metabolic compensation.

The onset of acute hypercapnia is associated with a reduction in pH, as only a small increase in plasma bicarbonate occurs as a function of cellular or tissue buffering. The metabolic compensation for a primary change in arterial PCO_2 thereafter pursues a characteristic time course over a number of days to weeks, depending upon the infant's renal adaptive mechanisms. (The transition from acute to chronic respiratory acidosis may be considered the point at which the renal compensation for a primary respiratory acidosis becomes manifest.) These adaptive responses stimulate renal tubular reabsorption of bicarbonate. Chloride stores are depleted as the increased acid excretion is largely in the form of ammonium chloride.

Tubular reabsorption of bicarbonate is fixed by the level of $PaCO_2$; a new steady state concentration develops and a predictable relationship exists between the degree of hypercapnia and the increased plasma bicarbonate level at which it has stabilized. It should be remembered that in the term infant in the first one to two days of life the normal bicarbonate is ± 20 mmol.l^{-1} and may be much lower in the preterm. Compensation with an increase in the serum bicarbonate leads to an increase over subsequent weeks. For each mmHg increase in PCO_2 the bicarbonate concentration increase is about 0.3 mmol. By about two weeks of age a urine pH of 4.5 to 5.3 can be achieved. It is important always to have the full arterial blood gas picture and not only the PCO_2 value, as lowering the PCO_2 abruptly in an infant adapted to chronic hypercapnia (e.g. an infant with BPD) may readily result in posthypercapnic metabolic alkalosis.

Assessment of acid-base status

Arterial blood pH represents the balance between hydrogen ion concentration and base substance availability for buffering. It is normally maintained within a narrow range by cellular, buffering, respiratory and renal mechanisms. In the normal term infant the pH is greater than 7.3 from one hour after birth and between 7.35 to 7.4 from 24 hours of age.

It is imperative to determine the primary nature of an acid-base disorder, i.e. whether it is respiratory or metabolic in origin. This requires knowledge of the full blood gases. In an acute respiratory acidosis reference to the $PaCO_2$/pH relationship will usually determine whether the pH is more acidic than anticipated for the PCO_2 and whether a degree of metabolic acidosis is also present.

The detection and management of a metabolic acidosis complicating the course of an infant with respiratory distress is an important component of management of these infants. Metabolic acidosis may increase pulmonary vascular resistance, impair surfactant synthesis and decrease cardiac output. The aetiology of a metabolic acidosis must therefore always be determined and managed appropriately. Causes include tissue hypoxia secondary to hypotension (hypovolaemia, excess intrathoracic pressure secondary to positive pressure ventilation, pneumothorax), excess work of breathing, PDA with congestive heart failure, asphyxia, severe anaemia, sepsis, intraventricular haemorrhage and hyperalimentation with excess protein intake.

A conservative approach to the management of a mild metabolic acidosis is usually sufficient if the cause is determined in a patient who is not severely ill. Occasionally pharmacologic intervention with slow infusion of sodium bicarbonate may be appropriate in a severely ill patient in whom the primary cause has been treated without correction of the pH. The use of sodium bicarbonate is contra-indicated in a primary respiratory acidosis as it may lead not only to hypercapnia but also to a decrease in PaO_2 and pulmonary perfusion.

Blood pressure monitoring

Infants with respiratory distress require close blood pressure monitoring; hypovolaemia with poor peripheral perfusion requires blood pressure support with appropriate volume expanders. Inotropic support may also be beneficial in improving the circulation, cardiac output and stroke volume and promoting a diuresis, although low dose dopamine does not appear to have a significant beneficial effect on respiratory parameters.[59]

Maintenance fluids

Maintainance fluid requirements require initiation of a peripheral intravenous infusion of 5–10 per cent dextrose solution to provide $\pm$ 60 ml.kg.$^{-1}$day. Fluid restriction is indicated for the first 48 hours or until diuresis occurs. Fluid requirements are dependent upon the status of the intravascular volume, blood pressure and serum electrolytes and restriction may not be possible in very low birthweight infants with excessive insensible water losses. The infant is not fed enterally in the early stages of respiratory distress.

Administration of antibiotics

As acute respiratory distress due to pneumonia and/or bacteraemia may occur in infants without a suggestive history, infants with more than minimal respiratory distress require appropriate specimens for culture (usually blood only in early onset sepsis) and initiation of antimicrobial therapy. Antibiotics are specifically indicated in an infant in whom respiratory distress develops after a period of hours to days during which time the infant was asymptomatic. Blood, CSF and urine cultures are usually all indicated.

Minimal handling and stimulation

The numerous interventions to which sick infants are subjected, e.g. tracheal suctioning, blood sampling, weighing, all tend to decrease arterial oxygen tension and should be kept to a minimum. Nursing the infant in the prone position tends to improve oxygenation and reduce the work of breathing.

Sedation/pain relief

Sedative or narcotic agents are being increasingly used as adjuncts to the management of the ventilated newborn. The recognition of the newborn's ability to perceive pain and the stress response induced by it have made it imperative that attention be paid to this aspect of care.[60,61]

While much can be done to assist the ventilated infant to acquire a calm, quiet state via non–pharmacologic means, e.g. positioning in a comfortable, flexed, prone position, the use of non–nutritive sucking, swaddling, decreasing environmental stimuli, etc., pharmacologic agents should be considered, particularly in postoperative infants, those with chest tubes in situ or those subjected to numerous procedures.

It is important to define the goal of such therapy, e.g. sedation only or analgesia or both. Sedation can be achieved with chloral hydrate (30 mg.kg^{-1}), benzodiazepines or barbiturates. However, sedative use remains controversial in ventilated infants and their administration has not been shown to permit lower levels of respiratory support.[62] In addition, these agents do not have analgesic activity; in fact both chloral hydrate and barbiturates have antalgesic properties, i.e. they may cause a greater perception of pain than if no drug were given.[63]

In addition to or instead of analgesia, most intubated babies require sedation and suitable drugs include diazepam or midazolam in a bolus dose of 0.2 mg.kg^{-1} followed by a continuous infusion of 0.4 μg.kg^{-1}.min.[64] For babies with intact enteral function chloral hydrate or one of its related compounds at 30 mg.kg^{-1} every 3–4 hours is an excellent sedative for intermittent use. This agent, even in higher doses, does not alter the CO_2 chemoreceptor drive in newborns, so is an ideal drug for sedation during weaning from the ventilator. Where pain is anticipated or suspected, narcotic analgesics such as morphine should be used. However, respiratory depressants should be used only in settings in which extremely close monitoring is available so that appropriate ventilatory support can be provided. Morphine provides effective analgesia: the onset of action is immediate and it may be given as 0.1–0.2 mg.kg^{-1} intravenously or intramuscularly 2–4 hourly or preferably via continuous infusion 0.01–0.02 mg.kg^{-1}.hr with the infusion rate titrated to clinical response.[65] The depression of respiratory drive is an advantage so that mechanical ventilation easily controls respiration at lower airway pressures. For the weaning process the administered dose can be reduced as is clinically appropriate, though a low dose in the range of 5–10 μg.kg^{-1}.hr may benefit the weaning from the ventilator. For babies with labile pulmonary vascular resistance (PVR) in whom morphine may cause rises in PVR and systemic hypotension, fentanyl is the preferred drug in doses of 1–5 μg.kg^{-1}.hr by continuous infusion. In addition to the infusion bolus doses of up to 20 μg.kg^{-1} may be given to obtund the reaction to physiotherapy and suctioning of the tracheal tube. Recently it has been suggested that non-surgical newborns intubated for mechanical ventilation with invasive monitoring should receive analgesia routinely.

Side effects include decreased gastrointestinal motility, respiratory depression, hypotension and occasionally urinary retention. Toxicity has rarely been reported in neonates. However, tolerance requiring escalation of doses to obtain an analgesic effect has been observed. The related physical dependence and adaptive state that is manifest by intense physical disturbances when the administration of the drug is suspended indicate that the drug should be tapered rather than discontinued abruptly once relief of discomfort and pain has been controlled for a period of time.

Neuromuscular paralysis

Consideration for neuromuscular paralysis via neuromuscular blocking agents such as pancuronium (0.05–0.1 mg.kg^{-1}) may arise in infants with strong (particularly expiratory) efforts, to reduce asynchrony with the ventilator. Relaxants are used in an attempt to improve oxygenation, reduce fluctuations in heart rate, blood pressure, intracranial pressure (ICP), cerebral blood flow velocity and thereby possibly decrease the incidence of pneumothorax, intraventricular haemorrhage (IVH) and barotrauma. There is often a significant immediate benefit in intractable hypoxaemic situations. The routine use of paralysis, however, is not recommended as it may affect heart rate and blood pressure in either direction, it may adversely affect ventilation requiring increases in ventilator parameters, and more negative haemodynamic effects of positive airway pressure may become evident. Its effect may be potentiated by acidosis, hypothermia and the concurrent administration of aminoglycosides. With prolonged usage fluid retention, oedema, jaundice and ileus (with loss of the radiographic abdominal gas pattern) may occur.

Paralysis removes the ability to make a clinical assessment of the central nervous system. It must also be appreciated by clinical staff that these agents have no sedative or analgesic effects. This therefore makes it imperative that infants described as 'agitated' or 'fighting the ventilator' be accurately assessed and that pain, hypoxaemia or hypercarbia be appropriately treated prior to initiating paralysis for asynchrony with a particular mode of assisted ventilation.

Surfactant replacement therapy

Following the demonstration that a lack of surfactant was central to the pathophysiology of respiratory distress syndrome (RDS), exogenous surfactant containing aerosolized dipalmitoyl phosphatidylcholine (DPPC), the major surface active phospholipid, given via the airways to prevent or decrease the severity of RDS has become widely utilized.[66–71] Numerous surfactant preparations have been produced: these include modified natural surfactants, human surfactant harvested from term amniotic fluid at the time of elective Caesarean section and artificial surfactants. Trials in which surfactant is given at birth are referred to as prophylactic trials and those in which surfactant is given to infants with RDS requiring ventilation, as 'rescue' therapy.

Analysis[72-74] of the numerous trials that have been conducted thus far shows that:

1. Surfactant is effective in improving oxygenation, reducing ventilatory support requirements and decreasing the incidence of pulmonary air leaks; there is a slower improvement in compliance and PCO_2 values. This has been seen in both prophylactic trials and with rescue treatment when surfactant has been used in babies up to 24 hours old. The improvement in oxygenation is demonstrated in most trials during the first three days, with less effect evident by seven days of age.

2. Multiple doses of surfactant may have short-term advantages over single doses, although the response to surfactant reflects, at least in part, the severity of the underlying RDS. The requirement for retreatment is generally associated with worse disease and a higher mortality. The recent OSIRIS trial provided no evidence that a regimen including the option of third and fourth doses when signs of RDS persist or recur is clinically superior to a regimen of two doses.[75]

3. Artificial surfactants appear comparable in efficacy to natural surfactants.

4. Surfactant has not reduced the incidence of necrotizing enterocolitis (NEC), ROP or sepsis; surfactant has been associated with an increased incidence of pulmonary haemorrhage. An anticipated decrease in the incidence of IVH has not thus far been borne out.

5. The effect on the incidence of patent ductus arteriosies (PDA) has been variable: in one study surfactant administration did not appear to alter the incidence nor affect natural closure or the magnitude of L-to-R shunting.[76] However, no trial has shown a significant reduction in PDA and in some rescue trials with natural surfactant an increase in the incidence of PDA was shown.

6. Significant improvements in survival rates have been shown in a number of studies. The effect on the incidence of bronchopulmonary dysplasia (BPD) is variable; a trend towards a decrease in BPD has been shown, but this has often required the combined endpoint of BPD or death during the first 28 days of life to be evaluated.

7. Follow up of infants has shown no adverse differences in growth, neurological or developmental parameters.[77-79]

A number of questions remain. Which surfactant preparation is optimal? Should surfactant be used as prophylaxis or rescue? This latter question raises the fact that with prophylactic therapy 20–40 per cent of low birthweight infants would be treated unnecessarily. While there may not be clinical justification for routinely using a prophylactic approach to surfactant therapy, the earlier the surfactant is used in the course of RDS, the more beneficial it appears to be.[80] The role of surfactant in respiratory diseases other than RDS is also beginning to be explored.[81]

Surfactant administration requires adherence to a unit protocol in which the indications are firmly established, the method, dose and frequency of administration determined, and the monitoring requirements defined. Monitoring requires close clinical assessment and use of transcutaneous oxygen, cardio-respiratory and blood pressure monitoring. Transient adverse effects include tracheal tube blockage and pulmonary haemorrhage, both of which require prompt detection and treatment. The period immediately following administration may also require rapid changes in ventilatory management.

The radiographic changes following surfactant administration vary from no significant differences between surfactant treated infants and saline treated controls to more impressive changes with clearing of the lung changes. In some infants a transient, diffuse interstitial process is seen.[82] The effect of surfactant administration in decreasing the immediate problems associated with mechanical ventilation is reflected radiographically in a decreased incidence of pulmonary interstitial emphysema and pneumothorax. In general, radiographic changes do not appear to correlate well with the clinical improvement seen with surfactant treatment.[83]

Management of Persistent Pulmonary Hypertension of the Newborn (PPHN)

The principles of management of PPHN complicating many respiratory disorders include:

1. Treatment of the specific cause of PPHN if present, e.g. polycythaemia, sepsis.

2. Prevention of hypoxia, acidosis and cold stress and avoidance of factors which may increase intrathoracic pressure and thereby decrease pulmonary blood flow, e.g. suctioning, excessive handling.

3. Decreasing pulmonary artery pressure by mechanical ventilation.

4. Volume expansion with frequent use of colloid to maintain BP. In addition, increasing systemic blood pressure to minimize right to left ductal shunting may be achieved with the use of inotropic agents such as dopamine and/or dobutamine. Cardiotonic agents are also used in those infants with evidence of cardiomyopathy or myocardial ischaemia, and if hypotension occurs during pulmonary vasodilator infusion.

5. Decreasing pulmonary artery pressures via pharmacologic agents (e.g. tolazoline). Tolazoline is a partial α-adrenergic blocking agent with other complex pharmacologic effects. It is occasionally used where adequate oxygenation ($PaO_2 > 50$ mmHg) is difficult to achieve and after hyperventilation has failed to decrease pulmonary vascular resistance. Side effects include systemic hypotension and GI bleeding. Other vasoactive agents, sodium nitroprusside, verapamil and nifedipine appear to decrease pulmonary and systemic vascular pressures and variable results have been reported. Nitric oxide has recently been used in a small number of infants as a selective pulmonary vasodilator.[84,85] This endothelially derived relaxant factor diffuses into underlying vascular smooth muscle, binds rapidly to haemoglobin and is inactivated. Concerns relate to the production of nitrogen dioxide (NO_2) and methaemoglobinaemia. Many questions remain with regard to its future use, including timing, dose and duration of administration and toxicity over time.

Management of pneumothorax

Evacuation of a pneumothorax is achieved via a thoracostomy tube inserted over the superior aspect of the fourth or fifth rib in the third or fourth intercostal space in the mid or anterior axillary line, following blunt dissection and pleural puncture with a curved haemostat. (The intercostal vessels course along the inferior border of the rib.) The thoracostomy tube is directed superiorly and anteriorly to the mid clavicular line. Anterior insertion of chest tubes in the second or third

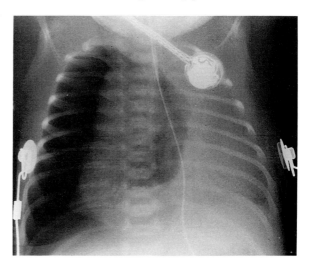

Fig. 5.2 Tension pneumothorax. AP radiograph of the chest shows large tension pneumothorax on the right shifting the mediastinum towards the left side. The heart size is difficult to assess because of the severe shift. Despite the tension, the right lung has not collapsed completely due to underlying diffuse pathology, as evidenced by the density of the lung and the air bronchiogram (RDS). The tension pneumothorax herniates across the midline to the left and has almost inverted the diaphragm.

intercostal space in the midclavicular line may also be performed (the nipple and breast bud must be carefully avoided to prevent scarring in this area).

The chest tube is connected to an evacuation device (pleur–evac). For most infants with lung disease on a ventilator, a negative pressure $\pm$ 10–20 cm H_2O is utilized; the pressure utilized should be assessed on the basis of the size of the air leak. A temporary substitute for an underwater seal evacuation device is the Heimlich one–way flutter valve. This is particularly useful for transport or delivery room care. Correct positioning of chest tubes should always be verified by AP and lateral chest radiographs.

Emergency thoracentesis may be achieved via a no. 21 or 23 scalp vein needle inserted at the superior edge of the third or fourth rib in the anterior or mid-axillary line. The needle is connected to an airtight three way stopcock and 20 or 50 ml syringe. Negative pressure is applied to the syringe as the needle is advanced. While needle aspiration may be therapeutic in an acute emergency situation, it should be discouraged as a means of diagnosing a pneumothorax and should ordinarily only be performed as a temporary

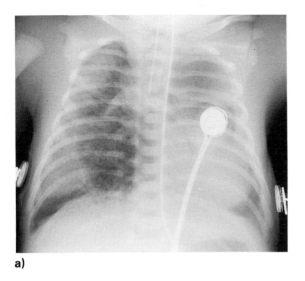

a)

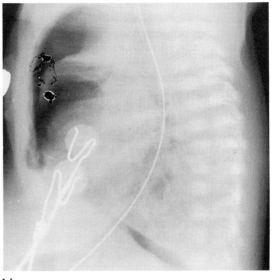

b)

Fig. 5.3 Pneumomediastinum. (a) AP and (b) lateral chest radiographs show large pneumomediastinum which clearly outlines the thymus on the right in (a) and anteriorly in (b). Visualization of the thymus helps to differentiate this air leak from a large anterior pneumothorax. There is an additional pneumothorax at the right base. (The lung shows typical changes of RDS.)

measure if a delay is anticipated in formal tube placement.

Complications of chest tubes include:

1. Misplacement outside the pleural cavity or across the mediastinum.
2. Subcutaneous emphysema secondary to a leak from the pleural insertion site.
3. Trauma to the lung (laceration or perforation) or haemorrhage from major vessels.
4. Recurrence of the pneumothorax if the chest tube is not removed correctly with closure of the skin site, or removed too early in the course of lung disease; (in general a chest tube is left in situ at least 12–24 hours after the tube has ceased to drain and negative pressure has been discontinued).
5. Infection at the skin site or systemically.

Ventilator management

Assisted ventilation is now a well established therapy for all forms of respiratory failure in the newborn. The large body of experience generated over the past 20 years has led to a significant increase in the survival of infants with respiratory distress. Improvement in survival has not, however, been achieved without a considerable incidence of

complications; continuous attempts are being made to improve mechanical ventilation so as to improve its efficacy and reduce these complications.

Specific goals of assisted ventilation

1. To maintain normal arterial O_2 tension/saturation.
2. To maintain normal $PaCO_2$ by improving alveolar ventilation.
3. To reduce work of breathing and overcome respiratory muscle fatigue.
4. To re–expand atelectatic lung segments.
5. To optimize pulmonary blood flow.

Definitions and physiological effects of common ventilatory parameters used in assisted ventilation of the newborn

Continuous positive airway pressure (CPAP)

CPAP implies that a constant distending pressure is applied to the airway during spontaneous breathing, during both inspiration and expiration. CPAP has been shown to increase functional residual capacity, increase oxygenation, reduce the work of breathing and stabilize the thoracic wall. CPAP may also influence the control of breathing via peripheral reflexes.

In RDS CPAP is considered to re–expand collapsed alveoli, increase the surface area of the lungs and reduce the right to left shunting. The PaO_2 will increase due to the increased surface area for diffusion and the reduction in intrapulmonary shunting. CPAP may be administered by tracheal tube (TT), nasopharyngeal tube (NPT) or a nasal prong. Both the NPT and nasal prong are less invasive than the TT. Normal physiological CPAP produced by the glottis is retained with both a nasal prong and NPT.

Excessive CPAP levels compromise cardiac output, pulmonary blood flow and contribute to hypercarbia. It is therefore critical that the work of breathing, blood pressure, peripheral perfusion, PaO_2 and PCO_2 be monitored closely during CPAP.

Nasal prongs and NPT may contribute to gastric distention and an orogastric tube must be placed as soon as possible following initiation. Improper positioning of the NPT may cause vagal stimulation with apnoea and bradycardia. There is a tendency for the NPT to block easily with secretions. CPAP is not appropriate in the unstable infant or in an infant requiring transport.

Intermittent mandatory ventilation (IMV)
IMV implies that positive pressure breaths are delivered at a set rate; fresh gas flow is provided between each positive pressure breath for spontaneous breathing. Most pressure–limited neonatal ventilators in the past have provided only this mode of ventilation.

Recently synchronized intermittent mandatory ventilation (SIMV) and assist control (A/C) modes have become available in pressure–limited neonatal ventilators. These sense the infant's inspiratory effort, either by abdominal movement or by detection of inspired directional flow at the proximal airway. It is anticipated that these newer modes will assist in reducing the work of breathing and the use of paralysing agents by promoting synchrony between the infant's respiratory effort and cycling of the ventilator. It appears that long–term patient triggered ventilation may be more appropriate in infants less than 28 weeks gestational age.[86]

Mean airway pressure (MAP)
MAP is the arithmetical calculation of the degree of lung distention. It is a result of the settings of the ventilator as well as the pressure waveform provided by the specific model of ventilator; the greater the magnitude and duration of the pressure transmitted to the lungs the greater the MAP. As MAP is increased, PaO_2 is increased. High MAP, particularly in the compliant lung, may cause decreased cardiac output and increased intracranial pressure. MAP can be approximated (if the ventilator does not offer a display) by the formula:

$$MAP = \frac{(PIP \times Ti) + (PEEP \times Te)}{Ti + Te}$$

Peak inspiratory pressure (PIP)
Pressure-limited, time–cycled neonatal ventilators are not designed to preset a tidal volume (VT) but rather a peak inspiratory pressure. PIP is the maximal pressure attained at the proximal airway during a controlled ventilator breath. On conventional neonatal ventilators this is controlled by the operator and determines the volume delivered per breath (tidal volume); the appropriateness of PIP must be assessed initially by observation of chest expansion and breath sounds. PIP affects PCO_2 by altering tidal volume and subsequently minute ventilation.

At a given PIP, tidal volume will be greater in a compliant lung than in a stiff lung. Alveolar overdistension occurs with excessive tidal volumes. PIP will improve oxygenation by increasing MAP; the degree to which this occurs will depend upon how rapidly the PIP is reached (flow-rate) and the inspiratory time. As compliance improves, a larger VT will result with the same level of PIP, leading to hyperventilation and low CO_2. Hyperinflation of the lung will increase barotrauma and the subsequent potential for pulmonary air leaks. Additionally, intra–alveolar pressure may be transmitted to the cardiovascular system leading to decreased cardiac output.

Positive end expiratory pressure (PEEP)
PEEP is the pressure maintained at the proximal airway between mechanical breaths; this assists in holding alveoli and terminal airways open at end–expiration, thereby improving the distribution of ventilation. PEEP increases MAP, resulting in improved oxygenation with pressure limited ventilators. An increase in PEEP without an increase in PIP will result in a decreased tidal volume and therefore increased PCO_2. If PEEP levels are excessive, potential overdistension with consequent decrease in compliance, increase in PCO_2, increase in pulmonary vascular resistance and decreased venous return may occur.

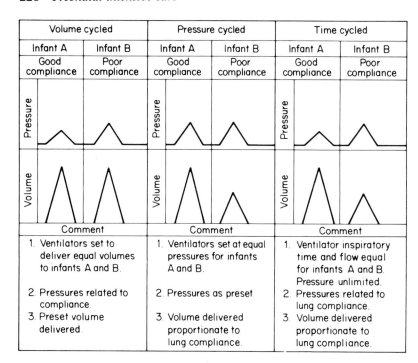

Fig. 5.4   The effect of pulmonary compliance on pressure and volume with volume-, pressure- and time-cycled ventilators. (Reproduced with permission from[87].)

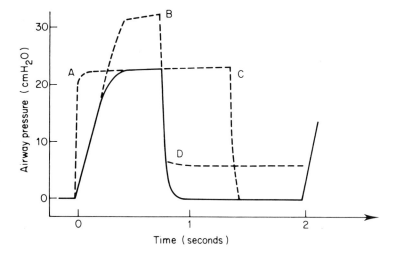

Fig. 5.5   Increases in mean airway pressure (area under the graph) with A, square wave form; B, increasing peak airway pressure; C, reversed I/E ratio; and D, constant distending pressure. (Reproduced with permission from[87].)

Inspiratory time (Ti)

Ti is the duration of the inspiratory time. Increased Ti allows for improved expansion of atelectatic alveoli; an increase in Ti will improve oxygenation by increasing MAP. Manipulation of Ti may also reduce asynchronicity. An excessively long Ti may lead to preferential alveolar hyperinflation and decreased pulmonary blood flow.

Expiratory time (Te)

Te is the duration of expiratory time. In some

ventilators, the Te is operator–adjustable so as to achieve the desired ventilator rate, while in others it will be the resultant product of the Ti and rate control. A longer Te allows more time for the infant's spontaneous respirations. A longer expiratory time may prevent pulmonary air leaks as a consequence of air trapping, particularly as compliance improves.

Ventilator rate

Rate or the frequency of positive pressure breaths

is operator-adjustable in some ventilators and the resultant product of the setting of the Ti and Te in others. At a fixed peak airway pressure, rate is the major control of $PaCO_2$; if by clinical assessment the PIP is sufficient to achieve good chest expansion, it may be less harmful to increase the ventilatory rate to assist in reducing CO_2 levels. Generally, the less compliant the lung, the faster the rate can be safely set. At higher rates, i.e. shorter expiratory times, there is a greater chance of air trapping particularly in the more compliant lung or the lung with increased airway resistance, e.g. meconium aspiration. High rates may therefore lead to incomplete expiration (inadvertent PEEP)leading to decreased compliance and potentially increasing the $PaCO_2$.

Hyperventilation, i.e. low CO_2 levels, may be desirable for its indirect effect of decreasing pulmonary vascular resistance and reducing right-to-left shunting in the treatment of PPHN. However, low CO_2 may reduce cerebral blood flow and hyperventilation may also result in unnecessary trauma to the lung.

Gas flow rate

The rate required is determined by the size of the infant, the leak around the TT, the tidal volume delivery, the inspiratory time, the mechanics of the ventilator and the volume of the ventilator circuit. In some ventilators increasing the flow will ensure PIP is reached earlier in the inspiratory cycle to allow for a more even distribution of gases; additionally, increasing flow may square off the pressure waveform, increasing MAP and PO_2. High flows have been identified as a contributing factor to necrotizing tracheobronchitis; particular attention therefore must be paid to the humidity level and temperature of the inspired gases when high flow rates are utilized. Excessively high flow rates may also lead to rapid pressurization of non–obstructed, non–atelectatic alveoli, increasing the potential for pulmonary air leaks.

Fractional inspired oxygen concentration (FIO₂)

FIO_2 may be controlled by adjustment of an air/O_2 blender either built into the ventilator or used as auxiliary equipment to power the ventilator. It is the main means of adjusting PaO_2.

Indications for mechanical ventilation

CPAP alone may be successfully used in infants with mild to moderate respiratory distress, where its early application may reduce the duration of oxygen requirements and enable lower airway pressures to be utilized, if subsequent mechanical ventilation is required. CPAP is also effective in the treatment of recurrent apnoea in the premature infant and in infants with pulmonary oedema and can be administered via a nasal prong.

In the earlier experience with mechanical ventilation strict criteria were advocated. These included:

1. Severe respiratory acidosis with pH < 7.25;
2. Severe hypoxaemia with $PaO_2 < 50$–60 mmHg despite $FiO_2 > 0.6$ to 1.0
3. Intractable apnoea.

Today less stringent criteria are generally accepted and mechanical ventilation is utilized in infants with evidence of deteriorating respiratory status, i.e. falling PaO_2 or rising CO_2 but with blood gas values which may still be outside those given above. IPPV is also initiated in extremely low birthweight infants at less severe or even normal blood gases, because of their structurally immature lungs, weak chest walls and tendency to hypoventilate with decreasing lung volumes.

Inital ventilatory parameters

Initial ventilator settings must be individualized for each infant with respiratory distress.

Pressures

At the outset the infant should be manually ventilated with a manometer in the bagging system line to monitor the pressures required to effect adequate chest expansion. The infant is then transferred onto a ventilator with the same pressures and rate as used when bagging. Initial settings for IPPV depend upon the severity of disease and the risk of acute lung injury. PIP in the 18–25 mmHg range and PEEP 4–5 mmHg are generally used. High PEEP would be detrimental to infants with meconium aspiration or air leaks.

Rate

For low birthweight infants a rate 30–60 min^{-1} (with corresponding Ti 0.5–0.4 sec) should be the initial desired rate. For very low birthweight infants a rate 60–80 min (corresponding Ti 0.4–0.25 sec) should be the initial rate. For infants without lung disease, e.g. neuromuscular disorders or immature lung syndrome, a rate of < 30 breaths per min (0.4 sec Ti) is chosen. An attempt is made to match the infant's own rate with the ventilator in order to optimize ventilation and reduce the risk of air leaks.

Inspiratory and expiratory time

In RDS with decreased compliance and therefore a short time constant, less time is required for expiration. In meconium aspiration a longer expiratory time is necessary because of increased resistance.

In summary, initial recommended settings are:

PIP   20–25 cm H_2O
PEEP   5 cm H_2O
RATE   40–60 breaths per minute
Ti   0.4–0.5 sec
FIO$_2$ as required to maintain transcutaneous PO_2 7–10 kPa (50–80 mmHg) and SaO_2 90–95 per cent
Gas Flow Rate   4–8 l.min^{-1}

Colour, oxygen requirements, chest expansion, breath sounds, retractions, synchronicity, blood pressure and perfusion must all be observed following the initiation of assisted ventilation. Arterial blood gases should be measured within 15–30 minutes of commencing assisted ventilation.

Table 5.4   Effects of parameter changes on blood gas values

Parameter	Effect on PaO_2	Effect on $PaCO_2$
FiO$_2$ ↑	↑	No change
PIP ↑	↑	↓
PEEP ↑	↑	↑ (if too high)
Ti ↑	↑	No change
Te ↑	No change	↑

To ↑ PO_2	↑ FiO$_2$
	↑ PIP
	↑ PEEP
	↑ Inspiratory time
To ↓ PCO_2	↑ Rate mainly by ↓ expiratory time
	↑ Tidal volume by ↑ PIP and/or ↓ PEEP

Decrease in oxygenation in the mechanically ventilated infant

A sudden deterioration in oxygenation in the mechanically ventilated infant may be due to:

Ventilator related problems

- Tracheal tube malposition
- Tracheal tube displacement
- Tracheal tube blockage
- excess leak around the tube
- excessive or loss of PEEP
- ventilator/circuit, electrical or mechanical malfunction
- excess condensation in tubing

Onset of a new problem

- PIE/Pneumothorax
- atelectasis
- pulmonary haemorrhage
- infection
- PDA
- IVH

Progression of the underlying disease process

This is usually a more gradual worsening of oxygenation than if due to ventilator related problems. This is commonly seen in:

- RDS in the first 24–48 hours
- infants with refractory PPHN
- infants struggling against the ventilator.

Interventions

Pulmonary and non pulmonary interventions and procedures. While some of these may be considered routine, e.g. tracheal suctioning, position changes, their potential in worsening of oxygenation must always be considered. (Suctioning is also associated with tracheal and bronchial mucosal trauma, microatelectasis and an increase in intracranial pressure and should therefore be kept to a minimum).

Management of deterioration during ventilation

If the deterioration in oxygenation is acute, the ventilator should be disconnected and manual ventilation commenced, whilst checking the ventilator settings. The tracheal tube should be suctioned and the position checked by auscultation and if necessary by direct visualization. Transillumination of the chest is indicated if a pneumothorax is suspected. This should be confirmed via chest radiograph.

A more gradual deterioration in oxygenation requires the assessment of the appropriateness of ventilator settings, the infant's status and other factors as described, e.g. infants in pain or struggling against the ventilator may require the use of morphine or muscular paralysis; suspicion of sepsis will require a septic work-up, etc.

Refractory Hypoxaemia

If the PaO_2 is intractable and remains below 7 kPa (50 mmHg) or respiratory acidosis cannot be managed by apparent appropriate manipulations using conventional ventilation,consideration may be given to high frequency ventilation or the use of extracorporeal membrane oxygenation if available.

High frequency ventilation (HFV)

High frequency low volume ventilation, delivering small tidal volumes at frequencies of about 4–15 Hz, has been utilized as short-term 'rescue' therapy to improve oxygenation when conventional mechanical ventilation (CMV) has failed, when pulmonary interstitial emphysema has developed or in an attempt to decrease the pertubations in intrathoracic pressure that occur with conventional mechanical ventilation that might adversely affect cardiac output, venous return and cerebral blood flow.[88–90]

A variety of mechanisms have been used: high frequency positive pressure ventilation (HFPPV) employs conventional pressure–controlled respirators cycled at rates of 60–150.min⁻¹; High frequency jet ventilation (HFJV) utilizes a small, high velocity jet of inspired gas delivered through a small bore to entrain a larger volume and augment the tidal volume; and high frequency oscillatory ventilation (HFOV) in which there is no bulk delivery of gas but a to–and–fro movement of the same volume of gas delivered by a reciprocating piston. In HFOV expiration is via active expiratory flow, while in the other techniques the nature of expiration is to allow passive recoil of the lungs and chest wall.

HFOV provides independent control over the mechanisms affecting oxygenation and CO_2 elimination. Recruitment of alveoli can be achieved by sustained inflation or a sigh; thereafter appropriate lung volume and oxygenation are achieved by alveoli remaining open continuously, as long as the infant receives oscillations at the set MAP. CO_2 elimination is achieved by the same factors as in CMV; tidal volume and frequency. With HFOV these can be altered without affecting pressure parameters: TV is adjusted with changes to the amplitude or peak–to–peak pressure that has been generated by the stroke volume of the piston. The usual frequency used during HFO is 15 Hz, delivering 900 breaths.min⁻¹. Although frequency can be altered to decrease $PaCO_2$, CO_2 elimination tends to reach a plateau at high frequencies.

Application of HFV in human infants has not yielded consistently beneficial results. Short–term improvements in gas exchange (more marked for CO_2 elimination than for oxygenation) have been achieved in infants with RDS using similar or lower MAP than used in the infants while on CMV. However, airway damage, greater gas trapping and alveolar pressures have occurred with this mode of ventilation.[91]

A controlled trial in premature infants with RDS which assessed the effect of high frequency oscillatory ventilation (HFOV) on morbidity, particularly BPD, found no difference between conventional ventilation and HFOV. There was, however, a higher incidence of the more severe grades of intracranial haemorrhage, and a greater incidence of periventricular lesions in the HFOV treated group of infants.[92]

Thus, while HFV may be effective under different research protocols, it is not used as an alternative in infants who can be managed with CMV.[91] It may have a role as 'rescue' therapy, particularly in infants with congenital diaphragmatic hernia, or as a preliminary manoeuvre to ECMO,[93] but is still considered an unproven form of ventilation in the newborn.[94]

Extracorporeal membrane oxygenation (ECMO)

ECMO is being used with increasing frequency in newborn infants with respiratory failure and hypoxaemia unresponsive to other forms of therapy.[95–97] ECMO or extra corporeal life support (ECLS) is essentially a heart and lung bypass technique whereby the circulation is diverted through a device permitting gas exchange across a permeable membrane. In the venoarterial bypass technique venous return from the internal jugular vein is diverted through an oxygenator and returned via the right common carotid artery to the aorta. Gas exchange across the lungs continues, although the ventilator rate, tidal volume and peak inspiratory pressures are markedly reduced; the lungs are therefore less subject to barotrauma and time is allowed for repair before weaning from bypass is attempted. Anticoagulation of the circuit and patient is required. The duration of ECMO support may be as short as 3–4 days for an infant with meconium aspiration or as long as 3–4 weeks for an infant with severe congenital diaphragmatic hernia (CDH).

Indications for ECMO have been based largely on a high predictive mortality ($\pm$ 80 per cent) for infants on conventional mechanical ventilation with certain measures of gas exchange, e.g. A–aDO$_2$ > 87 kPa (610 mmHg) for eight consecutive hours or an oxygenation index (OI) > 40 where OI = mean airway pressure $\times$ FIO$_2$ $\times$ 100/PaO$_2$.

ECMO has been used in infants generally over 37 weeks gestational age with birthweights > 2.5 kg, with reversible lung disease and without intracranial haemorrhage, congenital heart disease or a bleeding tendency. The specific conditions for which ECMO has been used include severe meconium aspiration syndrome (MAS), HMD, CDH, sepsis and PPHN.

Outcome
Statistics reported from the neonatal ECMO registry consistently show survival rates in excess of 83 per cent; the best outcomes are those in infants with MAS (> 90 per cent) while infants with CDH have a 62 per cent reported survival (Table 5.5).

Table 5.5 Neonatal aggregate survival by diagnosis: n = 3528. (Reproduced with permission from[98])

MAS	93% (1262/1356)
HMD	84% (446/532)
CDH	62% (364/585)
Sepsis	77% (321/416)
PPHN	86% (414/480)
Other	77% (120/156)

The effectiveness of ECMO in the treatment of the PPHN in CDH is inconsistent and the overall benefit and appropriate selection criteria in this clinical situation remain controversial.[98–99]

Morbidity from ECMO has been predominantly CNS injury, including seizures, cerebral infarction and haemorrhage. Neurologic follow–up studies have reported normal outcomes in up to 80 per cent of infants at $\pm$ 12 months of age.[100–101] There are, however, no readily available control groups to compare these figures with and it is also evident that clinical events in sick infants prior to their undergoing ECMO may be at least partly responsible for suboptimal outcome.

Two prospective studies attempted to compare ECMO with conventional mechanical ventilation.[95,102] Although both showed an increased number of survivors in the ECMO–treated groups, the numbers of infants enrolled were small and strict randomization was not used, such that the methodological strategies have been subject to criticism.[103,104]

The major issue facing the use of ECMO today is to determine its indications more precisely. The previously cited indications, based on an 80 per cent predicted mortality using historical controls, are no longer valid as the mortality from neonatal respiratory failure without ECMO has declined.[105] Improved understanding of the pathogenesis of neonatal lung disease, pursuing other forms of ventilation, making adjustments to conventional therapy and utilizing surfactant, may all further affect mortality and morbidity from neonatal respiratory failure. ECMO, too, will continue to undergo improvements; alternatives to carotid artery ligation may decrease the neurological morbidity (e.g. using venovenous access, a single venous catheter using tidal flow, or repairing the carotid artery at the time of decannulation); improvements in managing the bleeding and haemolytic complications (using non- thrombogenic surfaces) and other modifications such as the use of *in–vivo* O$_2$ saturation monitoring catheters, will also ameliorate the technical difficulties with the procedure.

There is no consensus at present as to whether further large controlled prospective randomized trials comparing ECMO and conventional therapy should be conducted to determine the future of ECMO.[106,107] There is also the question of whether this costly and invasive procedure is required at all, based on the low number of infants who might benefit from it.[108] While it is clear that a small number of infants' lives can be saved by ECMO, it should continue to be viewed as innovative and not yet as standard therapy. This is consistent with both the Australian and UK consensuses that ECMO be restricted to specific centres and then only as an innovative technique,[109] and with the recommendations by the American Academy of Paediatrics regarding the development of ECMO centres.[110]

Weaning from assisted ventilation

The decision to extubate an infant and discontinue mechanical ventilatory support is based on clinical and blood gas criteria. With adequate respiratory effort and an improving pulmonary status, PIP, Ti, FIO_2 and ventilator rate are gradually decreased. As the rate is reduced the inspiratory and expiratory ratio must be assessed such that the Ti is not excessively long, and a longer expiratory time is allowed for the infant to take more spontaneous respirations. From a low rate ± 5/min and PIP $16–18/3–4$ cmH_2O, infants can usually be successfully extubated, either to oxygen via headbox or nasal or NPT CPAP (particularly in infants < 1 kg). Weaning to CPAP is also commonly practiced. There is a view that the presence of the tracheal tube may increase resistance and dead space, making, successful extubation less likely, though this is not borne out in practice. The availability of new patient triggered ventilators may prove superior to conventional ventilation in weaning infants from assisted ventilation.[111]

Important factors that impact upon the success of weaning and extubation include:

1. The adequacy of central respiratory drive particularly in premature infants or infants who have been sedated. Inadequate central drive manifests in apnoea or hypercarbia within hours of extubation. The use of methylxanthines has been shown to increase the success of extubation in low birthweight infants.

2. The occurrence of postextubation lobar atelectasis, particularly the right upper lobe in low birthweight infants. The use of nasal CPAP postextubation may decrease the incidence of this complication.

3. The presence of upper airway obstruction, particularly laryngeal or subglottic oedema. Prophylactic systemic corticosteroids may occasionally be utilized in this situation although the effectiveness of this therapy remains controversial.

4. Vocal cord injury with incomplete apposition of the vocal cords may lead to aspiration. Enteral feeds are temporarily withheld prior to extubation and for a number of hours thereafter.

5. The cardiovascular status may limit the ability to wean an infant due to fluid overload, congestive heart failure or low cardiac output. These need to be addressed directly and may require the continued use of mechanical ventilation, particularly PEEP.

6. The nutritional status of the infant may limit weaning. The energy supply and the ability of the muscles to extract oxygen and substrates are an important consideration in the infant who has required prolonged ventilatory assistance. Energy requirements may exceed supply due to the increased work of breathing and adequate nutritional support must be provided.

7. Respiratory muscle fatigue or dysfunction occurs with a decrease in the strength and efficiency of the inspiratory muscles, particularly in premature infants and those with prolonged assisted ventilation. Muscles may fail to generate inspiratory force even though central respiratory drive is appropriate to the demand and the chest wall is structurally and mechanically intact. Methylxanthines may improve the contractility of the diaphragm, especially when fatigued.[112] Theophylline may be given in a dose of $6–8$ $mg.kg^{-1}$. by slow intravenous injection followed by a maintenance dose of 0.8 $mg.kg^{-1}hr$ intravenously.

Bronchopulmonary dysplasia (BPD)

BPD is a chronic respiratory disease of infancy resulting in most instances from the unresolved acute lung injury associated with oxygen therapy and mechanical ventilation in low birthweight infants with respiratory distress syndrome. While it occurs most commonly in very low birth weight (VLBW) infants following the treatment of RDS, it is also seen in other acute respiratory disorders, e.g. following mechanical ventilation for meconium aspiration, pneumonia, tracheo-oesophageal fistula and apnoea. Other chronic lung disorders e.g. Wilson–Mikity syndrome of pulmonary dysmaturity or the pulmonary hypoplasia associated with congenital diaphragmatic hernia and other causes of oligohydramnios, also lead to chronic lung disease. It is characterized by persistence of the clinical features of respiratory distress (tachypnoea, retractions, rales); the need for supplemental oxygen to maintain $PaO_2 > 7$ kPa (50 mmHg) beyond the first 28 days of life; and an abnormal chest radiograph.

The classic radiographic description of severe chronic BPD by Northway *et al.*[114] was one of overexpanded lungs which appear nonhomogeneous with focal areas of hyperlucency alternating with irregular dense, sharply outlined strands of opacification. This is only rarely seen today. More commonly, a radiographic picture emerges gradually, with more homogeneous or occasionally patchy opacification in both lungs (predominantly perihilar), with less emphysema and without coarse reticulation.[114] The presence of a PDA, pulmonary haemorrhage or infection may confound the interpretation of the chest radiograph in such infants and clinical correlation must be sought. The haze of density is usually fixed and persistent and unaffected by treatment of BPD with diuretics or antibiotics.

BPD has become the major cause of mortality and morbidity in extremely low birth weight (ELBW) infants, exerting great emotional and financial pressure on parents and care-givers. Incidence figures tend to vary markedly due to differences in diagnostic criteria, patient population and clinical management;[115] however the inverse relationship of the incidence of BPD with gestational age and birthweight is underscored in all studies, with figures as high as 85 per cent in infants < 800 gm and 5 per cent at 1300 gm.

The principal risk factor is the degree of prematurity and its related structural and functional pulmonary immaturity. Barotrauma from positive pressure ventilation and oxygen therapy lead to abnormal lung endothelial and epithelial protein permeability. Toxic oxygen metabolites (free radicals) are generated by pulmonary parenchymal cells, granulocytes and alveolar macrophages, and contribute to the development of lung injury, as endogenous antioxidants are lacking in the premature infant. Other clinical factors associated with the development of chronic lung disease include pulmonary air leaks, infection, fluid overload and left-to-right shunting through PDA. Atelectasis secondary to extremely underdeveloped lungs, the weak chest wall and any degree of hypoventilation, particularly in ELBW infants, also leads to chronic lung changes. The clinical evolution of the disease is one of continued respiratory insufficiency in an infant requiring prolonged oxygen and positive pressure ventilation, despite strategies aimed at reducing the concentration of FIO_2 and ventilatory parameters (particularly PIP) as rapidly as possible.

BPD is progressive, initially involving the distal airways and followed subsequently with development of abnormalities in all parts of the lung architecture. Infants with established BPD have abnormal pulmonary function due to oedema, fibrosis, airway distortion, and non-homogeneous inflation of the lungs.

Treatment of BPD

The first priority of treatment is to maintain satisfactory pulmonary O_2 and CO_2 exchange using supplemental oxygen alone or assisted ventilation at the lowest possible parameters.

The general principles of oxygen management are similar to those of acute lung disorders, i.e. to increase oxygen delivery (utilizing the lowest FIO_2 possible and red cell transfusion where appropriate) and to decrease oxygen consumption by careful thermal control and reduction in the amount of handling of the infant. Once infants are extubated, oxygen can be successfully delivered by low flow 100 per cent oxygen via nasal catheters to decrease the physical restriction of such infants to a head box or isolette and to facilitate their interactive behaviour. Oxygen requirements are determined in each infant using saturation monitoring during sleep, activity and feeds. Oxygen saturation is generally maintained at 90–95 per cent.

Ventilator support is redirected to that of a more chronic disorder in which respiratory acidosis and hypercarbia is not as vigorously pursued, as long as adequate compensatory metabolic alkalosis occurs and the pH is maintained > 7.25.

Increased oxygen consumption during BPD, as well as the requirements for growth, requires sufficient nutritional support with the goal of delivering $\pm$ 120 kcal.kg^{-1}.day. This often requires a combination of parenteral and enteral routes of delivery. It is important to appreciate that intravenous alimentation with a high ratio of carbohydrate to fat may stimulate CO_2 production and contribute to the hypercarbia, tending to overestimate the degree of respiratory acidosis.

Intercurrent nosocomial infections are particularly common in LBW infants with ventilator dependency, impaired mucociliary function and the continued requirement for i.v. lines, parenteral nutrition, etc. It is often difficult to determine the clinical significance of bacterial, viral or mycoplasma cultures from tracheal tubes and tracheal aspirates. These are normally considered significant only when associated with a positive blood culture and/or clinical deterioration in the infant; however, the prevention of superimposed pneumonia in an already compromised infant with BPD tends to lead to initiation of treatment with the earliest suggestive signs of infection.

Diuretic therapy

The role of long–term diuretic therapy in infants with BPD has yet to become well established.[116] While studies have demonstrated their short–term effect on lung mechanics and mobilization of pulmonary interstitial water and longer term effect on decreasing airway resistance and increasing pulmonary compliance, these effects have been inconsistent. Diuretics, therefore, are not considered routine therapy in infants with BPD: short–term courses are reserved for the treatment of pulmonary interstitial oedema in infants who deteriorate secondary to acute volume overload; longer term therapy is considered where resolution of lung injury has reached a plateau, or infants are unable to receive optimal fluid and caloric intake because of fluid restriction.

The potential benefit of diuretic therapy must also be evaluated in terms of side effects. These include electrolyte and mineral imbalance, hypochloraemia and metabolic alkalosis, nephrocalcinosis and bone demineralization and ototoxicity, particularly with chronic furosemide use.

Frusemide is given at 1 mg.kg^{-1}.day intravenously for a short 3–5 day course or as alternate day therapy; supplementation with potassium and chloride is required at 2–3 mmol.kg^{-1}.day.[117] Hydrochlorathiazide and spironolactone may be considered in the more chronic BPD situation, as they have less urinary losses of calcium, sodium and potassium than frusemide. Close monitoring of electrolyte and acid base status is required; where frusemide is used on a long–term basis bone demineralization (via wrist X–ray), and nephrocalcinosis (via renal sonography), should be sought.

Bronchodilator therapy

As premature infants have been shown to have sufficient bronchial smooth muscle to respond to bronchodilator stimuli, systemic and inhaled bronchodilators are occasionally used to treat airway hyper-reactivity and improve the air flow characteristics of infants with BPD. They are generally only used in those infants in whom a bronchospastic component to their clinical symptoms can be recognized and in whom unequivocal improvement or reversal can be demonstrated following acute therapy.

Short–term use of nebulized β_2 agonists are preferred to methylxanthines because of their more pronounced bronchodilatory effects. A short 2–3 day course is instituted if acute symptomatology improves and only continued in infants who respond to repeated administrations. While short–term therapy may show improvement in pulmonary mechanics, there is no evidence that long–term bronchodilator therapy improves resolution or outcome from BPD.

Corticosteroid therapy

Corticosteroids are increasingly being used in BPD because of demonstrated short–term improvement in pulmonary function. The mechanism of action of corticosteroids in infants with BPD is unclear; amongst the many potential mechanisms proposed are a modification of the inflammatory response to tissue injury, stabilization of cell and lysosomal membranes, increase in surfactant synthesis and a decrease in pulmonary oedema.

A number of randomized controlled trials have examined the role of dexamethasone in BPD.[118–22] Most studies have shown short–term benefit such as weaning from the ventilator and an early, but not sustained, decrease in O_2 requirements. None of the studies , however, aside from Cummings,[122] has shown a sustained beneficial effect with respect to mortality, length of hospitalization or duration of oxygen therapy. Recognized side effects of dexamethasone include increased rate of infection, systemic hypertension, cardiac biventricular hypertrophy, hyperglycaemia, glycosuria, intestinal perforation, adrenal suppression and impaired growth.

Different dosing regimens, durations of treatment and different outcome variables all make it difficult to make definitive recommendations with regard to corticosteroid therapy in infants with BPD.[116] The lack of nearly all the clinical trials' ability to demonstrate sustained beneficial effect, the emergence of potentially serious side effects and the possible adverse effect of corticosteroids in exacerbating the development of lung fibrosis, raise the issue of whether long–term dexamethasone treatment in this clinical setting should continue to be used.[123–5]

Other treatment modalities that may affect BPD include the use of antioxidants, vitamin A and E and superoxide dismutase. There is no definitive role for these agents at present in the management of BPD.

Apnoea

Apnoea is defined as the cessation of breathing for

more than 20 seconds or a briefer episode associated with bradycardia (< 100 beats per min) and/or cyanosis or pallor. In some preterm infants while only bradycardia may be recognized, polygraphic recordings show these episodes to be preceded by or simultaneous with apnoea.

Apnoea may be central (40 per cent) with no respiratory movement for more than 20 seconds or obstructive (10 per cent) in which breathing effort continues but airflow ceases because of obstruction in the upper airways, or a mixed central and obstructive picture (50 per cent) in which obstruction is followed by central apnoea or vice versa.

Periodic breathing is defined as brief respiratory pauses of 3–10 seconds, followed by effective periods of breathing for at least three cycles. Periodic breathing is not associated with bradycardia and is a normal respiratory pattern in premature infants.

Apnoea is considered primary if due to prematurity alone and secondary when a definitive cause can be determined.

Primary apnoea or apnoea of prematurity has the following characteristics: it is not present on day one; it usually ceases by 34–36 weeks gestational age; it occurs mostly during active sleep; and although it is not due to organic disease, the tendency to apnoea is exacerbated by hyperthermia, mild hypoxaemia, feeding or laryngeal secretions.

Apnoea in term or near term infants may be an early manifestation of many serious disorders and requires prompt investigation and management. The causes of secondary apnoea include:

1. Pulmonary disease: commonly RDS and pneumonia.
2. Upper airway obstruction: excess oral secretions, laryngeal and pharyngeal stimulation or anatomic obstruction.
3. Decreased tissue oxygen delivery: secondary to hypoxaemia of any cause, anaemia or congestive heart failure, PDA in particular.
4. Sepsis: bacterial or viral acquired sepsis, e.g. NEC, meningitis.
5. Feeding: related to vagal stimulation or the passage of an NG tube, the presence of gastrointestinal reflux or gastric distension.
6. Metabolic disorders: hypoglycaemia, hypocalcaemia, hypo and hypernatraemia.
7. CNS causes: ICH, seizures, asphyxia, drugs, cerebral malformations.
8. Other causes: increased environmental temperature, excessive handling, discomfort or pain.

Management of apnoea of prematurity

Premature infants (less than 32 weeks gestational age) are normally monitored via heart rate and/or respiratory (usually electric impedance) monitors. Heart rate monitors are preferred because respiratory monitors alone will not detect obstructive apnoea. In addition, continuous oxygen monitoring is required to detect the frequency of desaturation episodes. It is important to note that apnoea of 15–19 seconds associated with drops in heart rate are common in healthy preterm infants and should not necessarily be considered an indication for treatment or long–term cardiorespiratory monitoring. The decision to initiate treatment in primary apnoea is based on the severity, duration and frequency of the bradycardic and/or hypoxaemic episodes.

The principles of treatment

1. Exclusion and treatment, if present, of any secondary causes of apnoea, e.g. sepsis, metabolic disorders.
2. Avoidance of triggering reflexes such as excessive suctioning, hyperinflation during bagging, cold stimuli to the face or nursing the infant in a high environmental temperature. Maintaining the infant in the lower range of the neutral thermal environment is generally utilized.

   Changing the infant's feeding schedule, volume of feed, site of tube (oro *vs* nasogastric) or the infant's position during feed may also ameliorate the frequency of apnoeic episodes. Occasionally trying the infant off oral feeds for 1–2 days or investigations to rule out gastro–oesophageal reflux may be required.
3. Treatment of hypoxaemia. Small increases in inspired oxygen often reduce the frequency of episodes; increasing the oxygen carrying capacity via RBC transfusion is also often beneficial[126]

   If these measures fail, increasing the alveolar pressure via CPAP (nasal prongs or nasopharyngeal tube or TT) appears to improve oxygenation and stabilize the respiratory rhythm. Unresponsive apnoea may require IPPV at slow rates of 6–10 breaths per minute.
4. Increasing afferent input. Simple measures such as tactile stimulation or kinesthetic stimu-

lation via oscillation or rocking water beds may be efficacious.

If these measures fail, the use of methylxanthines is considered. Studies have shown a reduction in the frequency and duration of apnoea and bradycardia spells with the methylxanthines, theophylline, aminophylline and caffeine. They appear to act via a number of different mechanisms, including stimulation of the respiratory centre, increasing CO_2 sensitivity and decreasing diaphragmatic fatigue. Caffeine is preferred because it produces fewer side effects and has a larger therapeutic index. Age and individual variations in xanthine metabolism require monitoring of plasma levels. Side effects include tachycardia, jitteriness and vomiting.

Cardiovascular support

The basis for support of the cardiovascular system is the monitoring of physiological parameters, both by careful and frequent clinical observations from nursing and medical staff and by direct monitoring of pressures, gas exchange, temperatures, etc. and flow charting of haematological and biochemical data.

Initial management of congenital heart disease

The aim of medical therapy is to stabilize the patient prior to surgery so as to decrease the burden on an already compromised neonatal circulation. Definitive treatment is possible only when precise anatomical and pathophysiological diagnoses have been established. Initial supportive measures include:

Administration of oxygen

Oxygen is administered to correct hypoxaemia and for maintenance of normal oxygen saturation. In R–L shunts oxygen administration may not be indicated as oxygen is a stimulant for duct closure; a PaO_2 in the high 20s or low 30s may be acceptable in cyanotic congenital heart disease in the absence of metabolic acidosis.

Maintenance of fluid and electrolyte homoeostasis

Normal calcium, magnesium and blood glucose levels, adequate caloric intake and a neutral thermal environment must be maintained.

Correction of metabolic acidosis

Acidosis promotes pulmonary vasoconstriction and decreases pulmonary blood flow and will also impair myocardial contractility and the effectiveness of inotropic agents.

Correction of hypovolaemia

Management of hypovolaemia is aided, where possible, by the assessment of myocardial function by two-dimensional echocardiography or the use of central venous pressure monitoring. An infant who is adequately ventilated, with a blood pressure below the mean and low CVP (< 5 cmH$_2$0), with poor cardiac output but normal myocardial contractility warrants volume expansion. Changes in vascular capacitance with the use of tolazoline or prostaglandins will also require volume expansion. Infants with low blood pressure, poor cardiac output and myocardial contractility, and a large heart or a high CVP (> 10 cmH$_2$O) require inotropic support and fluid restriction.

Assisted ventilation

Assisted ventilation is usually indicated for any abnormality in cardiovascular function that may lead to pulmonary insufficiency, e.g.:

Congestive heart failure/pulmonary Oedema
Pulmonary and systemic congestion leads to increased pulmonary venous and capillary pressure. This results in pulmonary oedema in which effective lung volume, pulmonary compliance and FRC are decreased; airway resistance is increased and V/Q mismatching occurs.

CPAP restores FRC which improves compliance and decreases airway resistance, either by a shift of the lung to a higher volume on the same compliance curve or by opening atelectatic areas and shifting the lung to a new curve entirely. CPAP alone may suffice if respiratory effort is adequate; in most instances IMV and PEEP are indicated.

Low cardiac output states

Ventilation, by decreasing the pulmonary vascular resistance, will improve pulmonary blood flow. Ventilation will also improve gas exchange and therefore the pH of infants who are markedly acidotic. It may also decrease metabolic demands by decreasing the work of breathing and oxygen consumption in a stressed neonate.

Arterial hypoxaemia/cyanotic CHD

In this clinical situation ventilation is not the primary means of support but is indicated for the correction of acidosis and to decrease the metabolic demands as in low cardiac output states. It may also be required in the infant on prostaglandin therapy to prevent apnoea, particularly in low birthweight infants.

Adverse effects of assisted ventilation on cardiac function

The potential adverse effects of assisted ventilation in congenital heart disease may be due to its effects on preload, contractility and afterload.

By increasing intrathoracic pressure venous return may be impeded; similarly the ability of the heart to fill may be impaired by the 'tamponading' effect of this increased pressure. Likewise, right ventricular afterload may be affected by the transmission of intra-alveolar pressure to the pulmonary capillary bed.

CPAP per se may increase the work of breathing and should be used with caution in low cardiac output states.

Hyperventilation resulting in lowered pulmonary vascular resistance (PVR) may be disadvantageous in a number of conditions with a balanced pulmonary and systemic circulation, e.g. in infants with hyperplastic left heart syndrome and truncus arteriosus. The pulmonary and systemic blood flows are in a precarious balance and hypo- or hyperventilation may result in dramatic changes in these circulations.

Monitoring

In the intensive care unit direct monitoring of arterial blood is required using a percutaneously inserted cannula in the radial, brachial, axillary, femoral or a foot artery. With care an arterial line may function for many days if a sterile procedure has been used for the insertion and a slow flush of heparinized saline provided (1 unit per ml O.9 per cent saline) at 1 ml per hour. Central venous pressure can be monitored via a single cannula in the internal jugular vein. Double or even triple lumen catheters are available for use in newborns (e.g. Cook 4FG 5 cm long) and are inserted into jugular, subclavian or femoral veins by the Seldinger technique. Swan–Ganz catheters, though available in sizes appropriate for small infants, are not routinely used and for babies having open heart surgery a left atrial line can be inserted by the surgeon directly into the heart. These have a low morbidity though the chest drains should be left in place until the left atrial line is removed.[127]

Pulmonary artery pressure is measured in babies with a risk for pulmonary hypertensive crisis and the catheter can be inserted directly into the PA by the surgeon. An alternative is to insert a 2O G catheter into the internal jugular vein and allow it to coil in the PA until the surgical repair is complete, after which the catheter tip can be fed into the PA by the surgeon.

Direct methods of assessment of cardiac output e.g. by thermodilution, are not routinely employed in newborns: there are technical difficulties and results are often hard to reproduce.[128] Though absolute values may be unreliable, serial measurements may reflect changes. With experience the anaesthetist can assess cardiac output using heart rate, arterial and venous blood pressure, core:peripheral temperature gradient, urine output and serial echocardiography with Doppler studies. A temperature gradient core:periphery greater than 2°C implies suboptimal cardiac output. Echocardiography gives crucial information on ventricular contractility and diastolic (relaxation) function and cardiac output.[129,130] Urine output of at least $1 \ ml.kg^{-1}.hr$ is considered to be a minimal result of a full cardiac output. To assess cardiac output accurately all the variables must be taken into account.

Specific measures

If it is estimated that the cardiac index is low the four determinants of cardiac output – rate, preload, myocardial contractility and afterload – can be manipulated.

Rate

An optimal cardiac rate in a newborn is between 140–160 and because stroke volume is relatively fixed, rates below this level imply a reduced cardiac output. Increases of heart rate up to 200 increase cardiac output. Isoprenaline in a dose between 0.01–0.5 μg.kg^{-1}.min is a very reliable chronotropic agent as well as a pulmonary vasodilator. However, vasodilatation and hypotension, tachycardia and an increase in myocardial oxygen consumption (subendocardial ischaemia) may limit its usefulness.[131]

Preload

Preload determines stroke volume according to the Starling–Frank law and the CVP and LA pressures are used as a guide to the filling pressures. The neonatal heart is working towards the peak of the Starling curve and thus filling pressures tend to be higher. Whichever pressure, right or left, is the higher usually sets the upper limit and as a general rule the minimum filling pressure for an adequate cardiac output is chosen. Often the left ventricle has a low compliance particularly after the 'arterial switch' operation and left atrial pressure should not exceed 10 mmHg. A very small volume load may cause such a ventricle to decompensate. Because the neonatal liver is so distensible CVP may not adequately reflect an excessive volume load. Adequate filling is usually with blood or plasma to maintain a haematocrit of approximately 0.4.

Contractility

Cardiac contractility can be improved if the preload has been raised to what is regarded as an optimal level and the cardiac output is still judged to be low. Increase in myocardial contractility is the result of increased intracellular calcium concentration following increased intracellular cyclic AMP concentration, so the serum ionized calcium level should be normal. The basis of improved contractility is the continuous and carefully monitored infusion of catecholamines either singly or in combination. Stimulation of β_1-receptors produces increased stroke volume and heart rate, but at the expense of increased oxygen consumption; β_2 stimulation causes systemic and pulmonary vasodilation whereas α-stimulation gives systemic and pulmonary vasoconstriction. Stimulation of dopamine receptors increases myocardial contractility and at lower doses renal and mesenteric vasodilation, but at higher doses α-activity (vasoconstriction) predominates[132]

The response to dopamine and dobutamine may be comparatively diminished in newborns because of the reduced myocardial contractile mass and also because of 'down regulation' of receptors which occurs very easily in this age group.

Dopamine is usually considered to be the drug of first choice at a dose starting at 4 μg.kg^{-1}.min (renal vasodilating dose) and not exceeding 15 μg.kg^{-1}.min. If the pulmonary vascular resistance is particularly labile, dobutamine in a similar dose may be preferable. It causes fewer tachydysrhythmias and has the additional advantage of being safe to infuse into a peripheral line. The combination of these two agents is often successful with dopamine at a low renal vasodilating dose plus dobutamine at a higher, inotropic dose. Dobutamine has no selective renal effect, but both agents cause tachycardia in high doses.

Adrenaline, which is a very potent catecholamine causing peripheral and pulmonary vasoconstriction,

Table 5.6 The adrenergic effects of catecholamines

Catecholamine	Beta$_1$	Beta$_2$	Alpha	Dopamine
Dopamine	+ +	+	+ +	+ + +
Dobutamine	+ + +	+	+	
Isoprenaline	+ + + +	+ + + +	0	
Adrenaline	+ +	0	+ + +	
Noradrenaline	+ +	0	+ + + +	

Table 5.7   Cardiac drugs with dosages

Drug	Dose
Dopamine 6 mg.kg^{-1} in 100 ml 5% dextrose	1 ml.hr = 1 μg.kg^{-1}.min Dose 5–10 μg.kg^{-1}.min
Dobutamine 6 mg.kg^{-1} in 100 ml 5% dextrose	1 ml.hr = 1μg.kg^{-1}.min Dose 5–10 μg.kg^{-1}.min
Adrenaline 60 μg.kg^{-1} in 100 ml 5% dextrose	1 ml.hr = 0.01 μg.kg^{-1}.min Dose 0.01–0.5 μg.kg^{-1}.min
Isoprenaline 60 μg.kg^{-1} in 100 ml 5% dextrose	1ml.hr = 0.01 μ.kg^{-1}.min Dose 0.01–0.5 μg.kg^{-1}.min
Noradrenaline 60 μg.kg^{-1} in 100 ml 5% dextrose	1 ml.hr = 0.01 μg.kg^{-1}.min Dose 0.01–0.5 μg.kg^{-1}.min
Enoximone – dilution 100 mg in 40 ml *water* (= 2.5 mg.ml^{-1})	Bolus 0.5–1 mg.kg^{-1} slowly i.v. Infusion 10–15 μg.kg^{-1}.min
Dextrose/insulin–2 gm dextrose: 1 unit insulin	0.5 gm.kg^{-1}
Calcium chloride	10–20 mg.kg^{-1}
Sodium nitroprusside 6 mg.kg^{-1} in 100 ml 5% dextrose	1 ml.hr = 1 μg.kg^{-1}.min Dose 0.5–5 μg.kg^{-1}.min
Nitroglycerine 6 mg.kg^{-1} in 100 ml 5% dextrose	1 ml.hr^{-1} = 1 μg.kg^{-1}.min Dose 0.5–5 μg.kg^{-1}.min

Table 5.8   Clinical usage of catecholamines

Drug	Standard dose (μg.kg^{-1}.min)	Dose range ((μg.kg^{-1}.min)	Indication	Comments
Dopamine	5.0	5–20	Mild-to-moderate dysfunction Use first	If dose > 15 μg.kg.min, consider adrenaline
Dobutamine	5.0	5–15	Mild-to-moderate myocardial dysfunction in patients with tachydysrhythmias or labile PVR	Combine with renal dose of dopamine if oliguria is present (5 μg.kg.min)
Isoprenaline	0.05	0.01–0.5	Right ventricular failure Pulmonary hypertension Systemic vasoconstriction Relative bradycardia	Avoid in patients with tachydysrhythmias and reactive outflow tracts
Adrenaline	0.1	0.05–0.8	Moderate-to-severe myocardial dysfunction Severe arterial hypotension	Combine with vasodilator once adequate arterial pressure is achieved; avoid in patients with PHT crisis
Noradrenaline	0.1	0.05–0.8	Severe arterial hypotension caused by phenoxybenzamine Low systemic resistance, circulatory failure (including sepsis) Hypoxic spells in Fallot's tetralogy	

is used in a dose range of O.O1–O.5 μg.kg^{-1}.min in those babies in whom dopamine and dobutamine are not sufficiently effective. Because of the vasoconstriction, adrenaline is usually combined with a vasodilator such as nitroprusside or nitroglycerine.

Noradrenaline, which is a potent vasoconstricting catecholamine, is reserved for babies with extreme hypotension, for example from septic shock, or to increase peripheral resistance in babies with hypercyanotic spells of Fallot's tetralogy.

Enoximone is a selective phosphodiesterase inhibitor causing increase in intracellular cyclic AMP and may potentiate the effects of, for example, adrenaline; it works independently of β-receptors. It also has a peripheral vasodilating effect and the lusitropic effect of ventricular relaxation to improve diastolic function. An initial bolus dose of O.5–1 mg.kg^{-1} is slowly given, followed by an infusion of 5–15 μg.kg^{-1}.min. Initial vasodilation may cause the blood pressure to fall and volume replacement is often necessary.

Standard dilutions of all the drugs are in 5 or 10 per cent dextrose in 5O ml syringes and are infused via a central vein. The use of digoxin is not usually an early consideration in cardiogenic shock because of its unpredictable onset of action, low efficacy, slow excretion and high incidence of toxicity.

Afterload

Newborn cardiac function is optimal because systemic vascular resistance is low. However, compensatory vasoconstriction associated with poor ventricular function or following profound hypothermia or surgical stress is a very active reflex. Active vasodilatation improves cardiac performance by both arterial and venous smooth muscle relaxation, allowing an increase in ejection fraction and decrease in left ventricular end diastolic volume.

Sodium nitroprusside (2–10 μg.kg^{-1}.min) is the most powerful agent, acting directly on vascular smooth muscle via the endothelial relaxing factor, nitric oxide. It is indicated after deep hypothermia or if blood pressure is high and peripheral temperatures are low. Too high concentrations and prolonged administration raise the possibility of cyanide poisoning. Nitroglycerine is a less powerful drug and also allows venous dilatation, shifting blood to the peripheries and reducing the diastolic volume of both ventricles, thus improving coronary filling.

When afterload reduction is required for longer periods and enteral function has been re-established, captopril, an ACE inhibitor, is used. Doses are gradually increased from 0.1 mg.kg^{-1} given 8-hourly to 0.5 mg.kg^{-1} per dose.

The combination of inotropic agent and vasodilator often improves cardiac output; an effect not obtainable with either drug alone. The progress of treatment is monitored by clinical signs of rewarming, etc. or by more objective measurements of cardiac output.

Prostaglandins (PG)

The E-type prostaglandins, E_1 and E_2, are powerful vasodilators of nearly all arterioles and act by direct relaxation of vascular smooth muscle. The ductus arteriosus appears to be unusually responsive to vasodilatation at doses below those which affect systemic or pulmonary pressure or resistance. Prostaglandins are highly effective in improving pulmonary or systemic blood flow in neonates with ductus arteriosus dependent critical congenital heart disease. This includes: right-sided obstructive lesions, severe tetralogy of Fallot, pulmonary atresia, tricuspid atresia, severe pulmonary stenosis, TGA and Ebstein's anomaly; left-sided obstructive lesions, aortic atresia, critical aortic stenosis, severe coarctation and interrupted aortic arch, and hypoplastic left heart syndrome. Reversal of post-natal ductal constriction, thereby increasing pulmonary and systemic blood flow and improving oxygenation and metabolic acidosis in these critically ill infants, significantly affects the outcome of their subsequent palliative or corrective surgery. Prostaglandins in TAPVD with obstructive venous return may increase the risk of pulmonary oedema[133] but this infrequent situation should not prevent the initial use of prostaglandins in all cyanotic newborns with congenital heart disease.

Prostaglandin administration

PGE_1 is administered at a dosage of 0.1 μg.kg^{-1}.min via either an i.v. or UA catheter. There is often a dramatic improvement within 10–15 minutes in the hypoxaemic, non–acidotic infant. Following an initial response, the PG infusion rate may be reduced to a maintenance dose of 0.05 μg.kg^{-1}.min and continued until the completion of surgery. The half-life of PGE_1 is 5–10 minutes and therefore the route of administration must be secure in any critically ill infant. Infants more than four days of age have a significantly poorer response, reflecting the decreased reactivity of the ductus arteriosus smooth muscle due to the postnatal involutional changes in the ductal wall.

Acute side effects of PGE_1 administration are frequent but relatively minor and include apnoea, particularly in low birth-weight infants, cutaneous vasodilatation, hypotension, jitteriness, irritability, diarrhoea and hyperthermia. Care should also be exercised in infants with a bleeding diathesis because of an effect on platelet adhesiveness.

Long-term administration of PGE_1 may be necessary in infants in whom growth of the pulmonary arteries must occur before surgical treatment can be undertaken. Bone changes resembling infantile cortical hyperostosis have been reported in a number of these infants[134]; these regress slowly after prostaglandin is discontinued with no residual bony abnormality.[135] In addition gastric antral hyperplasia with feeding problems has been seen with long-term prostaglandin administration.

Diuretic therapy

Diuretics alleviate some of the congestive signs in heart failure by decreasing preload; some diuretics may have direct vasodilating effects and improve ventricular performance by reducing after-load as well. They are indicated when fluid and sodium restriction alone is insufficient to control the signs of congestive failure. Intravenous frusemide is extremely useful in acute congestive heart failure. It decreases extracellular fluid volume and venous return rapidly and acts as a vasodilator; diuresis within 30 minutes is usually seen, but variability in response is seen in low birthweight infants and those with renal impairment or poor cardiac output.[136] The usual starting dose is 1–2 $mg.kg^{-1}.day$ and may increase up to 2–4 $mg.kg^{-1}.day$.

Thiazide diuretics, or potassium–sparing diuretics, particularly spironolactone, are moderately effective and used when a less rapid effect is desired or for chronic administration in infants with congestive heart failure. These diuretics are less effective in infants with significantly decreased glomerular filtration rate.

Complications of diuretics include electrolyte abnormalities (hyponatraemia, hypokalaemia, hypocalcaemia) which may precipitate digitalis toxicity, acid-base abnormalities (metabolic alkalosis) and hyperglycaemia. Diuretics also have the potential for inducing hypovolaemia and dehydration. Longer term effects include hypercalciuria, nephrocalcinosis and osteopaenia of prematurity.

Acute treatment of supraventricular tachycardia

The first manoeuvre tried in the newborn is the firm placing of an ice-cold cloth or bag of ice over the infant's entire face for a few seconds. Thereafter, if unsuccessful the following acute measures are tried:

1. Adenosine 0.05 $mg.kg^{-1}$ i.v. This may be repeated at 2-minute intervals at increasing doses of 0.05 $mg.kg^{-1}$ increments, given as a bolus up to a maximum of 0.25 $mg.kg^{-1}$. Complete heart block results at the therapeutic dose and lasts less than 15 seconds.
2. Synchronized cardioversion 0.25–1.0 $joules.kg^{-1}$. Cardioversion should be the first choice if there is severe haemodynamic compromise.

Other agents may be used, including neostigmine, edrophonium or phenylephrine, but are not first choice agents in this situation.

Pulmonary hypertensive crisis

A reactive pulmonary vasculature is a feature of neonatal physiology, but it is seen particularly after correction of ventricular septal defect, total anomalous pulmonary venous connection, transposition of the great arteries VSD, TAPVD, TGA and truncus arteriosus, in the first few weeks of life. A greater reactivity of the precapillary arteriolar region is caused by a persistent fetal type of muscularity of the arterioles or an actual increase in the amount of smooth muscle in the media of these vessels. If an increase in pulmonary vascular resistance occurs and fetal channels have been closed surgically so that right-to-left shunting cannot take place, then a low cardiac output state ensues. Acute failure of the right ventricle severely affects left ventricular function by interfering with septal function and coronary blood flow as well as by reducing the volume of blood returning to the left side. There is a sudden rise in CVP, peripheral temperature falls and the baby becomes hypoxic.

The systemic pressure falls as both ventricles fail together in infants, the peripheral temperature falls and the patient becomes hypoxic. At this stage the condition becomes self-reinforcing because hypoxia causes further pulmonary vasoconstriction.

The pulmonary hypertensive crisis – which is likely to be fatal – can not be suspected unless the pulmonary artery or right ventricular pressure

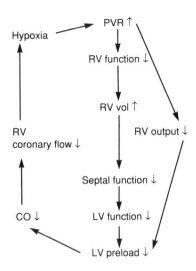

Fig. 5.6 Vicious cycle of falling cardiac output after increase in pulmonary vascular resistance.

is monitored, when the cause of the problem may be identified. This is now routine for this type of patient: a catheter is either placed directly into the pulmonary artery (PA) by the surgeon or is placed in the right atrium using a Seldinger technique via the right internal jugular vein. The catheter is then threaded into the pulmonary artery by the surgeon after the surgical correction but before cardiopulmonary bypass is discontinued.

The mechanism is the same as for persistent pulmonary hypertension of the neonate and the treatment patterns are similar. A major crisis is characterized by suprasystemic right-sided pressures, severe fall in cardiac output and hypoxaemia, but more minor events occur frequently with precipitating factors such as hypoxia, hypercarbia, acidosis, restlessness and tracheal suctioning. Phenoxybenzamine, the long-acting α-adrenergic blocking agent, is used intraoperatively (1 mg.kg^{-1}) in many centres for newborns and other high risk babies to reduce the reactivity of the pulmonary vasculature to potent constrictive stimuli such as a rising $PaCO_2$. It is, however, no help in treating a crisis once established. Phenoxybenzamine is continued postoperatively 1 mg.kg^{-1}.day in two divided doses for at least 48 hours until weaning from the ventilator has been started. Patients at risk are ventilated with a high FiO_2 to a $PaCO_2$ below 4 kPa (30 mmHg), while paralysis is maintained and an infusion of fentanyl (4–8 μg.kg^{-1}.h) is given to reduce stress responses. Further boluses of fentanyl (up to 25 μg.kg^{-1}) may be required before suctioning.[137,138]

Sedation and manual hyperventilation with 100 per cent oxygen are the first line treatments for a crisis, but if the PA pressure remains high an infusion of a pulmonary vasodilating agent is necessary. In the past many drugs have been used for this purpose, e.g. chlorpromazine and aminophylline, but only nitroglycerine, tolazoline and prostacyclin have any part to play in the treatment of a pulmonary hypertensive crisis. Nitroglycerine has some degree of pulmonary specificity and is useful as a background infusion.[139] Tolazoline (1 mg.kg^{-1}.h) may have a profound effect on the systemic resistance, causing a disastrous fall in blood pressure.[140] This drug is a histamine agonist and will cause gastric erosions and haematemesis unless antacids and an H_2 blocker such as ranitidine are also administered. Prostacyclin is the most effective and potent drug given intravenously. It is infused starting at 5 ng.kg^{-1}.min but the dose can be rapidly increased up to 20 ng.kg^{-1}.min.[141] After the situation has been brought under control a period of stability for at least 24 hours is desirable after which $PaCO_2$ is allowed to rise. If the PA pressure remains stable at normal levels of $PaCO_2$, paralysis is stopped, fentanyl dosage reduced and the patient is slowly weaned from the ventilator. Prostacyclin in a minimal dose is continued until the baby has been extubated.

The continuing requirement for a low $PaCO_2$ and high doses of pulmonary vasodilating agents is a poor prognostic sign and there is a considerable mortality in patients who develop major crises early and who require very aggressive treatment.

Since nitric oxide has been used increasingly in human subjects this agent will probably become the first choice for use in babies with labile pulmonary vascular resistance[142]; 20–40 parts per million are introduced into the inspired gases.

Nutrition

Feeding practices in the newborn are aimed at providing nutritional requirements for appropriate postnatal growth while avoiding harmful imbalances and with the least stress on immature or altered intestine and enzyme systems. Recommendations, particularly in the low birth weight or sick infant, are difficult to define and even when they are made, can often not be met due to the limitation of immaturity and physiological instability of these infants. Nevertheless, nutrition must be provided as soon after birth as possible via enteral and parenteral routes, as suboptimal nutrition may not only compromise the newborn's ability to overcome acute stresses but may also affect long-term brain growth and development.[143]

Nutrition Requirements

Energy

A number of factors affect energy requirements:

1. Decreased endogenous reserves of fat and carbohydrate. This is especially important in the premature infant where low stores are compounded by immaturity of the metabolic pathways in the oxidation of the primary metabolic fuels.
2. Thermal stress. A major factor determining increased energy requirements is the high rate of evaporative water loss. Increasing the supply of energy as heat by maintaining the neutral thermal environment is routine. However, if the lower range of the thermal neutral zone is used this may lead to a negative energy balance with failure to grow.[144]
3. Underlying illness increases basal energy requirements, particularly in infants with fever, sepsis, congestive heart failure, bronchopulmonary dysplasia or large intestinal losses.
4. The route of feeding affects energy requirements. Parenteral feeding requires less than enteral feeding (85–100 *vs.* 100–120 kcal.kg^{-1}.day) because of the lower energy costs of gastrointestinal absorption and metabolism and lower fecal energy losses with parenteral nutrition.[145]
5. The nature of the diet and the amount of weight gain also affect the energy requirements for synthesizing the absorbed nutrients into fat, protein and carbohydrate stores. Reichman showed that infants fed their own mother's milk required less energy than formula fed infants for each gram of weight gain (3.09 kcal.gm^{-1} weight gain *vs.* 4.26 kcal.gm^{-1}).[146]

Guidelines for energy requirements in the newborn range from 100 kcal.kg^{-1}.day in the term to 120 kcal.kg^{-1}.day in the premature infant. Higher energy requirements (130 kcal.kg^{-1}day) may be required in very low birthweight infants.[147] However, generalizations about energy requirements are difficult because of the marked variation between infants, e.g. AGA and SGA infants. SGA infants have higher resting metabolic rates and lower postprandial thermogenesis than AGA infants.

The caloric density of human and formula milks ranges from 680–810 kcal.l^{-1} and is able to provide these energy requirements. The energy is generally provided as carbohydrate 40–50 per cent, fat 35–40 per cent and protein 15 per cent of total calories. Fat may be a greater source of energy in growing premature infants. In enterally fed infants if energy requirements cannot be met, the caloric density of oral feeds can be increased by the addition of carbohydrate in the form of glucose polymers or caloreen, which do not increase solute load, as well as by the addition of fats such as corn oil, microlipid or medium chain triglyceride (MCT) oil. On occasion weight gain is greater than the rate of increase in length; disproportionate weight gain probably represents deposition of large amounts of fat. There does not appear to be any convincing reason to produce weight gain in excess of that appropriate for length.[148]

The above guidelines are essentially for infants on full oral feeding and can seldom be achieved in the first few days of life, not only because of the limitation on enteral feeding but also because of the high fluid volumes required. Thus, i.v. glucose in sick or premature infants provides the major energy source in the first few days of life with the gradual introduction of protein and fat thereafter. Glucose alone can usually only provide ± 40 kcal.kg^{-1}.day. (Maintenance energy requirements without weight gain can be achieved with ± 64 kcal.kg^{-1}.day.)

Protein

Protein requirements are determined by the high growth rate in the newborn in general and by the catabolic state of sick and low birthweight infants in particular. Protein is generally well absorbed in term and premature infants; the premature infant, however, is limited in both synthetic and degradative aspects of amino acid metabolism. The inability to synthesize makes certain amino acids semi-essential (e.g. tyrosine, cysteine and taurine) and the inability to catabolize excess amino acids may lead to metabolic imbalances. Protein synthesis with its major contribution to renal solute load is also curtailed in the presence of immature or altered renal function.

Intakes of 2.5–3 gm.kg^{-1}.day of amino acids and 100–120 kcal reliably produce weight gain of 10–15 gm.kg^{-1}.day and nitrogen accretion of 200–300 mg.kg^{-1}.day.[150]

Higher protein intakes (3.8 gm.kg^{-1}.day) may lead to metabolic abnormalities, metabolic acidosis, hyperosmolality, and an increase in the extracellular volume in extremely low birthweight infants.[148] Recent studies in extremely low birthweight infants suggest that early administration of amino acid (2 gm.gm^{-1}.day i.v. starting as early as day two) may be tolerated and be more beneficial than was previously thought in ameliorating protein catabolism with earlier positive nitrogen balance and weight gain in these infants.[150]

In the term infant term breast milk or formula provide these protein requirements; in the premature infant premature formulas provide the estimated protein requirements when appropriate volumes can be given; preterm breast milk may require protein supplementation with breast milk fortifiers after the first few weeks of life to meet the protein recommendations.

Carbohydrate

Carbohydrates are the main source of energy for the newborn; glucose and its isomer dextrose are the preferred carbohydrates in peripheral intravenous nutrition in the first few days of life. Carbohydrate in breast milk is in the form of the disaccharide lactose; premature formulas contain lactose and non-branched glucose polymers in a 50:50 mixture, so as not to overload the lactase capacity and to decrease the osmolality of feeds. Generally preterm infants tolerate lactose well without clinical problems; where the brush border of the small intestine has been affected by infection or hypoxia–ischaemia, lactase activity may be decreased and lead to an osmotic diuresis.

Lipids

Triglyceride is the most abundant of the dietary fats and is a major source of energy. Digestion and absorption of lipids requires hydrolysis by lingual, gastric and pancreatic lipases and solubilization of the products of the lipases by bile acids. In the premature infant this process is limited by low pancreatic lipase activity and low bile salt concentrations. This results in a degree of fat malabsorption which may also limit absorption of vitamin E and calcium.

Fats should comprise 35–40 per cent of the caloric content; essential fatty acids should supply at least 4 – 5 per cent of the total calories in the form of linoleic acid and about 1 per cent as linolenic acid. The absorption of fatty acid and acquisition of essential fatty acids is facilitated by breast milk and by formulas in which part of the milk fat has been substituted by MCT or a mixture of MCT and vegetable oils rich in polyunsaturated fatty acids. Higher energy density feeds, where the principal energy source is fat may increase energy expenditure and not increase growth rates.

Sodium

Sodium and chloride are essential for growth. Requirements are determined mainly by the degree of immaturity of the renal tubules such that the premature may require up to 6 mmol.kg^{-1}.day or even greater, whereas term infants grow well with sodium intakes of 1–2 mmol.kg^{-1}.day. Sodium homoeostasis is generally well maintained over a fairly wide range of intake provided that renal function is normal.

Breast milk contains sufficient sodium concentrations in the first four weeks of lactation; thereafter sodium supplements may be required to prevent late hyponatraemia. Premature formulas may also not contain sufficient sodium; supplementation may therefore be required in the formula-fed small premature infant.

Calcium and phosphorus

Calcium and phosphorus are required in the premature infant to compensate for the loss of rapid skeletal growth which occurs in the last trimester of pregnancy and also to replace obligatory fecal and urinary losses. Urinary losses are increased with the use of diuretics and sodium and glucose loads.

The intestinal absorption of calcium is dependent upon the infant's vitamin D status, the degree of malabsorption and fecal loss of fat and calcium, and the calcium:phosphorus ratio of the diet. Phosphorus absorption is also dependent upon the dietary composition. Its intestinal transfer is relatively independent of calcium transport processes, but dependent upon calcium and nitrogen retention. Absorption is inhibited by phytates (soy formulas) and by antacids containing aluminium and magnesium.

Breast milk provides less calcium and phosphorus than fetal accretion rates, but appears to be adequate for the term infant. Standard and preterm formulas contain higher levels to allow for less efficient absorption and retention. The fortifying of preterm human milk does enable higher levels of calcium and phosphorus to be achieved (in the ratio of calcium:phosphorus of 1.8:1) and this improves retention and bone mineralization. However, this may be associated with problems of sedimentation, impairment of fat absorption, milk bolus obstruction and phosphate overload.[147] The range of calcium requirements suggested by Bremer *et al*[151] is 70–140 mg.100 kcal^{-1} and for phosphorus 50–90 mg.100 kcal^{-1}.

Vitamin D

Current recommendations are 400 IU to 1000 IU per day. Infants receiving preterm human milk or premature formula usually require supplementation. There is no consensus on whether higher doses may be required; in a randomized study in which very low birthweight infants received oral supplementary vitamin D_2, 400 IU or 2000 IU per day, although higher serum levels of 25-hydroxyvitamin D were obtained, serum osteoclastic levels and radiographic evidence of bone disease were comparable.[152]

Trace metals

Deficiencies in trace minerals, zinc and copper, may develop, in particular in premature infants with low body stores and where parenteral nutrition does not contain these minerals. Premature formulas contain zinc, copper and other trace metals (manganese, cobalt, selenium, molybdenum). A solely breastfed premature infant may develop zinc deficiency by 2–4 months postnatal age; this will respond rapidly to supplementation.

Enteral feeding

Premature Formulas

To facilitate digestion and absorption of nutrients in preterm infants, premature formulas have been adapted in the following manner:

1. Protein concentration is higher in preterm than term formulas and is whey predominant. (However, much of this is β lactoglobulin which is present in only small amounts in human milk; human milk whey is in the form of lactoalbumin.)
2. Carbohydrate is provided by lactose and glucose polymers, the latter being theoretically more easily digested and absorbed; lactose is generally well tolerated and glucose polymers may not be necessary.[144]
3. The fat composition contains a variable proportion of medium chain triglycerides (MCT) which are thought to be better absorbed than long chain triglycerides (LCT) and improve nitrogen and calcium retention; however, a recent study has shown that preterm infants can efficiently digest and absorb formula fat containing as much as 98 per cent long-chain fatty acids.[153]
4. Preterm formulas also contain Na, Ca and phosphorus supplements to meet increased requirements.

Human milk

Human milk has a more balanced amino acid composition and solute load than formulas; there is also better absorption of protein, fat and minerals. Furthermore, the importance of breast milk in host defence is being increasingly recognized[154] (see Table 5.9).

Preterm breast milk

Preterm milk is nutritionally different in composition from mature human milk for the first 2–4 weeks of lactation. This may approximate to the nutritional requirements of the preterm infant as there are higher caloric, fat, protein, sodium, chloride, magnesium and secretory IgA concentrations and lower calcium, phosphorus and lactose concentrations. After the first four weeks concentrations of calcium, phosphorus, sodium and possibly iron, copper and zinc in preterm milk are considered less adequate for the preterm infant. Breast milk fortifiers have been developed for addition to preterm milk; their use has shown improvement in weight, length and bone mineralization.[156–8] The introduction of human milk protein fortification earlier than four weeks appears to be safe and may be advantageous in the sick preterm infant during the early intensive care course.[159]

Table 5.9 Components of breast milk and immunological function. (Reproduced with permission from[155])

Protein	
Casein subunit	Potentially enhances growth of *Lactobacillus bifidus*
Whey proteins	
Lactoferrin	Inhibits coliform, fungal growth by binding iron
	Bactericidal in combination with secretory IgA (SIgA)
	Anti-inflammatory properties
	Comprises 20 per cent of breast milk protein (only trace amounts present in cow's milk)
Lysozyme	Bactericidal vs. coliforms in conjunction with SIgA
	Anti-inflammatory agent
Secretory IgA	Inhibits adherence and proliferation of bacteria at epithelial surfaces
	Confers 'environmental specificity' to breast milk because IgA antibodies derived from entero- and bronchomammary pathways reflect antigenic and micro-organism exposure of mother
	Comprises 90 per cent of IgA and 10 per cent of total protein in breast milk
	Concentration probably increased in preterm vs. term breast milk
Carbohydrate	
Oligosaccharides	Analogous in structure to bacterial receptors, potentially inhibit binding of bacteria to cell surfaces
	Promote growth of *Lactobacillus bifidus*
	Comprise 15–20 per cent of total carbohydrate in breast milk
Lymphocytes	Secrete immunoglobulins

Pooled or banked human milk has lower concentrations of energy, protein and minerals and is generally not used; premature infants have been shown to grow more slowly than those fed their own mothers' milk.[147] Pasteurization of human milk inactivates lipases and this contributes to lipolysis of triglycerides and also destroys the heat labile humoral factors in human milk. Freezing, the most common method of storage of human milk, may also destroy certain cellular elements.

Promotion of breastfeeding
The promotion of breast milk feeding in the NICU has often not been actively pursued for a number of reasons: the logistic difficulties in obtaining milk from mothers at great distances from their infants in regional centres, the ready availability of premature formulas, fears of engendering guilt in mothers who may have chosen not to breastfeed, the necessity for prolonged manual expression for mothers of very lowbirth weight infants, fears of transmission of infection from mother to infant via breast milk, and some uncertainty about the adequacy of breast milk as a nutrient source in the extremely low birthweight infant. With the increasing recognition of the nutritional, immuno-logical and psychological benefits of breastfeeding, its potential role in ameliorating NEC, and the availability of supplementation of breast milk with fortifiers in extremely lowbirth weight infants, it is important that a strong case be made for the active promotion of breastfeeding in the NICU. A philosophy and attitude amongst the staff to support breastfeeding is essential to overcome the many difficulties that may be encountered. This includes:

1. Providing specific information to the staff about pumping, storage and handling of breast milk and the effect of diet, rest and anxiety upon milk production; the use of breast milk should not be delayed and dependent upon an infant's recovery if the mother is to be successful at breastfeeding.
2. Recognizing that staff highly trained in technical procedures may not have sufficient knowledge about breastfeeding to be supportive to mothers and may require other resources or role models to provide this information.
3. Standardizing procedures for safe handling and storage and ready provision of appropriate containers for mothers at any distance from the regional centre.

4. Providing mothers with comprehensive lists of community resources, clinics, help lines, etc.
5. Teaching alternative methods of feeding, e.g. finger feeding, which simulates breastfeeding and promotes the successful transition from gavage to breastfeeding. This can easily be accomplished by parents or nurses without altering the infant's suck pattern or the effort required to feed.

Initiating enteral feeds

Whenever possible feeding should be via the gastro-intestinal tract. However, a number of factors have to be considered prior to the initiation of feeds in the postoperative, sick or low birthweight infant.

The risk of necrotizing enterocolitis

Infants asphyxiated at birth or those with ongoing hypoxia, acidosis or hypotension are not fed for one to three days or until symptoms resolve. The presence of umbilical catheters, while a potential risk for NEC, is not an absolute contraindication to enteral feeding. If breast milk is the form of milk to be introduced it may be used slightly earlier than formula; similarly, dilute formula may be used initially if the predisposition to NEC is moderately high.

A large PDA with a significant diastolic run-off and the potential for shunting blood away from the splanchnic bed may lead to the withholding of feeds until haemodynamic stability is established. This is particularly important if indomethacin is to be used as this has been associated with gastrointestinal perforation.

Anastomotic function

Anastomotic function and intestinal motility must be established. This implies the absence of disten-sion and ileus, the presence of bowel sounds and the passage of meconium or stools. Infants who require muscle paralysis for assisted ventilation are not enterally alimented until peristalsis is restored.

Mechanical ventilation

Concern about the potential for gastro-oesophageal reflux and aspiration while on assisted ventilation has led to conservative feeding practices in infants receiving assisted ventilation; however, Newell[160] has demonstrated less reflux in infants during assisted intermittent positive pressure ventilation than during normal breathing. These studies would tend to support the practice of the enteral feeding of ventilated infants.

Respiratory status

A decrease in dynamic lung compliance, increase in minute ventilation, decrease in FRC and increase in diaphragmatic work resulting in apnoea has been described in some infants after gavage feeding.[161]

In addition, nasogastric feeding may affect respiratory gas exchange with a decrease in PaO_2 and an increase in $PaCO_2$; thus enteral feeds are usually not commenced until respiratory status is relatively stable.

Benefits of enteral feeding

Attempting enteral feedings, even with minimal amounts, appears to have many beneficial effects:

1. Prolonged deprivation of enteral feeds over time adversely affects gastrointestinal structure and function and a degree of atrophy may occur.
2. The introduction of enteral feeds leads to the release of gut hormones (increase in gastrin motilin and other GI hormones).[162]
3. The secretion of various intestinal hormones may also augment insulin action and improve the glycaemic response to glucose alimenta-tion.[163]
4. Local intestinal hormones may also enhance enterocyte growth and stimulate bile flow, enhancing the tolerance of enteral feeds.
5. Early feedings are associated with achieving full enteral nutrition earlier,[164] less indirect hyperbilirubinaemia and TPN-induced chole-stasis, and improved calcium metabo-lism.[165,166] Brown[166] fed infants with either standard TPN or amino acid-free i.v. nutrition with enterally delivered whey protein; the latter group had no signs of cholestasis as compared to 58 per cent in the solely TPN group.
6. The postprandial motor response of the small intestine of preterm infants is enhanced by exposure of the gut to enteral feeds.[167]

    Two controlled trials have failed to show that early feeding increases the incidence of NEC.[165,168]

In summary, although there is no consensus regarding the optimal time to initiate enteral feeds, and no single feeding regimen can be prescribed, it appears that the early institution of enteral feeds is both safe and of benefit in low birth weight infants and should be actively encouraged.[169]

Methods of feeding

Infants < 32 weeks are fed via nasogastric or orogastric tube because of the immaturity and incoordination of the suck-swallow and breathing mechanism. Beyond that age feeds may be tried orally dependent upon maturation of these mechanisms and the respiratory status of the infant.

Intermittent feeds are generally preferred. Continuous feeds may be considered if the infant is not thriving on intermittent feeding or in infants with gastro–oesophageal reflux or severe chronic lung disease, in short bowel syndrome or occasionally a priori in extremely low birthweight infants.

Transpyloric feedings to prevent reflux and aspiration are seldom used because of the difficulties in placing and securing them and also because of reports of impaired fat absorption (bypassing lipolytic activity in the stomach), alteration of the intestinal flora, and duodenal or jejunal perforation without any obvious nutritional benefit having been demonstrated.[155]

Parenteral nutrition

Parenteral nutrition has made a major contribution to the survival of post-operative surgical and premature infants. It is indicated in infants who are unable to meet their nutrient requirements via the enteral route; thus it is recommended for all surgical newborns who cannot be enterally fed for periods longer than 3-5 days.[145] In addition, it has become widely used as either a total or supplemental source of nutrition in ill and low birthweight infants who are not expected to tolerate full enteral feedings within a few days of birth. In general parenteral nutrition in low birthweight infants is initiated on about day three as soon as fluid, renal and metabolic stability has been achieved.

The essential features of TPN (Table 5.10) are to provide protein and an energy source, predominantly glucose, to meet the nutritional needs for appropriate postnatal growth plus the demands that specific infants may have because of tissue damage or disease.

The amount of calcium is inadequate for optimal skeletal mineralization. However, providing greater calcium concentration without decreasing phosphate is likely to result in precipitation of calcium phosphate.[149] Sodium and potassium acetate or lactate may be considered in patients with metabolic acidosis. Vitamins and trace elements including zinc and copper should also be provided as well as other essential trace minerals in infants on long-term parenteral nutrition.

Lipid emulsions

Intravenous lipid emulsions are used in parenteral nutrition to increase the caloric intake and to prevent the development of essential fatty acid deficiency. Intravenous fat solutions are triglyceride emulsions from soybean oil (or soybean plus safflower oil) stabilized by the addition of egg yolk phospholipid. They are hydrolyzed by lipases (lipoprotein plus hepatic) and release free fatty acids (FFA) which are available for oxidation in tissues or for the synthesis of stored triglyceride in fat. Circulating FFA are bound to albumin; they may be cleared by the liver and oxidized or incorporated into lipoproteins.

Ten and 20 percent emulsions are available (i.e. 10 or 20 $gTG.dL^{-1}$). Both contain linoleic and linolenic acid in quantities sufficient to satisfy recommended requirements. The 10 per cent solution leads to a greater rise in triglyceride, total cholesterol, phospholipid and low density lipoprotein than 20 per cent intralipid because of the higher phospholipid:triglyceride ratio of the 10 per cent emulsion.[170] It is uncertain whether these differences are of long-term clinical significance. Twenty per cent lipid emulsion may be useful in fluid-restricted infants.

The usual starting dose is 0.5–1.0 $gm.kg^{-1}.day$. This dose is sufficient to prevent essential fatty acid deficiency, but only provides 5–10 $kcal.kg^{-1}.day$. An increased caloric intake is obtained by increasing lipid emulsions up to a maximum of 2 $gm.kg^{-1}.day$ in premature infants and 3 $gm.kg^{-1}.day$ in older infants.[171] The amount of triglyceride infused into low birthweight premature infants may exceed this upper limit, as long as an emulsion that is rapidly cleared is administered. Further studies are needed to determine the safety of higher doses.[172]

Tolerance of lipid solutions is quite variable and monitoring for hyperlipidaemia is required. Measuring serum turbidity via visual inspection or nephelometry is a poor predictor of hyperlipidaemia[173]; thus direct measurement of TG, FFA and/or cholesterol is required. It is advisable to maintain triglyceride < 1 $mmol.l^{-1}$.

Table 5.10   The composition of the TPN formula used at the Hospital for Sick Children, Toronto

Composition of VAMIN-N based standard solutions (per litre)*

	P-5/'7.5	P-10	PI-10	I-10/20**
Protein (gm)	15.0	20.0	20.0	30.0
Glucose (gm)	50.0/75	100.0	100.0	100.0/200.0
Energy (kcal)	248.0/340.0	455.0	455.0	495.0/870.0
Na (mmol)	20.0	14.3	30.0	30.0
K (mmol)	20.0	18.9	30.0	30.0
Cl (mmol)	21.1	15.7	31.3	32.1
Ca (mmol)	9.0	9.0	9.0	9.0
P (mmol)	9.0	9.0	9.0	9.0
Mg (mmol)	3.0	4.0	4.0	4.0
Zn μmol)	46.0	46.0	46.0	46.0
Cu (μmol)	6.3	6.3	6.3	6.3
Mn (μmol)	1.8	1.8	1.8	5.0
I (μmol)	0.47	0.47	0.47	0.47
Cr (μmol)	0.076	0.076	0.076	0.076
Se (μmol)	0.25	0.25	0.25	0.25
Fe (μmol)***	–	–	–	18.0

*'P' solutions are standard for premature infants who are not fluid restricted. 'I' solutions are for premature infants who are fluid restricted and for children and infants
**I-20 is intended for central venous line therapy only
***Iron can be included in the 'P' solutions in neonates who have been receiving TPN for one month or more

If microtechniques are not available or available only on a restricted basis, visual inspection or nephelometry should be done, particularly with the initiation of lipid infusion or in conditions which are likely to interfere with the hydrolysis of triglyceride such as infection.[149] Infusion should be continuous over 18–24 hours via peripheral or central line, either as a separate i.v. or via a Y-connector to the parenteral amino acid/glucose line. Particular attention to the infusion rate is essential in very low birth-weight infants who have a limited capacity to metabolize triglyceride and free fatty acids (lower levels of heparin-releasable lipoprotein lipase) and who are thus at greatest risk of hypertriglyceridaemia.

Adverse effects of lipid emulsions have been described. These include:

1. Impaired oxygenation in premature infants.[174] In addition, experimental studies suggest that lipid may increase pulmonary vascular resistance, possibly by increasing production of the vasoconstrictor thromboxane B_2.[175] Thus lipid may not be advisable in hypoxaemic conditions associated with an elevation of pulmonary artery pressure, particularly RDS and PPHN.
2. Decreased bilirubin binding to albumin as FFA compete with bilirubin for binding.
3. Hyperglycaemia.
4. Alterations in lipid metabolism/deposition. Although lipid emulsions contain adequate amounts of essential fatty acids, linolenic and linoleic acid, they do not contain the longer-chain more unsaturated fatty acids of either family. Deficiency of these parent fatty acids may possibly relate to aberrations in the developmental fatty acid pattern of tissue lipids, particularly in the brain and eye.[144,176]
5. The possibility of impaired neutrophil and/or platelet function. In addition, lipid emulsions

have been associated with an increased incidence of sepsis due to coagulase-negative staphylococci.[177]

6. Intralipid microemboli have been described with the use of lipid emulsions.[178]

Most of the potential complications associated with lipid emulsions can be minimized by alterations in dose and duration of infusion or the timing of initiation of lipid as part of parenteral nutritional support.

The optimal timing for the initiation of lipid in the infant with respiratory distress and decreased oxygenation is uncertain. Although Gilbertson[179] showed no deleterious effect on gas exchange in ventilated very low birth weight infants after intravenous lipid was introduced in a step-wise manner from day one to a maximum of $0.15 \text{ gm.kg}^{-1}.\text{hr}$ in the first week of life, the findings of Hammerman[180] would appear to justify a more cautious approach, specifically in the first days of life when the calories derived from lipid are not felt to be critical.

I.v. lipid therapy utilizing MCT in the emulsion has been introduced in Europe. The potential advantages of MCT over LCT include more rapid hydrolysis, less displacement of unconjugated bilirubin from albumin plus the potential ability to be cleared more rapidly, even in the presence of hypoalbuminaemia. The safety and efficacy of these emulsions needs to be established.[172]

Methods of parenteral nutrition

The choice of route for parenteral nutrition is based on the patient's clinical condition, the nutritional status and the anticipated duration of parenteral nutritional requirement.

Peripheral venous lines

The most common form of parenteral nutrition is that provided through peripheral venous lines. This is used in normally nourished infants who are likely to commence enteral feeds within one to two weeks. Although this limits glucose concentration to 10 per cent and may involve frequent site changes, peripheral TPN has been very successfully used, with low rates of infection and the ability to provide up to $90 \text{ kcal.kg}^{-1}.\text{day}$.

Silastic catheters inserted percutaneously through a peripheral vein and threaded into the SVC may last longer than a single peripheral vein site and allow a more concentrated infusate to be used.

Central lines

Silastic catheters may be placed surgically in the superior vena cava just above the right atrium in infants who require higher concentrations of infusate and in whom the duration of therapy is likely to be greater than two weeks. Silastic catheters are preferred to polyvinyl catheters as they are less thrombogenic. The position of the catheter must be confirmed radiographically. Because of the greater incidence of infection with these lines they should be used only for nutrient infusion and not for blood transfusion or sampling.[181]

Complications of parenteral nutrition

Complications include those related to the technique itself and those that result from the nature of the infusate. The former include infection, thrombosis (particularly with central lines in SVC), thrombophlebitis and intravenous skin and subcutaneous 'burns' secondary to the infiltration of hypertonic solutions. Metabolic imbalances tend to occur when attempts are made to increase the nutrient intake: hyperglycaemia with an osmotic diuresis, abnormal plasma aminograms plus azotaemia and other electrolyte disorders are encountered. Most of these complications are simply managed by an alteration in the concentration of the various components in the solution.

Frequent monitoring for complications and calculation of the actual intake of the various nutrients is mandatory. Monitoring includes daily fluid balance and urine glucose; CBC, BUN, P, Ca, Mg, albumin, bilirubin, liver function tests and creatinine on initiation, and weekly thereafter; electrolytes, glucose and acid–base status at initiation and once to twice per week thereafter (Table 5.11). Lipid levels should be measured, particularly on initiation and thereafter with any suspicion of sepsis. Monitoring includes the assessment of growth parameters, weight daily, length and head circumference weekly.

The incidence of liver dysfunction, i.e. TPN induced cholestasis, is not infrequent with long-term TPN but usually resolves without residua. Cirrhosis and hepatic failure may occasionally occur. The incidence of cholestasis is considered a function of the duration of the TPN therapy and secondary to a number of factors including low birthweight, prematurity, the composition of TPN solution (higher amino acid load) and the duration of enteral starvation.

Table 5.11   Scheme for monitoring complications of TPN)

Complication	Monitored by	Frequency
Inadequate or excessive intake	Body weight	Daily
	Fluid balance	Daily
	Urea	Weekly
Protein depletion	Serum albumin	Weekly
Hypo/hyperglycaemia	Urine glucose	Daily
	Blood glucose	Daily–2 × week
Electrolyte imbalance	Serum Na, Cl, K	Daily–2 × week
	Urine Na, Bl, K	As necessary
Mineral imbalance	Serum Ca, P, Mg	Weekly
Iron depletion	Blood count with smear	Weekly
Acid-base imbalance	Blood gases	Weekly
Lipid overload	Exogenous lipids	2 × week
	Triglycerides	2 × week
Hepatic cholestasis	Liver function tests	2 × month

Renal failure

Acute renal failure is a clinical syndrome following an acute decrease in renal function of sufficient magnitude to result in retention of nitrogenous waste products. Renal failure is suspected when either oliguria (urine volume < 0.5 ml.kg.hr^{-1}) is present for 8–12 hours after day one, or the serum creatinine is greater than 100 mmol.l^{-1} or rising more than 20 mmol.l^{-1} per day.

Prerenal acute renal failure

The most frequent causes of renal failure in the newborn are prerenal in origin; these include perinatal asphyxia (particularly secondary to antepartum haemorrhage), respiratory distress syndrome, congestive heart failure and sepsis. A decrease in renal perfusion occurs as a consequence of hypotension, hypovolaemia or hypoxaemia alone or more usually in combination.

Increasing renal perfusion via volume expansion and/or vasodilatory agents may dampen the fall in GFR. The use of inotropes should be considered in infants with poor myocardial function once any volume deficits have been corrected. Of the inotropic agents, dopamine appears to be a unique sympathomimetic agent with α- and

β-adrenergic effects as well as dopaminergic effects. The dopaminergic system is particularly active within the kidney; the response to dopamine administration is dose dependent and directly related to the activation of specific receptor types.[182] At low dosages (2 μg.kg.min^{-1}) dopaminergic effects predominate, resulting in decreased renal vascular resistance, increased renal blood flow and the promotion of diuresis. Cuevas'[183] study in preterm infants with RDS suggests that low doses of dopamine exert beneficial effects on GFR and urine volume only in patients with oliguria and impending renal failure and/or hypotension and should not be routine in other circumstances. At higher doses an adverse effect on renal function is noted because of activation of α-adrenergic receptors in the kidney; this may result in vasoconstriction and decreased sodium and water excretion.[182]

If the prerenal aetiology is not recognized and managed appropriately it will predispose to the development of intrinsic renal failure.

Careful examination of the indices of renal function differentiates prerenal from intrinsic renal failure (Fig. 5.12).

In prerenal azotaemia, the urine SG and osmolality are high, urine sodium concentration

Table 5.12 Indices of intrinsic and extrinsic renal failure

	Prerenal	Renal (intrinsic)
Urine specific gravity (H_2O)	> 1.012	< 1.015
Urine osmolality (mosm.kg^{-1} H_2O)	(High) > 400–500	(Low) < 400
Urine Na+ (mmol.l^{-1})	< 10	> 20
Urine:plasma osmolality	> 1.3	< 1.1
creatinine	High	Low
urea	High	Low
FENa (per cent)	< 1	> 2–3
Response to volume (± frusemide)	Increased urine output	No effect

is low, the urine to plasma ratios of osmolality, creatinine and urea are high (indicating a concentrated urine and the necessity to increase fluid intake) and serum urea is increased out of proportion to the increase in serum creatinine. In intrinsic renal failure the urine SG and osmolality are low, urine sodium is high and the urine osmolality and urine to plasma ratio of osmolality, creatinine and urea are low (indicating a defect in urinary concentrating ability). The FENa may also help to distinguish prerenal from intrinsic renal failure after the first few days of life, particularly if frusemide has not been administered in the preceding 24 hours (t-half 18–24 hr).

If the distinction between prerenal and intrinsic renal failure cannot be decided, a fluid challenge is indicated, both as a diagnostic and possible therapeutic manoeuvre. 10–20 ml.kg^{-1} over one hour of an electrolyte solution, usually normal saline, is given, often in two infusions; the response is assessed in terms of urine output and frusemide 1–2 mg.kg^{-1} given if urine output does not improve. The frusemide dose after a second fluid challenge is usually doubled. If urine output fails to exceed 1 ml.kg^{-1}.hr a diagnosis of intrinsic acute renal failure is presumed and managed accordingly.

Intrinsic renal failure

Is commonly secondary to:

1. acute tubular, cortical or medullary necrosis;
2. renal vascular conditions (arterial or venous thrombosis), or
3. congenital abnormalities of the kidney, including renal agenesis, dysplasia, polycystic kidney disease or infection.

Post-renal renal failure

Renal failure following an obstruction to urine flow is usually reversible. However, longstanding obstruction may lead to irreversible parenchymal damage. This is particularly seen secondary to posterior urethral valves and ureteropelvic junction obstruction. Renal failure in this situation may occur with a normal or even increased urine output. Non-oliguric acute renal failure has a better prognosis and is more easily managed medically than oliguric acute renal failure.[184]

Surgery and renal failure

Infants who undergo surgery in the newborn period are particularly prone to the development of renal failure and should be very carefully assessed preoperatively, during the surgery and in the postoperative period.

Preoperative
Factors which predispose infants to the development of acute renal failure include low birthweight, hypoxaemia, metabolic acidosis, episodes of bradycardia and hypotension, low cardiac output states particularly coarctation of the aorta and other left ventricular outflow tract obstructions, cyanotic congenital heart disease and preoperative studies with contrast material.[185]

During surgery

Any episode of hypoventilation, hypoxaemia, arrhythmia or hypotension during the surgery may predispose to the development of postoperative renal failure.

Postoperatively

An episode of hypotension secondary to left ventricular dysfunction, hypovolaemia, cardiac arrest or bleeding makes the infant prone to the development of renal failure. The use of diuretics, particularly frusemide in the presence of a contracted blood volume will also exacerbate the development of renal failure.

Ongoing postoperative losses must be assessed and replaced frequently to avoid the development of dehydration. This is particularly important in infants with obstructive uropathy who have a marked postobstructive diuresis with enormous urinary losses resulting in hyponatraemia, dehydration and acidosis. Careful monitoring of the urine output, electrolytes and other parameters of renal function are essential for the first 24–48 hours, particularly if renal impairment was present prior to the relief of the urinary obstruction.

Management of Acute Renal Failure

Systemic

Systemic measures include: the treatment of acidosis, anaemia, hypertension, infection and hypocalcaemia if present. If left ventricular dysfunction is documented, inotropic support is indicated. Drug dosages and the frequency of drug administration must be adjusted for renal failure.

Fluid

Fluid requirements consist of insensible water loss plus replacement ml for ml of any urine produced with a solution containing NaCl or KCl equal to urine values for the electrolyte. Strict attention to fluid management with replacement of fluid for urine output is maintained until a diuresis occurs. This usually occurs within a few days with a progressive increase in urine output thereafter.

Nutrition

The nutritional objectives are to provide a minimum of 50 calories per kilogram per day. Provision of calories from carbohydrate and fat sources should be maximized with calories derived from protein at the lower end of normal requirements. The caloric intake is limited by fluid restrictions as long as the patient remains oliguric.

Dialysis

Dialysis is considered in the newborn with acute renal failure in the following clinical situations:

1. inadequate urine flow with symptomatic uraemia, resistant to frusemide 5 mg.kg^{-1};
2. symptomatic electrolyte disturbance/intractable hyperkalaemia;
3. congestive heart failure or fluid overload;
4. intractable acidosis.

Peritoneal dialysis is preferred over haemodialysis in the newborn because it is relatively safer, technically less demanding and similarly effective.[186] A P–D catheter is placed 1–3 cm below the umbilicus using an aseptic technique based on the Seldinger principle and its final position confirmed by an abdominal X–ray. Dialysis is usually started with 'isotonic' dialysate (No. 61 Diaflex solution has a sodium content of 140 mmol.l^{-1} and 1.36 per cent glucose) plus heparin 200 units.l^{-1} in hourly cycles of 20–30 ml.kg^{-1}.cycle. For babies that are haemodynamically compromised, 'minidialysis' of 10 mg.kg^{-1} per cycle every 30 minutes may be satisfactory.

Ten ml 50 per cent glucose added to one litre increases glucose concentration by 0.5 per cent, and to increase removal of fluid, concentrations up to 3.86 per cent can be used. Specially prepared bicarbonate dialysis is used in babies who have an intractable acidosis. Potassium, up to 4 mmol.l^{-1}, is added depending on the serum K$^+$ levels.

Complications include bleeding, fluctuation in serum glucose and sodium concentrations, perforation, hydrothorax and infection, but are rare. Continuous arterial–venous haemofiltration may occasionally be tried if peritoneal dialysis is not effective or if the infant is unstable or unsuitable for peritoneal dialysis (e.g. postabdominal surgery). It is also felt to be preferable in the removal of circulatory fluid overload.

Management of neurological disorders

Asphyxia in term infants

Despite advances in antepartum and intrapartum fetal monitoring, perinatal asphyxia occurs with sufficient frequency (3–6 per 1000 term births) that full details of the effects of labour and delivery and a full neurological assessment should be performed in any infant for whom surgery is contemplated.

Any condition that interferes with fetal gas exchange may result in perinatal asphyxia. This includes:

1. altered placental exchange (e.g., abruption, placenta praevia, prolapsed cord, 'placental insufficiency', postmaturity);
2. altered maternal blood flow to the placenta (e.g. maternal hypo- or hypertension, abnormal uterine contractions);
3. altered maternal arterial oxygen saturation (e.g. maternal hypoventilation, hypoxaemia or cardiopulmonary disease).

Abnormal respiratory gas exchange results in hypoxaemia, hypercapnia and acidosis. Severe hypoxaemia results in systemic hypotension, thus creating the potential for multiorgan hypoxic–ischaemic injury.

Perinatal asphyxia may result in fetal heart rate abnormalities, the passage of meconium, low umbilical cord pH, low Apgar scores, delay in the onset of spontaneous respiration, the need for resuscitation at birth and abnormal neonatal neurologic signs. Although various parameters, either alone or in combination, have been used to define birth asphyxia, a precise definition remains difficult as many of these parameters, e.g. fetal heart rate abnormalities, fetal acidosis or low Apgar scores correlate poorly with outcome. In clinical practice the signs of asphyxial encephalopathy and seizures are usually taken as conclusive evidence of an asphyxial event in term infants.

Despite the fact that significant injury has often occurred prior to the arrival of the infant in the NICU, there is evidence to suggest that postasphyxial management can markedly affect the outcome for that infant. Functional assessment of all systems is required, as a broad spectrum of organ dysfunction is observed, the most frequent being renal (50 per cent), CNS (30 per cent) and cardiovascular and pulmonary (25 per cent).[187]

Systemic Manifestations and Management

Renal

The kidneys are one of the first organ systems to be affected, resulting in renal failure with acute tubular, medullary, cortical or papillary necrosis. There may also be a delay in spontaneous voiding of urine following asphyxia.

Early appreciation of renal damage is often difficult because of the low urine output normally seen on day one and the fact that serum creatinine reflects maternal serum levels at this age. Nevertheless oliguria is a particularly useful indicator of both renal and neurologic impairment and particular attention to urine output is essential.[188] Judicious fluid and electrolyte management must attempt to avoid aggravating both hypoperfusion and fluid overload.

Cardiovascular

Hypovolaemia, suggested by peripheral vasoconstriction, low mean arterial blood pressure and metabolic acidosis, requires volume replacement, usually with colloid 10–20 ml.kg^{-1} initially. While hypotension may further decrease cerebral perfusion pressure (mean arterial blood pressure–intracranial pressure (MABP–ICP)), rapid changes in blood pressure or hypertension should be avoided in a cerebral circulation which is likely to be pressure–passive following the loss of autoregulation secondary to asphyxia.

Other cardiac complications of asphyxia include tricuspid insufficiency secondary to papillary muscle necrosis, cardiac failure and dysrhythmias. ECG and two-dimensional echocardiographic functional assessment of the heart is usually indicated in severe asphyxia.

Treatment of tricuspid valve insufficiency, suggested by a systolic murmur, hepatomegaly and cardiomegaly involves improving oxygenation and correcting acidosis. Inotropic support (dopamine initially at 5 μg.kg^{-1}.min) and/or volume replacement may be required for a low cardiac output.

Respiratory

Respiratory complications include respiratory distress secondary to ischaemic damage to alveolar lining and surfactant production, pulmonary haemorrhage, meconium aspiration and persistent pulmonary hypertension of the newborn. Postnatal asphyxia and acidosis increase the likelihood of the infant developing a picture of PPHN.

The required treatment involves improving oxygenation, correction of acidosis, maintenance of normal blood pressure and achieving physiologic acid–base balance. Respiratory support is usually required for all of the respiratory complications of perinatal asphyxia, whether it be transient postasphyxial respiratory distress due to ischaemic lung injury or more severe meconium aspiration and PPHN.

Hyperventilation and the induction of an alkalosis may be required to improve oxygenation in PPHN; this however, may lead to further brain ischaemia by decreasing cerebral blood flow. Because of concerns that CBF may be compromised in hypoxic–ischaemic encephalopathy,[189] the $PaCO_2$ is generally maintained between 30–40 mmHg.

CNS

Neurological signs of perinatal asphyxia include decreased level of consciousness, muscle tone, degree of spontaneous activity, deep tendon reflexes and complex reflexes (suck, Moro, oculovestibular); an altered respiratory pattern (apnoea, periodic breathing to respiratory arrest) and other brainstem functions including pupillary reactivity, extraocular movement and impaired suck and swallow mechanism, the presence of seizures and signs of raised intracranial pressure. The latter may occur between days one and four with a tense or bulging fontanelle and relative bradycardia.

CNS management is aimed at providing adequate oxygen and glucose to the brain, decreasing energy demands, controlling seizures and limiting cerebral oedema.

Seizures Rapid control of seizures once they occur is imperative as seizures may compromise respiration and add further insult to pre-existing injury. Seizures of metabolic origin are treated by correction of the deficient agent. Once this has been excluded, vigorous but safe anticonvulsant therapy is attempted with a loading dose of 20 mg.kg^{-1} of phenobarbitone. If control is not achieved further phenobarbitone up to a total of 30–40 mg.kg^{-1} or a second anticonvulsant, e.g. phenytoin 20 mg.kg^{-1}, is added. Seizures may be resistant to treatment and require an escalating number of drugs to be utilized, including lorazepam and/or paraldehyde (the latter given as a 5 per cent solution at 3 ml.kg^{-1}.hr over two hrs).

Although there are no clinical studies to date that demonstrate conclusively that clinical seizures per se are damaging to the newborn brain as long as systemic cardiovascular and metabolic homoeostasis is maintained, it seems prudent to continue to treat vigorously all seizures occurring in the newborn infant.[193] Whether a comatose and ventilated infant showing subtle or purely electrical seizures should be vigorously treated with anticonvulsants is not certain.

The interval following the asphyxial insult and prior to the onset of clinically overt seizures has led to trials of prophylactic treatment with phenobarbitone. Studies, however, have not shown any beneficial effect with the use of prophylactic phenobarbitone or pentobarbitone in severe perinatal asphyxia.[194,195]

Table 5.13 Correlation of severity of hypoxic-ischaemic encephalopathy and outcome[190], (based on Finer[191] and Sarnat and Sarnat[192])

Severity	Clinical features	Outcome (per cent abnormal)
Mild (Stage I)	Hyperalertness, jitteriness, exaggerated Moro and stretch reflexes, duration $\leq$ 24 hours	0
Moderate (Stage II)	Lethargy/stupor, hypotonia, suppressed reflexes, seizures	20–40
Severe (Stage III)	Coma, hypotonia, seizures, abnormal brainstem and autonomic function, increased intracranial pressure	100

Cerebral Oedema Signs of cerebral oedema may occur 24–72 hours following the hypoxic–ischaemic injury. The role of cerebral oedema in aggravating postischaemic encephalopathy is unresolved; infants may demonstrate severe encephalopathy and a poor outcome without evidence of raised intracranial pressure.[196,197] The variable findings in these studies have not made ICP monitoring techniques suitable for clinical decision–making.[198] In general, fluids are restricted to maintenance requirements to control cerebral oedema; this is obviously dependent on the adequacy of the renal and cardiopulmonary status.

Other interventions to reduce elevated ICP have included diuretics, glucocorticoids and hyperosmolar agents. There is, however, no evidence that these interventions improve neurologic outcome.[190,193]

Hyperventilation may decrease intracranial pressure via its effect on decreasing cerebral blood flow; however, it may be contraindicated when brain oedema is associated with normal or decreased cerebral blood flow.

A variety of neuroprotective agents to limit the biochemical events following asphyxia are being investigated. Of particular interest has been the role of the excitatory amino acid neurotransmitter L–glutamate. Activation of glutamate receptors involves calcium influx and a series of deleterious events resulting in the generation of free radicals and delayed cell death.[199] While therapy aimed at limiting the biochemical cascade following an asphyxial event may hold promise for the future, none of these agents can currently be recommended. (In one study the use of the water soluble calcium channel blocker nicardipine led to the development of hypotension).[196]

GI tract
As GI function is often impaired and ischaemic mucosal damage predisposes the infant to necrotizing enterocolitis the introduction of oral feeds is usually delayed.

Metabolic disorders
Correction of metabolic disorders and maintenance of electrolytes, serum glucose, calcium, magnesium, etc. within the normal range are required. Temperature must be maintained within the thermoneutral zone.

Haematopoietic involvement
Haematopoietic involvement may lead to disseminated intravascular coagulopathy.

Endocrine abnormalities
Endocrine abnormalities following perinatal asphyxia include adrenal haemorrhage, transient hypoparathyroidism and the syndrome of inappropriate antidiuretic hormone production.

Monitoring

Monitoring of asphyxiated infants requires:

1. serial clinical neurologic examination;
2. maintenance of an adequate cerebral perfusion pressure (CPP=MABP-ICP);
3. monitoring of the functional status of organ systems, plus the quantitation of damage, e.g.:

- *renal*: urine output, electrolyte balance, renal function tests, drug excretion
- *CVS*: cardiac output, BP, ECG, enzymes
- *respiratory tract*: arterial blood gases
- *Liver*: bilirubin, drug metabolism
- *Metabolic status*: glucose, calcium, magnesium, ammonia, lactate

4. monitoring of the functional/electrical activity of the brain, e.g. EEG, evoked potentials;
5. monitoring of the anatomical status of brain structure, e.g. CT scan, ultrasound.

Diagnosis of perinatal asphyxia

While repeated clinical neurological examination is the mainstay of the diagnosis and prognosis of perinatal asphyxia, a number of imaging, electrodiagnostic and other techniques performed in conjunction with the evolution of the clinical status of affected infants are extremely useful measures. These become particularly important when detailed clinical examination is not possible because of mechanical ventilation, the use of anticonvulsants or paralysing agents.

Imaging techniques
In the term infant with hypoxic ischaemia encephalopathy (HIE) cranial ultrasound is a useful screening method and is usually the first imaging investigation. Diffuse neuronal necrosis may be suspected with diffuse increased echodensity; localized increased echoes suggest focal infarction. It may require repeat studies after day two to demonstrate these increases in echodensity.

An early CT scan is performed when the

sonogram does not adequately explain the clinical status of the infant (e.g. to rule out ICH). A CT scan on day two to four correlates with maximal increased intracranial pressure and cerebral oedema; scans performed between days four to seven are more predictive of outcome than earlier phase scans. The extent of decreased tissue attenuation on CT correlates well with outcome. Later scans may demonstrate focal or generalized atrophy or diffuse encephalomalacia, evidence of a very poor prognosis.

MRI has been used in severe asphyxia with good correlation between abnormal scans and subsequent neurological abnormalities.[200-2] MRI findings are similar to those seen on the CT scan but may demonstrate better anatomical definition of the different types of infarct and accurate evaluation of myelination.

Phosphorus magnetic resonance spectroscopy studies have shown specific biochemical alteration of spectra patterns at various moments of HI injury, which are of both diagnostic and prognostic significance.[203-5]

Cerebral blood flow studies in infants with HIE have included Doppler ultrasound (CBF velocity), positron emission tomography (regional perfusion and metabolism), and more recently single photon emission computerized tomography (regional CBF) and near infrared spectroscopy (cerebral oxygen delivery, blood volume and tissue oxygen utilization).[189,196,207] At present these techniques remain essentially research tools providing insight into the responses of the cerebral circulation following a hypoxaemic–ischaemic injury.

Electroencephalography (EEG)

EEG is an essential part of the evaluation of the asphyxiated newborn. A pattern of evolution from slow and reduced amplitude to a burst suppression pattern with further deterioration to an isoelectric pattern parallels the severity of the clinical picture. Studies have emphasized that the degree and duration of abnormality is strongly predictive of an unfavorable neurological outcome.[192,208]

Electrodiagnostic techniques

Evoked potentials particularly visual (VEP), and somatosensory potentials are useful adjuncts to the clinical and neuroradiologic investigations in perinatal asphyxia; serial testing reflects the evolution and extent of brain injury. Multimodal testing enhances the reliability of these techniques, which have recently been shown to have an extremely high predictive power.[209,210]

Outcome

In the group of term infants who develop HIE in the newborn period following intrapartum asphyxia, the clinical picture does correlate closely with outcome.[191,192,211,212] In general, in mild encephalopathy the signs subside within 24–48 hours and the long–term prognosis is very good. Moderate encephalopathy carries a 25–40 per cent risk of abnormal outcome, particularly if signs persist longer than 5–7 days. Severe HIE has a significant mortality and very high incidence of severe morbidity in survivors. Specific features of the clinical picture also aid in predictability, i.e. the earlier the onset of seizures and the stronger the refractoriness to anticonvulsant medication or evidence of increased intracranial pressure, the more severe the neurologic sequelae. In addition, the extent of decreased tissue attenuation on CT scan, abnormal VEP and somatosensory evoked potentials and EEG findings, allows an accurate prediction of outcome.[190,210,213]

Brain injury in premature infants

Intraventricular/periventricular haemorrhage (IVH/PVH) and periventricular leukomalacia (PVL)

Preterm infants are particularly susceptible to haemorrhagic and ischaemic cerebral insults; IVH/PVH and PVL constitute the most common of these and will be briefly discussed.

IVH/PVH occurrs in 20–25 per cent of infants < 1500 gm.[215,219] Less than 10 per cent of preterm infants who do not require mechanical ventilation or those requiring mechanical ventilation but with minimal respiratory distress, demonstrate IVH.[216] The incidence of IVH, particularly of the more severe grades of haemorrhage appears to have decreased over the past decade. It is difficult to attribute this decrease in incidence to any specific intervention and incidence figures must be cautiously interpreted as this has not been a universal finding.[217]

Pathogenesis

Bleeding typically originates in the rich capillary bed of the subependymal germinal matrix, a transition zone which is the site of neuronal and glial proliferation. The immature capillary network, with less basement membrane than in capillaries of more mature brain, is both poorly supported and subserved by an abundant arterial supply, making these capillaries particularly vulnerable to rupture.

Disturbances in cerebral blood flow have been considered the major pathogenetic mechanism of IVH in the premature infant: hypoxia, hypercarbia and acidosis disturb the normal autoregulatory vascular response of the arterioles leading to a pressure–passive cerebral circulation. Increased blood flow in infants with impaired autoregulation may thus lead to bleeding from the arteriolar–capillary network. The strong clinical associations of IVH are prematurity, asphyxia, RDS, mechanical ventilation, alterations in blood pressure and pneumothorax. These disorders all share the capability of increasing pertubations of CBF,[187] via systemic effects on cardiac output, arterial blood pressure and central venous pressure. In addition, systemic coagulation disorders and fibrinolytic activity within the germinal matrix may be involved in the pathogenesis of bleeding.

PVH (periventricular haemorrhage) refers to haemorrhagic necrosis in periventricular white matter. The haemorrhages are usually asymmetric and are seen in association with IVH in 80 per cent of cases, with the parenchymal lesions invariably on the same side as the larger amount of IVH.[218] Previously considered an extension of IVH into brain parenchyma, PVH is now considered more likely to represent venous infarction secondary to IVH and its associated germinal matrix haemorrhage, with haemorrhage leading to obstruction of the medullary and terminal veins resulting in venous infarction.[218–220]

While a single aetiological factor is unlikely to account for IVH, appreciation of the premature infant's limited cerebral autoregulatory capacity has led to a number of clinical mechanisms to minimize alterations in systemic BP and CBF:

1. Continuous PO_2, PCO_2 and blood pressure monitoring, careful intubation, suctioning and minimal handling techniques.
2. Mechanical ventilation to avoid the effects of hypercarbia, hypoxia and acidosis on CBF. In addition, careful attention to ventilatory parameters to avoid the complication of a pneumothorax and its potential effects on cerebral venous pressure. Achieving synchrony between ventilator and infant may allow lower ventilator pressures to be used. The use of muscular paralysing agents in the ventilated

preterm infant has shown a reduced risk of IVH in one study.[221] The use of narcotic analgesics such as morphine sulphate in ventilated infants may also eliminate fluctuations in arterial blood pressure.[214,222]

The decreased incidence of IVH seems to have preceded the advent of surfactant replacement therapy and may have resulted from the greater awareness of IVH and its predisposing and aggravating factors. Although it was anticipated that surfactant, by decreasing ventilatory parameters and the incidence of pneumothorax, would further decrease the incidence of IVH, conclusions from the surfactant trials conducted thus far have shown that only 25 per cent of both prophylaxis and rescue trials demonstrate a reduction in the incidence of any IVH, and surfactant has not significantly reduced the incidence of the more severe grades of IVH.[223] Further information from ongoing studies about the epidemiology and aetiology of IVH will define whether reducing the risk for RDS and its complications will have a more prominent effect on IVH than has been found thus far.[223]

3. Avoidance of sudden increases in cerebral perfusion pressure, e.g. via slower volume expansion in infants with possibly impaired autoregulation or the slow infusion of bicarbonate so as to minimize the induction of hypertonicity in the cerebral vessels.
4. At present no pharmacologic agent is considered to decrease the incidence or severity of IVH consistently.[224] Drugs which have been studied include phenobarbitone, indomethacin, ethamsylate and vitamin E (?decrease CBF, enhance autoregulatory ability, stabilize vascular endothelium or minimize oxidative damage from increased oxygen free radicals). Postnatal phenobarbitone has not shown a consistent beneficial effect; indomethacin has the potential risk of ischaemic brain injury due to a decrease in CBF; evidence for ethamsylate use is also not sufficient and larger studies in the use of vitamin E are required before recommending its use.[225]
5. Increasing knowledge about the impact of routine caregiving practices on ICP and CBF, e.g. the amount of handling, suctioning, vigour of resuscitation measures, ventilatory parameters, etc. In addition, new techniques to monitor cerebral haemoglobin

oxidation–reduction status and cerebral blood volume continuously at the bedside may in the future also provide an increased awareness factor in the routine care practices of the NICU.

6. Prenatal interventions including vitamin K or phenobarbitone to the mother have not proved consistently beneficial. The role of caesarean section to prevent IVH is also not clear. The prevention of prematurity and perinatal asphyxia remain the most important, yet the most elusive, of all the factors implicated in the pathogenesis of IVH.

Clinical aspects

The diagnosis of IVH should be suspected in any preterm infant in an intensive care unit, particularly one with a history of asphyxia, difficult delivery or significant respiratory distress requiring mechanical ventilation. The clinical signs include a change in tone or degree of spontaneous activity, seizures, fall in haematocrit, full fontanelle, metabolic acidosis and hyperglycaemia. The signs are usually evident within the first 12–72 hours although signs may appear earlier in extremely low birthweight infants. Parenchymal lesions tend to have a peak occurrence at four days, slightly after that for lesser grades of IVH.[219] Routine ultrasound of all low birthweight infants has shown that IVH may be asymptomatic in a large number of infants.

Diagnosis

Cranial ultrasound is the imaging procedure of choice. It identifies all grades of IVH and PVH from which prognostic considerations can be made. See Fig. 1.17 (p. 50)

Management

Infants with IVH are followed with serial ultrasound examinations at weekly to ten day intervals to document progressive ventricular dilatation. This evolves over a number of weeks and is due to early obstruction to CSF outflow or a more gradual obliterative arachnoiditis in the subarachnoid space. Three patterns of dilatation are described:

1. progressive ventricular dilatation with subsequent arrest and thereafter spontaneous regression in ventricular size;
2. severe progressive ventricular dilatation with-

out clinical signs of raised intracranial pressure;
3. progressive development of hydrocephalus with symptomatic increased intracranial pressure.

The indication for ventriculoperitoneal shunt insertion is based on demonstrating increasing ventricular size, usually with clinical evidence of raised intracranial pressure. Direct measurements of ICP, Doppler assessment of cerebral vascular resistance or assessment of CSF dynamics are not routinely performed. Early shunting is usually not required as the majority of infants show regression in the size of the ventricles and there is a relatively high incidence of shunt complications if performed early. With increasing head circumference (> 2 cm per week), clinical signs of increased intracranial pressure, and progressive ventriculomegaly, ventricular shunting is performed, usually after 3–4 weeks of life. Lumbar punctures are only used occasionally to determine the opening pressure or CSF status of the infant and generally not as temporizing manoeuvres prior to shunt placement, as the practice of performing serial LPs to prevent shunt placement has not proven beneficial.[227,228]

The requirement for V–P shunting for posthaemorrhagic hydrocephalus is infrequent today, ± 4 per cent of infants < 35 weeks gestational age.[229] Late hydrocephalus may occur in infants with ventriculomegaly and these infants need to be followed for months after discharge from the NICU.

Outcome

The acute mortality from IVH/PVH is substantial. It is dependent upon several factors, including the size of the haemorrhage, the degree of immaturity of the infant, mechanical ventilatory requirements and complications, any associated disorders and the philosophy prevailing in any particular neonatal unit with regard to the aggressiveness of supportive measures for infants with documented severe IVH. Infants with small (grade I) haemorrhage with few or no acute symptoms show no or only mild neurologic abnormalities on follow–up examination; haemorrhages of grade II and III severity (IVH with or without ventricular dilatation) may produce few residua, but are associated with mild to moderate abnormalities in as many as 40 per cent of infants. Severe IVH with extensive parenchymal haemorrhage and the development of intraparenchymal echodensities (Grade IV),[236] is associated with major motor deficits and almost invariably cognitive deficits in the majority of infants. The development of posthaemorrhagic hydrocephalus complicating IVH increases the ultimate neurologic morbidity over that of IVH alone, particularly if shunt complications supervene.

Periventricular leukomalacia (PVL)

PVL is the neuropathological consequence of ischaemic injury to periventricular white matter. It may occur as a separate lesion or more commonly in association with IVH. In fact the extent of ischaemic injury may be more important in determining neurodevelopmental outcome than the degree of haemorrhage. The incidence of PVL in recent years has been approximately 25–40 per cent of very low birth weight infants.[224] This appears to increase with the duration of postnatal survival and with the frequency and severity of cardiorespiratory disturbances.[232]

Pathogenesis[225]

Pathogenesis relates to three principal factors.[224]

1. Periventricular vascular anatomical factors: PVL is considered a watershed infarction as it occurs in the border zone between ventriculopetal and ventriculofugal arterioles.
2. The enhanced vulnerability of actively differentiating and/or myelinating periventricular glial cells.
3. A pressure–passive cerebral circulation due to impaired autoregulation secondary to immaturity alone (deficient musculature in cerebral arterioles and the narrow range of the normal regulatory plateau

in premature infants[232,233] and/or secondary to hypercarbia and hypoxaemia following asphyxia, respiratory distress, sepsis, PDA, apnoea spells, etc. The premature infant is thus susceptible to decreases in CBF and injury to the periventricular white matter with hypotension. While close monitoring of such infants may prevent episodes of hypotension, the prevention of PVL is limited by the maturation–dependent deficiencies of the periventricular microcirculation.[224]

Diagnosis

There are no specific early clinical signs of PVL. Detection during life is dependent upon ultrasound scanning which demonstrates increased echodensities adjacent to the external angle of the lateral ventricles. These may occur early, often within a few days of birth. The characteristic evolution of the echodensities of PVL is the formation of small cysts, often multiple, occurring two to three weeks after the appearance of echodensities. In order to assess the significance of early parenchymal lesions, serial scans should be performed until at least 40 weeks postconceptual age.[234] With relatively circumscribed cysts the lesions may disappear, at least ultrasonographically, after 1–3 months.[224] Later diagnosis of PVL via CT or MRI will assess the degree of white matter atrophy.[235]

Prognosis is dependent upon the extent and site of the lesions; infants with sonographic changes confined to the frontal cortex or with only transient 'flares' usually develop normally; those with more extensive and persistent frontoparietal or frontoparietal–occipital coarse changes, or cystic cavitation are associated with major neurological sequelae, especially cerebral palsy with spastic diplegia and to a lesser extent, intellectual deficits.[224,236-8]

Sepsis and infection control

The newborn, and in particular the premature infant, is considered an immunocompromised host, with deficiencies in all arms of the immune system that generally parallel the degree of immaturity. It is the recognition and possible prevention of

the further compromise of host factors by many of the current techniques of neonatal intensive care that may improve morbidity and mortality from infection in infants in the neonatal intensive care unit. Prevention of these infections requires a multifaceted approach, including meticulous patient care techniques, elimination of inappropriate antibiotic administration to avoid further alteration of the colonizing bacterial flora and particular attention to all aspects of infection control. Further improvements may result from increasingly accurate and sensitive methods of the early detection of sepsis and possibly with the use of genetically engineered products that enhance the newborn's response to infection.

Sepsis may be congenital or acquired; the former will not be discussed in this chapter as the congenital infections (CMV, Rubella, herpes, toxoplasmosis, syphilis) generally have little impact on newborns with surgical conditions. Acquired infections may occur early, within the first 48 hours of life, or later, usually nosocomial or hospital acquired, after one or more weeks of hospitalization. It is this latter group of acquired infections that have a major impact on infants undergoing surgery in the neonatal period.

Incidence rates vary widely; 1–8 cases per 1000 live births are affected by early onset infection; nosocomial infection rates also vary widely, from 5–25 per cent of infants in NICUs,[239] and with an inverse correlation with birthweight.

Early onset sepsis

The maternal risk factors for early onset infection in the newborn are additive, and include prolonged rupture of membranes for > 24 hr, maternal colonization with group B streptococci, maternal fever, urinary tract infection or chorioamnionitis (maternal fever, uterine tenderness, foul smelling amniotic fluid, fetal tachycardia) and unexplained premature delivery. The common organisms leading to infection are those within the birth canal and include group B streptococci, *E. coli* and other coliform organisms.

The signs of sepsis are protean and non-specific; they include lethargy, hypothermia, fever, apnoea, cyanotic spells, respiratory distress, jaundice, poor perfusion, shock, abdominal distension, poor feeding, ileus, irritability, jitteriness, seizures, petechiae and purpura.

Diagnosis

Isolation of bacteria from blood or other body fluids is standard and specific. The blood culture should preferably be from a fresh umbilical arterial catheter or via venepuncture. The decision to do more than a blood culture and complete blood count, specifically whether to perform a lumbar puncture or urine examination, is often difficult in the light of the non-specificity of symptoms; it is based on clinical judgement, the likelihood of a positive yield and the ability to interpret cell counts and biochemistry. In general there is a low yield for both CSF and urine examination in early onset sepsis.[240] Detection of group B streptococcal antigen via the latex particle agglutination test from urine, serum or CSF usually warrants its use in the specific diagnostic work–up for group B streptococcal disease, although contamination of bag specimens of urine may produce false positive results,[241] and the utility of a urine latex test is not considered equivalent to a positive blood culture.[242]

Despite the blood culture being the 'gold standard', cultures are often negative in infants with clinical signs or in infants who subsequently die from sepsis. The white blood count and differential cell count remain the most consistent adjunctive test for early onset (< 72 hr) sepsis, particularly neutropenia (< 2000 mm^3) in the absence of maternal pre-eclampsia or other known causes of neutropenia, and an immature to total neutrophil ratio of > 0.2.[243] Other signs of sepsis on the peripheral blood smear include toxic granulations and neutrophil vacuolization.

Acute phase reactants, e.g. C-reactive protein, micro ESR, haptoglobin and fibronectin have limited usefulness and provide little additional sensitivity or predictive value. The use of the nitroblue tetrazolium test and Gram stain and culture of the gastric aspirate has tended to decrease, except as indicators of chorioamnionitis.

Late onset or nosocomial infection

Signs of infection usually appear during the hospital stay, generally after 1–4 weeks of life, but may occasionally appear as early as day three or four, or after discharge from the NICU. The most common organisms responsible for nosocomial infection in the NICU are coagulase negative staphylococci; other organisms include fungi and viruses.

The infant may be infected by various routes, either by human carriers or via contaminated materials and equipment. Human sources include droplet spread (e.g. respiratory virus), hand carriage of organisms (e.g. staphylococcal or streptococcal species), or direct contact with infectious lesions (e.g. Herpes simplex virus and *Staph. aureus*). A number of gram negative bacteria are known to flourish in aqueous environments (e.g. pseudomonas species, *Serratia marcescens*) and contamination of solutions used in nebulization, room humidifiers and hand cleaning agents have all been described.

The most common route of infection is via invasive procedures in the care of the newborn, particularly umbilical arterial and venous lines central venous lines, and V–P shunts. Factors influencing the rate of infection related to catheters include the type of catheter, the catheter material, its location, the use of lipid emulsions, the duration of placement, the use of topical agents, the dressing material and colonization via organisms on the skin at the catheter exit site (Table 5.14). Acquisition of cytomegalovirus (CMV), hepatitis B or C, or human immune virus (HIV) via blood products must still be considered, despite screening programmes.

Table 5.14 Risk factors for nosocomial infection

1	VLBW infants
2	Prolonged hospitalization
3	Prior antibiotic therapy
4	Indwelling device, catheter, shunt
5	Major surgery
6	Parenteral nutrition, fat emulsions

Two specific nosocomial infectious agents that are important in infants who have undergone surgical procedures are:

1. Coagulase negative staphylococci (CNS):

Twenty-one species of Gram positive staphylococci are coagulase negative, of which *Staph. epidermidis* is most commonly associated with nosocomial infections in the newborn.[244,245] They account for approximately 80 per cent of the bacteraemias encountered each year in the NICU. These organisms are normal residents of neonatal skin; colonization of the skin, upper respiratory and GI tract is usually established by the first week of life.[246]

The virulence of these organisms appears to be related to their production of a mucoid substance, slime, an extracellular glycocalyx material which promotes adherence and growth of organisms on the surfaces of the synthetic polymers used in the production of catheters and shunts, and which tends to protect against antimicrobial activity and phagocytosis.[247,248] Other virulence factors including an adhesion factor and a delta–toxin, possibly associated with necrotising enterocolitis (NEC), have been described.

A case control study noted a six–fold increase in CNS bacteraemia in those infants who received lipids as part of their parenteral nutrition. The following pathogenesis has been suggested: after colonization of the skin and mucosa by coagulase negative staphylococci during the first days of life, these organisms adhere to the outside of the percutaneous intravascular catheter and gain access to the interior of the catheter through cutaneous or haematogenous routes; microcolonies of staphylococci which are protected by the slime layer develop within the catheter. Rapid bacterial growth is stimulated when lipids are introduced, ultimately leading to the invasion of the bloodstream as the organisms reach an inoculum of sufficient size.[249]

The major question arising from documentation of a bacteraemia due to a coagulase negative staphylococcus is whether it is a contaminated skin culture or a true pathogen. A number of studies have attempted to clarify this issue by the association of the bacteraemia with various clinical criteria, using more than one consecutive positive culture, or quantitating CNS together with haematologic parameters.[246,250] In general, it is the level of clinical suspicion of sepsis in the high risk infant that determines whether the bacteraemia is regarded as significant or not and this judgement will dictate the readiness to initiate antibiotic therapy. Unnecessary treatment certainly has its potential deleterious effects, i.e. alteration of normal flora, medication errors, requirement for an i.v. and possible removal of catheters in addition to the emotional set–back to parents of chronically hospitalized infants. Treatment, therefore, is usually initiated only with sufficient clinical evidence of infection in infants with one or more underlying risk factors.

Signs of CNS sepsis are often indolent and non–specific in nature: temperature instability, an increase in ventilatory requirements, apnoea or an alteration in gastrointestinal function. Signs may occasionally be more fulminant or focal. The latter include infective endocarditis, meningitis, an NEC–like picture, pneumonia and omphalitis. Although the mortality from CNS appears much lower than that with group B streptococcal infection or Gram negative enteric bacteria, treatment should be initiated upon clinical suspicion without waiting for a second culture to exclude potential contamination. Other adjunctive tests for sepsis, e.g. CBC, should be performed but are often not helpful.

Identification of strains within the coagulase negative staphylococcus species is usually not necessary; it is occasionally indicated to determine the clinical significance of an isolate if two or more systemic isolates are found in an individual patient or in assessing the likelihood of transmission from one patient to another from a common source or via a common mechanism.[247,250]

Treatment

A number of strains of nursery acquired CNS are sensitive to the penicillinase-resistant penicillins and therefore methicillin or cloxacillin or a cephalosporin may be used. CNS may be resistant to the β-lactam agents in up to 40 per cent of cases.[247] Treatment therefore may be initiated with cloxacillin, and vancomycin is used if there is clinical failure to respond to this agent. Many recommend vancomycin as the drug of first choice[244,247] as it has shown consistent efficacy against coagulase negative staphylococci, although resistance of CNS to vancomycin has also been rarely described.[252] Vancomycin can be used either alone or with gentamicin. Removal of an indwelling catheter or shunt may be necessary, particularly if recurrent bacteraemia is demonstrated, an exit site infection fails to clear or there is evidence of thrombosis or persistent thrombocytopaenia.

If there is improvement after the initiation of treatment the child is generally treated for seven days. Once the organism is identified the infant is treated as per susceptibility. If the suspicion of sepsis has been low, and cultures are negative after 48–72 hours, antibiotics are often discontinued.

2. Candidiasis

Systemic or focal candidiasis is becoming of increasing concern in the low birthweight or postoperative surgical patient, correlating with the improved survival and chronic hospitalization of these patients.[253,254] Colonization, particularly of the lower gastrointestinal tract with *C. albicans* and *M. furfur* has been identified within ten days of life in patients in the NICU.[255] The relationship between colonization and invasive disease has not been well studied. Predisposing factors to fungal infection are similar to those for CNS and include the use of broad spectrum antibiotics, prolonged intubation, indwelling catheters, the use of total parenteral nutrition with hypertonic glucose and fat emulsions and major surgery requiring prolonged invasive monitoring. Haematogenous dissemination may lead to the seeding of multiple organs including the brain, heart, kidney and the eye. The majority of infections are due to *Candida albicans*, but other yeast species are also reported including *Malassezia furfur* (particularly associated with the use of lipids in TPN).[256]

Signs of infection

Signs of systemic or focal candidiasis can be recognized if a high index of suspicion is maintained in those infants with predisposing factors. The clinical picture resembles bacterial sepsis and the diagnosis is often only considered with persistence of symptoms after the exclusion of bacterial infection.

Focal signs of candida infections include:

1. *GI tract*: abdominal distension and feeding intolerance mimicking NEC.
2. *Respiratory tract*: pneumonia, difficult to differentiate from bronchopulmonary dysplasia but suggested by an unexpected increase in oxygen requirements.
3. *Renal tract*: infection may be clinically silent or lead to renal failure. The renal involvement may be detected via ultrasound in which echogenic fungal balls are seen within the collecting system; a parenchymal abscess or signs of obstruction with dilatation of the pelvicalyceal junction may also be seen. There are potential pitfalls in relying on sonography in the management of infants with renal candidiasis.[257]
4. *Cardiovascular system*: infected thrombi may be seen in the aorta or vena cava; occasionally right atrial intracardiac masses can be documented on two-dimensional echocardiography.
5. *Meningitis*: difficult to diagnose because of the low concentration of organisms in the CSF but should be suspected if the CSF glucose is low in the absence of intraventricular haemorrhage.
6. *Eye involvement*: endophthalmitis; any suspicion requires indirect ophthalmoscopy to detect the chorioretinal fluffy white lesion and hazy vitreous.

Diagnosis

Fungi may be seen in the buffy coat smear of the

blood; often multiple cultures of blood, urine or CSF are required to establish the diagnosis.

Treatment

Treatment of systemic candidiasis is not undertaken lightly because of the toxicity of the agents available. Nevertheless, if candida is cultured or if clinical signs are highly suggestive, amphotericin B is used as the agent of choice. It should be administered intravenously over 4–6 hours in a dextrose solution; the high incidence of toxicity requires monitoring of renal and hepatic function. The concurrent use of 5-fluorocytosine is occasionally considered, particularly if there is neurological involvement.[253] Removal of a catheter or shunt is undertaken if a fungal infection is documented or suspected.

Other organisms responsible for nosocomial infection include Gram negative enteric bacilli and respiratory viruses, particularly the respiratory syncytial virus which has a significant morbidity in newborns who require prolonged assisted ventilation.

Examples of late manifestations of perinatally acquired infection from the birth canal include chlamydia involving the eye (conjunctivitis) and lung (pneumonia), and genital mycoplasmas, *U. urealyticum* and *Mycoplasma hominis*, associated with chronic lung disease.[258]

An infant suspected of nosocomial infection should have a complete physical examination with special attention to the catheter sites, skin, perianal area, fundi and oropharynx. Cultures from various sites include central line and peripheral blood cultures; urine, drainage and tracheal tube cultures.

Antimicrobial agents

If sepsis is probable immediate treatment is imperative without prior identification of the organism or documentation of antimicrobial agent sensitivities. Initially all antibiotics are administered intravenously; the choice is based upon the suspected organism and its antibiotic sensitivity within each individual NICU. Ideally antibiotics in which the pharmacokinetics have been adequately evaluated in the newborn should be used. Empiric antibiotic therapy is based on common organisms and known antibiotic sensitivity as suggested in Table 5.15. Specific therapy should be guided by clinical response to initial therapy and final culture and sensitivity data.

Table 5.15 Empirical Antibiotic Selection

Suspected sepsis/site	Empiric therapy
Bacteraemia	Ampicillin and aminoglycoside (gentamicin or tobramycin) or Ampicillin and cefotaxime; add cloxacillin if risk for *S. aureus*
Meningitis	Ampicillin and aminoglycoside or Ampicillin and cefotaxime
if shunt related	Vancomycin and cefotaxime; cefotaxime and aminoglycoside if Gram negative bacilli or coliform
Pneumonia	Ampicillin and aminoglycoside
Soft tissue and bone/joint	Cloxacillin and aminoglycoside
NEC	Ampicillin and aminoglycoside; clindamycin if perforation

Other measures

Other measures for the treatment of sepsis include appropriate electrolyte and fluid management, oxygen therapy, monitoring of glucose and acid–base status and the use of blood and blood products where necessary.

In infants with fulminant sepsis, and particularly those with a neutrophil count of $< 3 \times 10^9.1^{-1}$ and evidence of a depleted marrow neutrophil storage pool, granulocyte transfusions (preferably prepared by automated leukopheresis) appear to be beneficial.[259-1] However, the small number of patients studied and their heterogeneity make it difficult to reach a consensus on guide–lines for granulocyte transfusion therapy.[262-3] It is also difficult to recommend a bone marrow aspirate to assess the myeloid reserve pool in sick infants to identify candidates for treatment. For these and other reasons, including the lack of rapid availability, the use of granulocyte transfusions appears to have declined recently.[263] Further studies will be needed to establish whether granulocyte transfusions offer any benefit over antibiotic therapy and supportive care.

Immunoglobulin has been administered to neonates with clinical signs of sepsis or as prophylaxis for infection. A variable response has been found and further trials are necessary before recommending their routine use in high risk infants.[254,264-6] One of the obvious concerns is the relative concentration of antibodies versus different pathogens, e.g. group B streptococci in early onset infection and against coagulase negative staphylococci in later onset nosocomial infection.

The recent identification of various haematopoietic colony stimulating factors and other cytokines suggests a method of increasing neonatal defence mechanisms.[267] This will require future evaluation before these factors become more readily used.

Infection control

It is extremely important that the NICU have strict infection control policies and guidelines. The surveillance team must fulfil a number of important functions: provide data on the antimicrobial susceptibility of organisms so as to guide initial or empiric therapy; identify different or new patterns of resistance early; and help create policies regarding issues such as isolation criteria, screening of staff, nursery routines, etc.

Principles of control

The principles of infection control in the NICU include:

1. Knowledge of the immunization status of the NICU personnel, e.g. against chickenpox, rubella and polio; the recommendation for immunization of susceptible staff; avoidance of patient contact for staff carriers of RSV, Herpes virus, etc.
2. Hand washing with chlorhexidine before and after every patient contact.
3. Adequate skin preparation for all i.v.s and blood cultures, and particularly for procedures involving indwelling devices.
4. Minimal to no use of intravascular parenteral nutrition lines for sampling purposes.
5. Prompt isolation of infants with suspected congenital infection, acquired viral illness, bloodborne infections, bacterial gastroenteri-

tis or infants colonized with multiply resistant organisms.

The current literature[268] does not support gowning as a means of infection control in the NICU; however, in specific nosocomial infections it may substantially reduce transmission rates, e.g. RSV infection.[269]

Prophylaxis against specific infections

Hepatitis B

If the mother is a known HbsAg carrier, hepatitis B immunoglobulin (HBIg) should be given to the infant within 12 hours after birth (this should be repeated after three months if vaccine is not given); 0.5 ml HBIg is given intramuscularly. Administration of both HBIg and HBV vaccine provide a level of protection superior to that obtained when either is used alone, therefore, hepatitis B vaccine (suspension of purified surface antigen protein) is given at the same time as the first HBIg injection as either Heptavax B 10 μg (0.5 ml i.m.) or Recombivax–HB 5 μg (0.5 ml i.m.). The vaccine should be given at a different site from HBIg (the anterolateral side of the thigh is preferable as suboptimal responses have been seen when vaccine is given in the buttocks). Subsequent doses of vaccine are given at one and six months of age.

Varicella

When maternal chickenpox occurs within five days before or two days after delivery, the newborn infant is at risk of severe disseminated disease. The incubation period is shorter than in normal chickenpox either because of the route of exposure, the dose of the virus or the immaturity of cellular immune defence mechanisms. There is thus significant risk of severe disease with dissemination to liver, lung, brain and other organs. Infants at risk should therefore receive varicella zoster immune globulins (VZIG) as soon as possible after birth; severe disease may occur despite the use of VZIG, and many authorities recommend that exposed infants receive acyclovir in addition.[270]

Routine immunization

Low birthweight infants or those with complicated neonatal courses may require hospitalization for a number of months. In these infants immunization against diphtheria, pertussis, tetanus and poliomyelitis as combined DPT-polio (inactivated polio virus [IPV]) should begin at the chronological age recommended for term infants, provided there are no contraindications to its use. Satisfactory antibody responses are attained and side effects are infrequent. Oral polio vaccine is not used in infants while in the NICU. If pertussis vaccine is contraindicated for any reason, DT and IPV are given separately. Prematurity per se does not constitute a contraindication to pertussis immunization.[271]

Perinatal HIV infection

The increasing incidence of perinatal HIV infection has clearly impacted on NICU routines; where appropriate, knowledge of the maternal HIV status may be important in the management of the newborn in an NICU. Transmission to the newborn occurs either during the intrapartum period with ingestion of maternal blood by maternal–fetal transfusion during labour and delivery or postnatally via breastfeeding. It appears that the timing of the mother's primary infection may be an important factor in the route of transmission[272,273]; prevention of transmission from an infected mother to the newborn will depend upon further studies defining more precisely how and when perinatal

HIV transmission occurs and the factors influencing it.

The diagnosis in the newborn involves the determination of specific HIV antibodies by ELISA, confirmed by Western blot analysis. This will not, however, distinguish an infected infant from an infant who has received passive transfer of antibodies from an infected mother. Therefore, other tests such as virus culture, detection of p24 antigen or the use of the polymerase chain reaction technique for the amplification of viral DNA in infected cells have been adapted for the early identification of HIV in newborn infants.[274]

Appropriate precautions must be taken by staff to avoid mucosal exposure to HIV infected blood. These include the concept of universal blood precautions in which all blood and bloody body fluids are considered potentially infectious. NICU practice should ensure proper adherence to HIV testing procedures (confidentiality, consent and counselling) and safe practice by staff in any procedures that involve blood, body fluids or other potential combinations of hazards.

Ethical considerations in the care of newborn infants

Abbyan Lynch, PhD

Appropriate clinical decision making is the goal of medical practice. Such decision making encompasses both a medical and a moral choice: 'What is to be done should be medically right for the presenting patient; what is to be done should also be good for the presenting patient.'[275]

This ethical aspect of medical practice is as old as medicine itself.[276-8] However, public and professional interest in medical ethics has mushroomed in recent years. There are a number of possible explanations for this phenomenon: greater public awareness of developments in science, technology and medicine has heightened interest in medical moral decision making, particularly when resources are limited.[279-83]

Growing recognition of patient rights and maturing public acceptance of ethical pluralism have focused public concern on the need for change in the older, more paternalistic forms of clinical decision making. Proliferation of health care professional groups, each pledged to do what is 'best' for the patient, has prompted a certain moral

confusion and thus an increased ethical concern among an increasing number of staff and patients.

These factors particularly affect the area of neonatal care: agreement on the legitimate moral interests of the newborn patient, the patient's parents/guardians, society and relevant practitioners will always be problematic. Such decision making within a therapeutic milieu also subject to research and educational demands can never be accomplished easily.[284-7] The particular uncertainties of newborn diagnosis and prognosis make this process still more difficult.[288-91] In addition, there are pressures of time and the need to attend to the emotional distress of the parents of acutely ill newborn children.[292] One unique challenge, quite different from that posed in the care of many critically ill adults, is the absence of any patient direction as to initiation or non–initiation of therapy so that the 'best interests' of the NICU infant must always be determined by others. All these various considerations underline the need for ethical consideration in the NICU context.

Resolution of ethical dilemmas arising in the provision of neonatal care

The moral choices accompanying every clinical encounter become ethical dilemmas when they involve conflicts of beliefs, values, obligations or loyalties. For example:

1. the physician may face a conflict between his obligations to the parents and his obligations to the patient if he foresees that frank disclosure of prognosis may so heighten parental anxiety that they will refuse the appropriate therapy for their child.
2. the physician may know that the pursuit of a particular therapeutic regimen will cure the pneumonia in an infant with severe bronchopulmonary dysplasia and a consideration of his obligation to the patient would seem to indicate that course as the correct one. Yet, if saved from death via pneumonia, that infant will continue on a longer but still fatal downhill course, incurring protracted parental suffering. The apparent conflict of values between provision of benefit and avoidance of harm here constitutes an ethical dilemma.

When such dilemmas exist, when good reasons can be given for following any one of a variety of value options and when it seems that not all options can be chosen or implemented at the same time, an orderly approach is called for: having established (a) that the dilemma faced is indeed an 'ethical' dilemma, it then follows (b) that those who are responsible for resolving it must be identified along with (c) all the relevant facts and options available to them. (d) The differing personal and professional values of those involved will need to be taken into account, and (e) in the light of all this, the options will be evaluated and the choice made on how to proceed.

When is a dilemma an ethical dilemma?

Many dilemmas need to be resolved in the medical setting: differences of opinion on labour management, interpersonal problems, failures of communication etc. But, as the examples given suggest, the ethical dilemma is recognizably different and involves reflection on such concepts as 'the quality of life', 'the rights and responsibilities of parents', 'the overall good of the patient', 'team loyalty', 'respect for a variety of religious and other beliefs'.

Whose dilemma is it?

At an early stage, ownership of the dilemma must be established. Does it 'belong' to the medical practitioner? To other health care staff? To administrators? To parents? The responsibility is a shared one, between parents or guardians on the one hand and, on the medical side, those with the relevant special knowledge and 'those health professionals with the most continuous committed and trusting relationship with [the patient or] the parents [who] should have primary responsibility in the health care domain for deciding and coordinating care' around whatever decision is made.[293]

What are the facts and what are the options?

Satisfactory choice relies on adequate knowledge. Knowledge of:

- the medical facts, e.g. diagnosis, prognosis;
- facts about the family, e.g. religion, status, any language barrier, past experience of illness, etc.;
- facts about relevant professional practice, e.g. legal or institutional policy considerations;
- the views of peers and colleagues in the medical team;
- facts of previous unit or institutional experience.

A careful and complete enumeration of the various possibilities for action is essential. As an example: in the case of the child with bronchopulmonary dysplasia who has developed pneumonia, life might be preserved with vigour, or life might be allowed to end, or semiaggressive measures could be used. Insufficient attention to identification of options can only limit the possibility of appropriate choices for resolving the difficulty. At the same time, the options identified must be realistic for this place and this time and these particular circumstances.

Where are the areas of possibly conflicting values?

The ethical choice is not made in a vacuum but within the framework of the attitudes and understanding of the people involved. A sensitive but clear appraisal of this framework is therefore essential and will entail such questions as: how do parents understand 'best interests of the child'? Is their understanding different from that of the neonatologist?[294–300] Is justice in the use of resources understood differently by different members of the health care team? Do staff vary in their attitudes to disclosure and confidentiality? What is the surgeon's general conviction as regards truthfulness, preservation of life, parental choice? What is the standpoint of the practitioner on 'the rights of the individual', on the tension between the benefit to one and the benefit to many, on the absolute nature of medical obligations regardless of possible social consequences?

Weighing the options; making the choice

Weighing one option against another is not unlike the process used by physicians when weighing evidence prior to determination of the right medication for the patient in a particular case. But where an ethical dilemma exists, the process of assembling reasoned arguments for and against each option has a twofold purpose: it is clearly the most likely route to a decision which is best for the patient but it also smooths the path to a harmonious joint or group decision, because it provides a specific argued response to a specific situation, rather than just a personal intuition on the one hand or the mere application of some general rule of thumb on the other. The group has a right to understand and, ideally, have confidence in the reasons for the practitioner's declared choice. As a minimum, an explanation is required if a decision contrary to the values of others is taken. Once the preferred option is established and, if necessary, a choice made between different methods of implementation, the final choice of whether to implement it or not can be reached. 'Patient good' is the continuing and over-riding goal.

Without underestimating the gravity of these matters nor the importance of measured steps in resolving them, the authors nevertheless regard the main ingredient of ethical reflection to be experienced common sense.

Negotiation of ethical agreement between medical practitioner and parents

As already noted, several individuals will be involved in the provision of care for the seriously ill newborn infant. Ideally, all will agree in the matter of any ethical decision to be made regarding the infant's care. In reality, however, such agreement may not be achieved so easily. A particular concern is the matter of agreement between the neonatologist or surgeon and the parents.[301]

It should be understood that it is the physician's professional prerogative to determine which of the available medical options should be pursued. Moreover, the physician may have a relevant personal ethical viewpoint. At the same time, parents, morally and legally, have primary responsibility for the decision made about the care of their child.[302–7]. Numerous arguments are made in support of that stance, e.g.,

> *Respect for the family and desire to foster the diversity which it brings; the fitness of giving the power to decide to the same people who created the child and have the duty to support and protect it . . . or simply the conclusion that the administrative costs of giving authority to anyone but the parents outweigh the risks for children and for society unless the parents are shown to be unable to exercise their authority adequately.*[296]

There are, however, two obvious limitations to parental discretion in deciding care for their children. First, parents are not ordinarily free to deny their child access to life–saving measures, nor access to those interventions which would prevent substantial, irreversible harm to their child. In those cases in which parents attempt to do this, society, via warning from the concerned practitioner or others, will intervene for protection of the child. Professional judgement constitutes a second limitation: the physician who will provide care for the child determines the therapeutic regimens to be offered parents in deciding about intervention/non–intervention in the case of their particular child. While parents may request various measures of therapy, the physician need not accede to such requests if they seem to the physician to be medically inappropriate. In the end, this means that parents may choose only from the interventions/options offered by the physician. If they wish to go beyond these modalities, they must enter negotiation with the physician, or change physicians, or move to some other type of intervention from that which is medically proposed.

Before any moves of this kind are initiated, however, it is well to remember that any difference here may be more apparent than real. For example, parents may not be able to make any ethical judgement about the care of their child, either because of their distressed emotional state or because they are unable to comprehend the information offered to them regarding their child's longer-range status by the physician. If appropriate assistance is offered, however:

> . . . most parents can overcome these difficulties and make decisions on the child's behalf in an appropriate fashion. In order to make good decisions, parents must be told the relevant information, including as accurate an appraisal or prognosis as possible. The medical information they receive, including its uncertainties, should be up–to–date. Their consideration of the situation may be helped by the opportunity to talk with other parents who have faced such decisions, with consultant medical specialists, and perhaps with religious advisors.[294]

Again, staff must provide empathy and understanding for parents.

Following attempts to accommodate differences, several other options might be pursued. For example, in the event that parents disagree with the medically proposed initiation/continuation of a 'life/health' therapeutic regimen, Rostain and Bhutani[308] propose the following: 'Attempt to persuade parents; obtain other medical opinions; obtain assistance from support services; consult with Bioethics Committee; consult legal advice; obtain court order'.

Committee for bioethics

Further to the role of a bioethics committee, the scheme suggested by the President's Commission[294] could be adapted to more general cases of ethical difference between parents and physicians. Using the Commission's 'best interests' standard (balance of potential benefit over potential harm or distress which could result from provision of a certain kind of treatment), the simplest responses compatible with the physician's assessments would thus be: 'provide treatment" when treatment is deemed 'clearly beneficial'; 'forego treatment' when treatment is judged to be 'futile'; 'provide/forego treatment' where the proposed treatment is seen to be 'ambiguous or futile', depending on parental wishes. When there is disagreement between parents and physician (the parents prefer treatment), treatment would be provided except when the physician declines to do so in the case of physician-determined futility. When there is disagreement between parents and the physician such that parents prefer to forego treatment, that

would be the practice except when the physician perceives that treatment to be clearly beneficial; in that case, treatment would be provided during the ethics review process.

Objections have been raised to the use of the bioethics committee in the matter of negotiating ethical differences between parents and physicians, however. It is thought that the committee might interfere with professional decision making; the committee could remove from parents their rightful responsibility for such decision making; the committee process can be lengthy and difficult in terms of emotional energy and lack of privacy within what is recognized to be a very intimate and personal decision making process. The use of a bioethics committee in this context is not common to all those institutions in which an NICU is located. More frequent is recourse to other medical opinions and/or support services. Bioethics consultation at an early stage of discussion is recommended as possibly obviating the need for the more formal approach to the bioethics committee.

Numerous objections can also be raised to the pursuit of negotiation of parental–physician ethical difference in the court room setting. Courts are slow in their determinations; the message provided is blunt; there is concern that there is insufficient knowledge on the part of judges concerning the practice of medicine; court interventions often result in heightened antagonisms between parents and the physician; family relationships may suffer as a result of court intervention just at the time when the most support among family members is required. On the other hand, it is also argued that court decisions are fairest, that they are reasoned on the basis of principle, that they can provide useful precedent.[309]

While ethical agreement between parents and physician is the goal, and while that goal may be reached by way of certain kinds of assistance, education, negotiation or even the passage of time, achievement of that goal may continue to elude those who pursue it. In that case, withdrawal by parents or physician seems the only suitable response.

Initiation/non-initiation of therapy for the newborn patient

We focus now on the ethical considerations proper to any decision on the practitioner's part regarding initiation/non-initiation of therapy. These considerations are looked at here in isolation, though in practice they will of course be reviewed in the broader context of the ethical questions and relationships already discussed.

There are a number of factors, some purely medical, some more general, which can be cited as a basis for further ethical reflection.

The diagnostic category assigned the infant

In common with other commentators, Weir and Bale[310] provide a listing of various neurological malformations which they consider untreatable, in the sense that physicians' best efforts cannot sustain the lives of such infants. Included in this first category are, for example, anencephaly, myeloschisis and multiple severe congenital anomalies requiring repeated efforts at resuscitation. Other somewhat less serious neurological disorders are still 'sufficiently serious that physicians and other decision makers should usually choose to allow a death'. Examples include trisomy 13, trisomy 18, Tay–Sachs, Canavan's disease. The authors believe that the vast majority of newborn infants should not be placed in either of the two preceding groups; rather, they should be treated to prolong and enhance their lives. This judgement obtains 'even when the prognosis for some of the infants includes the likelihood or certainty of physical or neurologic abnormalities'. Included in this latter group are, for example, 'most prematurity, hydrocephalus, most cases of neonatal intraventricular haemorrhage, most cases of myelomeningocele, trisomy 21'.

Rhoden's[311] approach elaborates a possible clinical response to the above-mentioned second category of infants with less serious neurological disorders. Thus, in a state of some uncertainty, the clinician could:

- wait until certain;
- act according to statistical information;
- develop an individualized prognostic strategy.

A variant of Rhoden's approach is proposed by Fleischman.[312] Speaking of uncertainty as regards the second category of infants he remarks:

> *American neonatology has evolved a decision-making strategy which deals with this uncertainty (prognosis regarding seriously ill newborns) by ranking the letting of an infant die who could have lived a reasonable life as far worse than saving an infant who becomes devastatingly disabled.*

In his view, while the vitalist and statistical approaches could be used, one should withdraw/withhold 'when death or a terribly impaired life seems inevitable'.

Cassady[313] offers a quite different perspective with regard to this second group of infant patients. Emphasizing the continuing uncertainty as to the 'best method' for their treatment, he advocates use of a truly randomized scientific trial of various modalities in their regard. Such randomization would provide the knowledge necessary to treat the many other future patients who will come within this group.

Ethically speaking, the categories proposed do not dictate medical or parental response. Any such response follows rather from the value espoused and the judgement of the diagnostic category as fulfilling or thwarting achievement of that value.

The infant's clinical status

The Canadian Paediatric Society[298] presumes the standard 'best interests of the child' and adds to it consideration of several specific categories of clinical presentation. These categories form exceptions to the general duty of providing life-sustaining or life-prolonging treatment:

- Irreversible progression to imminent death;
- Treatment which is clearly ineffective or harmful;
- Instances where life will be severely shortened regardless of treatment and where non-treatment will allow a greater degree of caring and comfort than the treatment;
- Lives filled with intolerable and intractable pain and suffering.

Each category proposed is open to the ever-present problems of uncertainty and variability of medical judgement, as well as to interpretation of terms, e.g.: 'imminent', 'ineffective', 'harmful', 'greater degree', 'intolerable', etc. Once again, ethical judgement as to appropriate action will rest on determination of relevant values and judgement of the identified medical conditions as achieving/thwarting the 'value goals'.

Specific weight/gestational age

Quite apart from the presence of severe abnormality in the newborn infant, neonatologists have particular concern regarding the prognosis and treatment of the extremely low birthweight infant. Campbell, Lloyd and Duffty[314] perceive quality of life here to be just as important as, if not more important than, the fact of life in determining treatment alternatives for children in this group. This position is defended by way of these criteria:

- Reasonable expectation of *healthy* survival;
- Complications of treatment like intermittent positive pressure ventilation (IPPV) do not appear to cause significant brain damage;

Or

- Where congenital abnormalities suffered by the baby alone or in combination do not seem seriously to impair the future functioning of the child's central nervous system.

This approach is based on a 'quality of life' perspective: 'Good prospects for the child achieving a cognitive, sapient and interactive life free from the kind of crippling disability that would prevent normal relationships and independence'.[314]

The infant's status as a 'person'

Some will query this criterion with regard to decisions regarding care of newborn infants. Among those who view the criterion as a critical element in such decision making are the following:

1. Tooley[315] e.g., denies personhood to all infants and young children on the grounds of non-self-identity. In consequence, newborn infants 'have no moral claim on society's services'. Further to this viewpoint, therapy might be provided to a newborn infant on the grounds of social well-being; but to refuse it, so long as such refusal does not entail pain, would not necessarily be considered ethically wrong. Consistent with this position, some could endorse the practice of active euthanasia in the NICU.[315–17]
2. Magnet and Kluge[318] recognize the newborn infant as a person, given the child's potential for development. As a person, the newborn infant has a right, but not a duty, to live; it also has a 'right to die' under certain conditions. Again, active euthanasia can be ethically acceptable within such a perspective.[318,319]
3. Engelhardt[320] supports the view that current or potential neocortical function (cognition, social interaction) is essential to personhood. Strictly speaking, newborn infants do not possess such

function; thus, they are not persons in the moral sense. They are persons socially speaking, however, which is to say that their claim to health care should be met, so long as the decision to provide such health care takes account of the needs of both the child and the family.

Best Interests of the child.

This is a familiar standard for neonatal practice, yet discussion continues as to the clinical and ethical content of the concept. According to Weir and Bale,[310] amongst the criteria considered in application of this standard are:

- Availability of curative or corrective treatment;
- Presence of serious neurological impairment;
- Extent of infant's suffering;
- Multiplicity of other serious medical problems;
- Life expectancy of the infant;
- Relative benefits to the infant of the treatment as against its burdens;
- Ontologic 'personhood' status;
- Future interests of the neonate (i.e. not to be harmed).

Once again, such criteria will not be applicable in the absence of reference to preferred values.

Brody and others[320] have explored such ethical ambiguity implicit in the 'best interests' standard. Thus, some will interpret 'best interests' as requiring preservation of physical life only; others understand 'best interests' to permit natural death in the case of serious physical or mental abnormality. Again, the standard of 'best interests' can be utilized in limiting a certain treatment for the child concerned, lest in attending fully to the one child, the family responsible for providing care to that child be seriously affected in the process. In this connection, the view that others should take over responsibility for this child might be defended. Finally, there will be difference as well in any discussion of 'best interests' when the question of long versus short-term benefit to the child is mentioned. Some will argue that current intervention to save a compromised child's life may be contraindicated unless adequate social arrangements for future protection of the compromised child can be foreseen.

Evidently, use of the 'best interests' standard is not conclusive in itself. Rather, it serves as a basis for the work of clarification of terms, leading to ethical resolution of the difficulty by referring to the values of importance of those conducting the discussion.

The practitioner's relationship to the team and to society

In theory, the ethical obligation of the neonatologist to the infant patient is well delineated: 'The well-being of the patient is my first concern.' As already noted, the implementation of that concept under the rubric, 'best interests of the child' is evidently less certain. This difficulty notwithstanding, development of a constructive relationship with the parents of the infant is of great importance and it must be established quickly as mutually trusting and supportive. The greater burden in this regard rests with the physician: the skilled, knowledgeable 'expert' who can 'empower' such parents by informing them, remaining in close communication with them, empathizing with them in their distress, consulting and collaborating with them throughout the time of the child's presence on that unit and exercising non-paternalistic protective imagination on their behalf.

Any success the neonatologist may have in these areas will be quite limited in the absence of a collaborative relationship with other necessary members of the NICU health care team. The physician must ensure the overall care of everyone in the unit, serving as a leader who shares responsibility with all other staff. In the model proposed, the contributions of nurses, respiratory therapists, nutritionists and social workers are not only welcome, they are actively sought. In this process, the whole becomes greater than the sum of its parts. Better patient care results from the team approach, which could be called 'team medicine'.[321] This is a particularly difficult mandate for the neonatologist, given the stress factors already noted as endemic to work in the NICU. 'Care for the caregivers', including the neonatologist, has thus been the subject of considerable comment in the literature.[322-4]

Already mentioned as a possible source of NICU team stress or 'burn-out' is the need for 'team agreement' in the matter of decision making and care of the newborn infant. One route for ameliorating possible difficulty, perhaps proactively, is continuing ethical education and ethics discussion within the unit.

There is also a need to reduce any such differences by way of some previously agreed guidelines or statements of protocol in the neonatal unit. One example of such a guideline, used at The Hospital for Sick Children in Toronto in the matter of deciding about the use of life-prolonging measures, has proved helpful on numerous occasions since its initiation in 1985. Given the unit's goal, i.e. compassionate medicine (a combination of objective data with sound and ethical human values), the guidelines identify as basic principles:

- Best interests of the child;
- Informed consent/consensus between physicians and parents;
- Respect for law.

Included in the guidelines are consideration of 'meaningful human life' ('life as benefit to the individual who lives it'), the need for consultation among experts and 'openness of discussion in difficult ethical issues'. The HSC statement identifies preference for withdrawal of treatment over its non-initiation and speaks to concern for truthfulness and the management of differences between parents and physicians as well as the need for emotional support for parents and communication and collaboration amongst all staff. The guidelines suggest that the 'physician's own value system' should not be imposed on others and allow for the possibility of nurses' conflicting loyalties, as well as warning to 'guard against the traditional hierarchical order of the doctor–patient relationship' and to set aside reference to 'the economic issues surrounding utilization of resources' because they 'should not be a consideration in clinical decision making'. Overall, the guidelines stress the need for a reasonable consensus in terms of making clinical decisions within the NICU.

It may well be that ethical difference among the team members is not easily resolved, either by way of proactive education or pursuit of such guidelines. In such a situation, the use of ethics consultation may be helpful, as may reference to an ethics committee.[294,296,326-29]

While attending to responsibilities regarding patients, parents, colleagues and staff, the neonatologist cannot ignore or neglect the very real social dimension of the activity at hand. This can be addressed with reference to three different perspectives: first, that neonatology be practised within the limits of law. In the more obvious sense, this will require knowledge and observance of such issues as regulation, statute and case law, with reference to child abuse/neglect, for example, and with reference as well to homicide, allowing death and euthanasia. Perhaps the neonatologist will be confronted with the increasing pressure of possible litigation further to the modalities used or unused in treatment of the seriously ill infant. 'Good' medicine can be identified as practice which is clinically, ethically and legally sound; still there is very real uneasiness among neonatal practitioners lest the threat of lawsuit endanger 'good' medicine. This might occur by way of overtesting so as to satisfy legal requirements, for example; it might occur by way of 'overcommunication', by way of putting legal distance between the physician and the potentially adversarial parent. Inclusion of 'law' in medical practice is necessary and desirable; at the same time, a 'letter of the law' approach, in contrast to a 'spirit of the law' approach, can be disadvantageous to all concerned.

From a second perspective, the neonatologist must be concerned with societal response and judgement regarding the care provided in the neonatal unit. Physicians are pledged to serve the public as they have a contract with society empowering and charging them to do so. While the formal view of society is expressed in law (and that will be derived and formulated differently in different jurisdictions), such a view is elaborated gradually over many years. Of more immediate concern in practice will be the local community standards influencing the care given in the local NICU. For example, what is the local practice in providing social benefits for the family with a severely handicapped infant? If the social acceptance of such children is negative, then even with the support of legislation, the physician and parents concerned may be uneasy in pursuit of vigorous treatment for such a child lest it be socially neglected in the longer term. More generally, what social pressure is there to reduce the costs of neonatal intensive care?

In those matters in which the law is not yet formulated, the force of social opinion may greatly influence the practice of neonatology. How is the physician to know such social concerns with accuracy and how to respond to them? Some clarification and respite is to be found in the hospital's statement of mission and in the profes-

sion's articulated standards of practice. However, there will be continuing social pressures specific to the care of newborn infants which cannot do other than impinge on neonatal practice as parallel or contrary to such statements. These pressures must be identified and a response made despite continually recurring ambiguity. Development of consensus statements/policies/guidelines, colleague support and constructive dialogue with community members have all been useful types of response to such pressures.

Thirdly, but not least of the neonatologist's responsibilities to society in general and to the newborn population and their parents in particular, is that of ethical leadership.[330] Some of this responsibility is met in terms of involving newborn infants in research, thus advancing knowledge concerning the care of these children. Such research engenders numerous ethical problems which are not easily surmounted. In the end, concern for prevention of harm to newborn infants and their claim to justice in treatment may modify the pursuit of scientifically sound and ethical research in this area.

Also of concern here is the matter of the education and the training of future neonatologists. Such activity poses certain ethical dilemmas, i.e. balancing the matter of possible short-term harm against long-term benefit for the population as a whole. Ethical justification here rests on the well-recognized claim of newborn infants for continuing, safe medical care.

It is possible that those who care for seriously ill newborn infants may also mould the public view of these children and the attitude to be expressed to their parents. Neonatologists set a standard of care and compassion for public imitation and emulation with regard to a small but highly visible part of the general population. The ethics of neonatologists may thus determine the future of their patients and of children generally. In this respect, what neonatologists *do* may be more important than what they *say* or the guidelines they follow. If for no reason other than this, those who practise neonatology must recognize the ethical dimension inherent in each of their everyday clinical decisions. They must identify it, teach it and put it into practice as part of their continuing professional responsibility.

References

Scope and organization

1. American Academy of Pediatrics/American College of Obstetricians and Gynecologists. *Guidelines for Perinatal Care*, 3rd edn. American Academy of Pediatrics, 1992.
2. Health and Welfare Canada. *Perinatal Intensive Care Units in a Perinatal Care Network, Guidelines*. Ottawa: Health and Welfare Canada, 1986.
3. Bergman AB, De Angelis CD, Feigin RD, Stockman JA. Regulation of working hours for pediatric residents. *Journal of Pediatrics*. 1990; **116**, 478–83.
4. Klein JD. Resident education, work hours and supervision: Time for change. *Journal of Pediatrics*. 1990; **116**, 484–6.
5. Bogdonoff MD. Suggested personnel additions to department of medicine training programs. *New England Journal of Medicine*. 1987; **317**, 765–6.
6. Honigfeld L, Perloff J, Barzansky B. Replacing the work of pediatric residents: strategies and issues. *Pediatrics*. 1990; **85**, 969–76.
7. Mitchell A, Watts J, Whyte R, Blatz S, Norman GR, Guyatt GH, Southwell D, Hunsberger M, Paes B. Evaluation of graduating neonatal nurse practitioners. *Pediatrics*. 1991; **88**, 789–94.
8. Mayfield SR, Albrecht J, Roberts L, Lair C. The role of the nutritional support team in neonatal intensive care. *Seminars in Perinatology*. 1989; **13**, 88–96.
9. Knaus WA, Draper EA, Wagner DP, Zimmerman JE. An evaluation of outcome from Intensive Care in major medical centers. *Annals of Internal Medicine*. 1986; **104**, 410–18.
10. Miles MS, Funk SG, Kasper MA. The neonatal intensive care unit environment: Sources of stress for parents. *Critical Care Nursing*. 1991; **2(2)**, 346–54.
11. Kennell JH, Slyter H, Klaus M. The mourning response of parents to the death of a newborn infant. *New England Journal of Medicine*. 1979; **283**, 344–9.
12. Pinch WJ, Spielman ML. The parents' perspective: ethical decision-making in neonatal intensive care. *Journal of Advanced Nursing*. 1990; **15**, 712–19.
13. Bok. *Lying: Moral Choice in Public and Private Life*. New York: Random House, 1978.
14. Perlman NB, Freedman JL, Abramovitch R, Whyte H, Kirpalani H, Perlman M. Informational needs of parents of sick neonates. *Pediatrics*. 1991; **88**, 512–18.
15. Bogdan R, Brown MA, Foster SB. Be honest but not cruel: Staff/parent communication on a neonatal unit. *Human Organization*. 1982; **41(1)**, 6–16.

16. Hardwig J. What about the family? *Hastings Center Report*. 1990; **20**, 5–10.
17. Raju TN, Kecskes S, Thornton JP, Perry M, Feldman S. Medication errors in neonatal and paediatric intensive care units. *Lancet*. 1989; **12(2)**, 374–6.
18. Stevenson RC, Pharoah PO, Cooke RW, Sandhu B. Predicting costs and outcomes of neonatal intensive care for very low birthweight infants. *Public Health*. 1991; **105**, 121–6.
19. Ewald U. What is the actual cost of neonatal intensive care? *International Journal of Technology Assessment in Health Care*. 1991; **7** (Suppl. 1), 155–61.
20. Vimpani GV. Resource allocation in contemporary paediatrics: The case against high technology. *Journal of Paediatric Child Health*. 1991; **27**, 354–9.
21. Gagnon DE. Managing the future: an examination of the neonatal intensive care unit. *Journal of Perinatology*. 1991; **11**, 168–71.
22. Tudehope DI, Lee W, Harris F, Addison C. Cost-analysis of neonatal intensive and special care. *Australian Paediatric Journal*. 1989; **25**, 61–5.
23. Sinclair JC. Economic evaluation of neonatal intensive care. Which variables have to be known? *International Journal of Technology Assessment in Health Care*. 1991; **7** (Suppl. 1), 146–50.
24. Torrance GW. Measurement of health state utilities for economic appraisal. A review. *Journal of Health Economics*. 1986; **5**, 1–30.
25. Ozminkowski RJ, Wortman PM, Roloff DW. Evaluating the effectiveness of neonatal intensive care. What can the literature tell us? *American Journal of Perinatology*. 1987; **4**, 339–47.
26. Perrault C, Coates AL, Collinge J, Pless IB, Outerbridge EW. Family support system in newborn medicine: Does it work? Follow-up study of infants at risk. *Journal of Pediatrics*. 1986; **108**, 1025–30.
27. The infant health and development program. Enhancing the outcomes of low-birth-weight, premature infants: a multisite, randomized trial. *Journal of the American Medical Association*. 1990; **263**, 3035–42.
28. Bennett FC. Neurodevelopmental outcome in low birth weight infants: The role of developmental intervention. *Clinical Critical Care Medicine*. 1988; **13**, 221–49.
29. Allen MC. Neurodevelopmental outcome and interventions. In: Jones MD, Gleason CA, Lipstein SU. (eds). *Hospital Care of the Recovering NICU Infant*. Baltimore: William & Wilkins, 1991; pp. 133–47.

30. Saigal S, Szatmari P, Rosenbaum P, Campbell D, King S. Cognitive abilities and school performance of extremely low birth weight children and matched term control children at age 8 years: A regional study. *Journal of Pediatrics.* 1991; **118**, 751–60.

31. Teplin SW, Burchinal M, Johnson-Martin N, Humphry RA, Kraybill EN. Neurodevelopmental, health, and growth status at age 6 years of children with birth weights less than 1001 grams. *Journal of Pediatrics.* 1991; **118**, 768–77.

32. Msall ME, Buck GM, Rogers BT, Merke D, Catanzaro NL, Zorn WA. Risk factors for major neurodevelopmental impairments and need for special education resources in extremely premature infants. *Journal of Pediatrics.* 1991; **119**, 606–14.

33. Doyle LW, Murton LJ, Kitchen WH. Increasing the survival of extremely-immature (24–28–weeks' gestation) infants – at what cost? *Medical Journal of Australia.* 1989; **150**, 558–63.

34. Hack M, Fanaroff AA. Outcomes of extremely low birth weight infants between 1982 and 1988. *New England Journal of Medicine.* 1989; **321**, 1642–7.

35. Benfield DG, Leib SA, Vollman JH. Grief responses of parents to neonatal death and parent participation in deciding care. *Pediatrics.* 1978; **62**, 171–7.

36. Kirk EP. Psychological effects and management of perinatal loss. *American Journal of Obstetrics and Gynecology.* 1984; **149**, 46–51.

37. Harmon RJ, Glicken AD, Siegel RE. Neonatal loss in the intensive care nursery: Effects of maternal grieving and a program for intervention. *Journal of the American Academy of Child Psychiatry.* 1984; **23**, 68–71.

38. Hodge DS, Graham PL. A hospital-based neonatal intensive care unit bereavement follow-up program: an evaluation of its effectiveness. *Journal of Perinatology.* 1988; **8**, 247–52.

39. Whitfield JM, Siegel RE, Glicken AD, Harmon RJ, Powers LK, Goldson EJ. The application of hospice concepts of neonatal care. *American Journal of Diseases of Children.* 1982; **136**, 421–4.

40. Schreiner RL, Gresham EL, Green M. Physicians responsibility to parents after death of an infant. *American Journal of Diseases of Children.* 1979; **133**, 723–6.

41. Jellinek MS, Catlin EA, Todres ID, Cassem EH. Facing tragic decisions with parents in the neonatal intensive care unit: Clinical perspectives. *Pediatrics.* 1992; **89**, 119–22.

Management of the airway

42. Brandstater B. Prolonged intubation: An alternative to tracheostomy in infants. *Proceedings of the First European Congress of Anesthesiology.* Vienna 1972, Paper 106.

43. Allen TH, Steven IM. Prolonged nasotracheal intubation in infants and children. *British Journal of Anaesthesia.* 1972; **44**, 835–40.

44. McDonald IH, Stocks JG. Prolonged nasotracheal intubation. *British Journal of Anaesthesia.* 1965; **37**, 161–72.

45. Thomas DV, Fletcher G, Sunshine P, Shafe IA, Klaus MH. Prolonged respirator use in pulmonary insufficiency of newborn. *Journal of the American Medical Association.* 1965; **193**, 183–90.

46. Aberdeen E, Glover WJ. Endotracheal intubation or tracheostomy? *Lancet.* 1967; **1**, 436–7.

47. Epstein BS, Rudman HL, Hardy DL, Downes H. Comparison of orotracheal intubation with tracheostomy for anaesthesia in patients with face and neck burns. *Anesthesia and Analgesia.* 1966; **45**, 352–9.

48. Fearon B, MacDonald RE, Smith C, Mitchell D. Airway problems in children following prolonged endotracheal intubation. *Annals of Otolaryngology.* 1966; **75**, 975–86.

49. Ratner I, Whitfield J. Acquired subglottic stenosis in the very–low–birth–weight infant. *American Journal of Diseases of Children.* 1983; **137**, 40–3.

50. Reid DHS, Tunstall ME. Treatment of respiratory distress syndrome of the newborn with nasotracheal intubation and intermittent positive pressure respiration. *Lancet.* 1965; **1**, 1196–1.

51. Quiney RE, Gould SJ. Subglottic stenosis, a clinico-pathological study. *Clinical Otolaryngology.* 1985; **10**, 315–27.

52. Hatch DJ. Prolonged nasotracheal intubation in infants and children. *Lancet.* 1968; **1**, 1272–5.

53. Abbott TR. Complications of prolonged nasotracheal intubation in children. *British Journal of Anaesthesia.* 1968; **40**, 347–52.

54. Stocks J. Prolonged intubation and subglottic stenosis. *British Medical Journal.* 1966; **2**, 1199–200.

55. Black AE, Hatch DJ, Nauth-Misir N. Complications of nasotracheal intubation in neonates, infants and children: a review of four years experience in a children's hospital. *British Journal of Anaesthesia.* 1990; **65**, 461–7.

Supportive measures and oxygen administration

56. Bucher H–U, Fanconi S, Baeckert P, Duc G. Hyperoxemia in newborn infants: detection by pulse oximetry. *Pediatrics.* 1989; **84**, 226–30.

57. Hay WH, Brockway JM, Eyzaguirre M, Neonatal pulse oximetry: Accuracy and reliability. *Pediatrics.* 1989; **83**, 717–22.

58. Langton JA, Lassey D, Hanning CD. Comparison of four pulse oximeters: effects of venous occlusion and cold–induced peripheral vasoconstriction. *British Journal of Anaesthesia.* 1990; **65**, 245–7.

59. Cuevas L, Yeh TF, John EG, Cuevas SD, Pildes R.S. The effect of low–dose dopamine infusion on cardiopulmonary and renal status in premature newborns with respiratory distress syndrome. *American Journal of Diseases of Children.* 1991; **145**, 799–803.

60. Anand KJS, Hickey PR. Pain and its effects in the human neonate and fetus. *New England Journal of Medicine.* 1987; **317**, 1321–9.

61. Editorial. *Lancet.* 1992; **339**, 275–6.

62. Kuban KC, Leviton A, Brown ER, Krishnamoorthy K, Baglivo J, Sullivan KF, Allred E. Respiratory complications in low–birth–weight infants who received phenobarbital. *American Journal of Diseases of Children.* 1987; **141**, 996–9.

63. Snodgrass WR. Selected aspects of pediatric intensive care unit clinical pharmacology. *Current Opinion in Pediatrics.* 1991; **3**, 314–18.

64. Silvas DL, Rosen DA, Rosen KR. Continuous intravenous midazolam infusion for sedation in the paediatric intensive care unit. *Anesthesia and Analgesia.* 1988; **67**, 286–8.

65. Koren G, Maurice L. Pediatric use of opioids. *Pediatric Clinics of North America.* 1989; **36**(5), 1141–56.

Surfactant replacement therapy

66. Soll RF, Hoekstra RE, Fangman JJ, Corbet AJ, Adams JM, James LS, Schulze K, Oh W, Roberts JD Jr., Dorst JP, Kramer SS, Gold AJ, Zola EM, Horbar JD, McAuliffe TL, Lucey JF and Ross Collaborative Surfactant Prevention Study Group. Multicenter trial of single–dose modified bovine surfactant extract (Survanta) for prevention of respiratory distress syndrome. *Pediatrics.* 1990; **85**, 1092–102.

67. Long W, Corbet A, Cotton R, Courtney S, McGuiness G, Walter D, Watts J, Smyth J, Bard H, Chernick V. A controlled trial of synthetic surfactant in infants weighing 1250g or more with respiratory distress syndrome. *New England Journal of Medicine.* 1991; **325**, 1696–703.

68. Meritt TA, Hallman M, Berry C, Pohjavuori M, Edwards DK, Jaaskelainen J, Grafe MR, Vaucher Y, Wozniak P, Heldt G, Rapola J. Randomized, placebo–controlled trial of human surfactant given at birth versus rescue administration in very low birthweight infants with lung immaturity. *Journal of Pediatrics.* 1991; **118**, 581–94.

69. Dunn MS, Shennan AT, Possmayer F. Single versus multiple–dose surfactant replacement therapy in neonates of 30 to 36 weeks gestation with respiratory distress syndrome. *Pediatrics.* 1990; **86**, 564–71.

70. Kendig JW, Notter RH, Cox C, Reubens LJ, Davis DM, Maniscalco WM, Sinkin RA, Bartoletti A, Dweck HS, Horgan MJ, Risemberg H, Phelps DL, Shapiro DL. A comparison of surfactant as immediate prophylaxis and as rescue therapy in newborns of less than 30 weeks gestation. *New England Journal of Medicine.* 1991; **324**, 865–71.

71. Horbar JD, Soll RF, Schachinger H, Kewitz G, Versmold HT, Lindner W, Duc G, Mieth D, Linderkamp O, Zilow EP, Lemburg P, von Loewenich V, Brand M, Minoli I, Moro G, Riegel KP, Roos R, Weiss L, Lucey JF. A European multicentre randomized controlled trial of single–dose surfactant therapy for idiopathic respiratory distress syndrome. *European Journal of Pediatrics.* 1990; **149**, 416–23.

72. Yee WFH, Scarpelli EM. Surfactant replacement therapy. *Pediatric Pulmonology.* 1991; **11**, 65–80.

73. Morley CJ. Surfactant treatment for premature babies – a review of clinical trials. *Archives of Disease in Childhood.* 1991; **66**, 445–50.

74. Soll RF, McQueen MC. Respiratory distress syndrome In: Sinclair JC, Bracken MB (eds). *Effective Care of the Newborn Infant.* Oxford: Oxford University Press, 1992; pp. 325–58.

75. OSIRIS Collaborative Group. Early versus delayed neonatal administration of a synthetic surfactant – the judgement of OSIRIS. *Lancet.* 1992; **340**, 1363–9.

76. Reller MD, Buffkin DC, Colasurdo MA, Rice MJ, McDonald RW. Ductal patency in neonates with respiratory distress syndrome. A randomized surfactant trial. *American Journal of Diseases of Children.* 1991; **145**, 1017–20.

77. Ware J, Taeusch HW, Soll RF, McCormick MC. Health and developmental outcomes of a surfactant controlled trial: follow–up at 2 years. *Pediatrics.* 1990; **85**, 1103–7.

78. Dunn MS, Shennan AT, Hoskins EM, Lennox K, Enhorning G. Two–year follow–up of infants enrolled in a randomized trial of surfactant replacement therapy for prevention of neonatal respiratory distress syndrome. *Pediatrics.* 1988; **82**, 543–7.

79. Morley CJ, Modey R. Follow–up of premature babies treated with artificial surfactant (ALEC). *Archives of Disease in Childhood.* 1990; **65**, 667–9.

80. Dunn MS, Shennan AT, Zayack D, Possmayer F. Bovine surfactant replacement therapy in neonates of less than 30 weeks gestation – a randomized controlled trial of prophylaxis versus treatment. *Pediatrics.* 1991; **87**, 377–86.

81. Auten RL, Notter RH, Kendig JW, Davis JM, Shapiro DL. Surfactant treatment of full–term newborns with respiratory failure. *Pediatrics.* 1991; **87**, 101–7.

82. Edwards DK, Hilton SvW, Merritt TA, Hallman M, Mannino F, Boynton BR. Respiratory distress syndrome treated with human surfactant: Radiographic findings. *Radiology.* 1985; **157**, 329–34.

83. Soll RF, Horbar JD, Griscom NT, Barth RA, Lucey JF, Taeusch HW. Radiographic findings

associated with surfactant treatment. *American Journal of Perinatology*. 1991; **8**, 114–18.

Management of persistent pulmonary hypertension

84. Roberts JD, Polaner DM, Lang P, Zapol WM. Inhaled nitric oxide in persistent pulmonary hypertension of the newborn. *Lancet*. 1992; **340**, 818–19.
85. Kinsella JP, Neish SR, Shaffer E, Abman SH. Low–dose inhalation nitric oxide in persistent pulmonary hypertension of the newborn. *Lancet*. 1992; **340**, 819–20.

Ventilator management

86. Mitchell A, Greenough A, Hird M. Limitations of patient triggered ventilation in neonates. *Archives of Disease in Childhood*. 1989; **64**, 924–9.
87. Goldsmith JP, Karotkin EH. *Assisted Ventilation of the Newborn*. Philadelphia: WB Saunders, 1981.
88. Carlo WA, Siner B, Chatburn RL, Robertson S, Martin RJ. Early randomized intervention with high frequency jet ventilation in respiratory distress syndrome. *Journal of Pediatrics*. 1990; **117**, 765–70.
89. Keszler M, Donn SM, Bucciarelli RL, Alverson DC, Hart M, Lunyong V, Modanlou HD, Noguchi A, Pearlmen SA, Puri A, Smith D, Stavis R, Watkins MN, Harris TR. Multicenter controlled trial comparing high–frequency jet ventilation and conventional mechanical ventilation in newborn infants with pulmonary interstitial emphysema. *Journal of Pediatrics*. 1991; **119**, 85–93.
90. Froese AB, Butler PO, Fletcher WA, Byford LJ. High–frequency oscillatory ventilation in premature infants with respiratory failure: A preliminary report. *Anesthesia and Analgesia*. 1987; **66**, 814–24.
91. Bancalari E, Sinclair JC. Mechanical ventilation. In: Sinclair JC, Bracken MB (eds). *Effective Care of the Newborn Infant*. Oxford: Oxford University Press, 1992; pp. 200–20.
92. The Hifi Study Group. High frequency oscillatory ventilation compared with conventional mechanical ventilation in the treatment of respiratory failure in preterm infants. *New England Journal of Medicine*. 1989; **320**, 88–93.
93. Carter JM, Gerstmann DR, Clark RH, Snyder G, Cornish JD, Null DM, deLemos RA. High frequency oscillatory ventilation and extracorporeal membrane oxygenation for the treatment of acute neonatal respiratory failure. *Pediatrics*. 1990; **85**, 159–64.
94. Milner AD, Hoskyns EW. High frequency positive pressure ventilation in neonates. *Archives of Disease in Childhood*. 1989; **64**, 1–3.

Extracorporeal membrane oxygenation

95. O'Rourke PP, Crone RK, Vacanti JP, Ware JH, Lillehei CW, Parad RB, Epstein MF. Extracorporeal membrane oxygenation and conventional medical therapy in neonates with persistent pulmonary hypertension of the newborn: a prospective randomized study. *Pediatrics*. 1989; **84**, 957–63.
96. Bartlett RH. Extracorporeal life support for cardiopulmonary failure. *Current Problems in Surgery*. 1990; **27**, 621–705.
97. Stolar CJ, Snedecor SM, Bartlett RH. Extracorporeal membrane oxygenation and neonatal respiratory failure: Experience from the extracorporeal life support organization. *Journal of Pediatric Surgery*. 1991; **26**, 563–71.
98. Atkinson JB, Ford EG, Humphries B, Kitagawa H, Lew C, Garg M, Bui K. The impact of extracorporeal membrane support in the treatment of congenital diaphragmatic hernia. *Journal of Pediatric Surgery*. 1991; **26**, 791–3.
99. O'Rourke PP, Lillehei CW, Crone RK, Vacanti JP. The effect of extracorporeal membrane oxygenation on the survival of neonates with high–risk congenital diaphragmatic hernia: 45 cases from a single institution. *Journal of Pediatric Surgery*. 1991; **26**, 147–52.
100. Adolph V, Ekelund C, Smith C, Starrett A, Falterman K, Arensman R. Developmental outcome of neonates treated with extracorporeal membrane oxygenation. *Journal of Pediatric Surgery*. 1990; **25**, 43–6.
101. Schumacher RE, Palmer TW, Roloff DW, LaClaire PA, Bartlett RH. Follow–up of infants treated with extracorporeal membrane oxygenation for newborn respiratory failure. *Pediatrics*. 1991; **87**, 451–7.
102. Bartlett RH, Roloff DW, Cornell RG, French Andrews A, Dillon PW, Zwischenberger JB. Extracorporeal circulation in neonatal respiratory failure: A prospective randomized study. *Pediatrics*. 1985; **76**, 479–87.
103. Ware JH, Epstein MF. Extracorporeal circulation in neonatal respiratory failure: A prospective randomized study. *Pediatrics*. 1985; **76**, 849–51.
104. Elliott SJ. Neonatal extracorporeal membrane oxygenation: how not to assess novel technologies. *Lancet*. 1991; **337**, 476–8.
105. Dworetz AR, Moya FR, Sabo B, Gladstone I, Gross I. Survival of infants with persistent pulmonary hypertension without extracorporeal membrane oxygenation. *Pediatrics*. 1989; **84**, 1–6.
106. Lantos JD, Frader J. Extracorporeal membrane oxygenation and the ethics of clinical research in pediatrics. *New England Journal of Medicine*. 1990; **323**, 409–13.
107. Short BL, Brans YW. Extracorporeal membrane oxygenation: Pro and con. *Current Opinion in*

Pediatrics. 1990; **2**, 308–14.

108. Greenough A, Emery E. ECMO and outcome of mechanical ventilation in infants of birthweight over 2kg. *Lancet.* 1990; **336**, 760.

109. Roberton DM. Pediatric ECMO – a consensus position. *Medical Journal of Australia.* 1990; **153**, 122–3.

110. AAP Committee on Fetus and Newborn. Recommendations on extracorporeal membrane oxygenation. *Pediatrics.* 1990; **85**, 618–19.

111. Chan V, Greenough A. Randomized controlled trial of weaning by patient triggered ventilation or conventional ventilation: *European Journal of Pediatrics.* 1993; **152**, 51–4.

112. Aubier M, DeTroyer A, Sampson M, Macklem PT, Roussos C. Aminophylline improves diaphragmatic contractibility. *New England Journal of Medicine.* 1981; **305**, 249–52.

Bronchopulmonary dysplasia

113. Northway WH, Rosan RC, Porter DY. Pulmonary disease following respirator therapy of hyaline–membrane disease. *New England Journal of Medicine.* 1967; **276**, 357–68.

114. Hyde I, English RE, Williams JD. The changing pattern of chronic lung disease of prematurity. *Archives of Disease in Childhood.* 1989; **64**, 448–51.

115. Avery ME, Tooley WH, Keller JB, Hurd SS, Bryan MH, Cotton RB, Epstein MF, Fitzhardinge PM, Hansen CB, Hansen TN, Hodson WA, James LS, Kitterman JA, Neilsen HC, Poirier TA, Truog WE, Wung J–T. Is chronic lung disease in low birthweight infants preventable? A survey of eight centres. *Pediatrics.* 1987; **79**, 26–30.

116. Rush MG, Hazinski TA. Current therapy of bronchopulmonary Dysplasia. *Clinics in Perinatology.* 1992; **19**, 563–90.

117. Rush MG, Engelhardt B, Parker RA, Hazinski TA. Double–blind placebo–controlled trial of alternate–day furosemide therapy in infants with chronic bronchopulmonary dysplasia. *Journal of Pediatrics.* 1990; **117**, 112–18.

118. Harkavy KL, Scanlon JW, Chowdhry PK, Grylack LJ. Dexamethasone therapy for chronic lung disease in ventilator–and–oxygen dependent infants: a controlled trial. *Journal of Pediatrics* 1989; **115**, 979–83.

119. Kazzi NJ, Brans YW, Poland RL. Dexamethasone effects on the hospital course of infants with bronchopulmonary dysplasia who are dependent on artificial ventilation. *Pediatrics.* 1990; **86**, 722–7.

120. Cummings JJ, d'Eugenio DB, Gross SJ. A controlled trial of dexamethasone in preterm infants at high risk for bronchopulmonary dysplasia. *New England Journal of Medicine.* 1989; **320**, 1505–10.

121. Collaborative Dexamethasone Trial Group. Dexamethasone therapy in neonatal chronic lung disease: an international placebo–controlled trial. *Pediatrics.* 1991; **88**, 421–7.

122. Yeh TF, Torre JA, Rastogi A, Anyebuno MA, Pildes RS. Early postnatal dexamethasone therapy in premature infants with severe respiratory distress syndrome: a double–blind controlled study. *Journal of Pediatrics.* 1990; **117**, 273–82.

123. Frank L. The use of dexamethasone in premature infants at risk for bronchopulmonary dysplasia or who already have developed chronic lung disease. A cautionary note. *Pediatrics.* 1991; **88**, 413–14.

124. Avery GB. Letter to the Editor. *Pediatrics.* 1991; **88**, 415–16.

125. Brownlee KG, Ng PC, Henderson MJ, Smith M, Green JH, Dear PRF. Catabolic effect of dexamethasone in the preterm baby. *Archives of Disease in Childhood.* 1992; **67**, 1–4.

126. Joshi A, Gerhardt T, Shandloff P, Bancalari E: Blood transfusion effect on the respiratory pattern of preterm infants. *Pediatrics.* 1987; **80**, 79–84.

Cardiovascular support:

127. Gold JP, Jonas RA, Long P, Elixon EM, Mayer JE, Castaneda AR. Transthoracic intracardiac monitoring line in pediatric surgical patients: a ten-year experience. *Annals of Thoracic Surgery.* 1986; **42**, 185–91.

128. Nadeau S, Noble WH. Limitations of cardiac output measurement by thermodilution. *Canadian Anaesthetists' Society Journal.* 1986; **33**, 780–4.

129. Alverson DC. Neonatal cardiac output measurement using pulsed Doppler ultrasound. *Clinics in Perinatology.* 1985; **12**, 101–27.

130. Tibballs J, Osborne A, Hochmann M. A comparative study of cardiac output measurement by dye dilution and pulsed doppler ultrasound. *Anaesthesia and Intensive Care.* 1988; **16**, 272–7.

131. George BL. Congestive heart failure. In: Nelson NM (ed). *Current Therapy in Neonatal–Perinatal Medicine 2.* Philadelphia: BC Decker, 1990.

132. Sumner E, Stark J. Postoperative care: In: Stark J, deLeval MR (eds). *Surgery for Congenital Heart Disease.* Philadelphia: Saunders, 1993.

133. Freedom RM, Olley PM, Coceani F, Rowe RD. The prostaglandin challenge. Test to unmask obstructed total anomalous pulmonary venous connections in asplenia syndrome. *British Heart Journal.* 1978; **40**, 91–4.

134. Ringel RE, Haney PJ, Brenner JI, Mancuso TJ, Roberts GS, Moulton AL, Berman MA. Periosteal changes secondary to prostaglandin administration. *Journal of Pediatrics.* 1983; **103**, 251–3.

135. Host A, Halken S, Anderson PE. Reversibility of cortical hyperostosis following long–term prostaglandin E1 therapy in infants with

ductus–dependent congenital heart disease. *Pediatric Radiology*. 1988; **18**, 149–53.

136. Guignard J–P, Goujon J–B. Body fluid homeostasis in the newborn infant with congestive heart failure: Effects of diuretics. *Clinics in Perinatology*. 1988; **15**, 447–66.

137. Hickey PR, Hansen DD, Wessel DL, Jonas RA, Elixson EM. Blunting of stress responses in the pulmonary circulation of infants by fentanyl. *Anesthesia and Analgesia*. 1985; **64**, 1137–42.

138. Hansen DD. Pulmonary circulation and pediatric anesthesia. *Current Opinion in Anesthesiology*. 1992; **5**, 387–91.

139. Kermode J, Butt W, Shann F. Comparison between prostaglandin E[1] and eposprostenol (prostacyclin) in infants after heart surgery. *British Heart Journal*. 1991; **66**, 175–8.

140. Monin P, Dubruc C, Vert P, Morselli PL. Treatment of persistent fetal circulation syndrome of the newborn: Comparison of different doses of tolazoline. *European Journal of Clinical Pharmacology*. 1987; **31**, 569–73.

141. Bush A, Busst C, Knight WB, Shinebourne EA. Modification of pulmonary hypertension secondary to congenital heart disease by prostacyclin therapy. *American Review of Respiratory Disease*. 1987; **136**, 767–9.

142. Blomquist H, Frostell C, Hedenstierna G, Zapol WM. Inhaled nitric oxide (NO): A selective pulmonary vasodilator reversing human hypoxic pulmonary vasoconstriction (HPV) (Abstract). *Circulation*. 1991; **89**, 91.

Nutrition

143. Lucas A, Morley R, Cole TJ, Gore SM, Davis JA, Bamford MFM, Dossetor JFB. Early diet in preterm babies and developmental status in infancy. *Archives of Disease in Childhood*. 1989; **64**, 1570–8.

144. Hay WW. Nutritional needs of the extremely low birth weight infant. *Seminars in Perinatology*. 1991; **15**, 482–92.

145. Pereira GR, Ziegler MM. Nutritional care of the surgical neonate. *Clinics in Perinatology*. 1989; **16**, 233–53.

146. Reichman B, Chessex P, Putet G, Verellen G, Smith JM, Heim T, Swyer PR. Diet, fat accretion, and growth in premature infants. *New England Journal of Medicine*. 1981; **305**, 1495–500.

147. Shaw JCL. Growth and nutrition of the very preterm infant. *British Medical Bulletin*. 1988; **44**, 984–1009.

148. Heird WC, Kashyap S, Gomez MR. Parenteral alimentation of the neonate. *Seminars in Perinatology*. 1991; **15**, 493–502.

149. Heird WC, Hay W, Helms RA, Storm MC, Kashyap S, Dell RB. Pediatric parenteral amino acid mixture in low birth weight infants. *Pediatrics*. 1988; **81**, 41–50.

150. Kashyap S. Nutritional management of the extremely low birth weight infant. In: Cowett RM, Hay WW (eds). *The Micropremi: The Next Frontier*. Report of the 99th Conference on Pediatric Research. Columbus OH, Ross Laboratories, 1990, pp. 1570–8.

151. Bremer HJ, Brooke OG, Orzalesi M, Putet G, Raiha NCR, Senterre J, Shaw JCL, Wharton BA. Nutrition and feeding of preterm infants. *Acta Paediatrica Scandinavica*. 1987; **76** (Suppl. 336), 2–14.

152. Evans JR, Allen AC, Stinson DA, Hamilton DC, Brown J, Vincer MJ, Raad MA, Gundberg CM, Cole DE. Effect of high dose Vitamin D supplementation on radiographically detectable bone disease of very low birth weight infants. *Journal of Pediatrics*. 1989; **115**, 779–86.

153. Hamosh M, Mehta NR, Fink CS, Coleman J, Hamosh P. Fat absorption in premature infants: Medium–chain triglycerides and long–chain triglycerides are absorbed from formula at similar rates. *Journal of Pediatric Gastroenterology and Nutrition*. 1991; **13**, 143–9.

154. Schanler RJ. Human milk for preterm infants: Nutritional and immune factors. *Seminars in Perinatology*. 1989; **13**, 69–77.

155. Hudak BH. Nutritional requirements of the preterm infants. In: Jones MD, Gleason CA, Lipstein SU (eds). *Hospital Care of the Recovering NICU Infant*. Baltimore: Williams & Wilkins, 1991.

156. Pettifor JM, Rajah R, Venter A, Moodley GP, Opperman L, Cavaleros M, Ross FP. Bone mineralization and mineral homeostasis in very low birth weight infants fed either human milk or fortified human milk. *Journal of Pediatric Gastroenterology and Nutrition*. 1989; **8**, 217–24.

157. Modanlou HD, Lim MO, Hansen JW, Sickles V. Growth, biochemical status, and mineral metabolism in very low birth weight infants receiving fortified preterm human milk. *Journal of Pediatric Gastroenterology and Nutrition*. 1986; **5**, 762–7.

158. Raschko PK, Hiller JL, Benda GI, Buist NRM, Wilcox K, Reynolds JW. Nutritional balance studies of VLBW infants fed their mothers' milk fortified with a liquid human milk fortifier. *Journal of Pediatric Gastroenterology and Nutrition*. 1989; **9**, 212–18.

159. Hagelberg S, Lindblad BS, Persson B. Amino acid levels in the critically ill preterm infant given mother's milk fortified with protein from human or cow's milk. *Acta.Paediatrica Scandinavica*. 1990; **79**, 1163–74.

160. Newell SJ, Morgan MEI, Durbin GM, Booth IW, McNeish AS. Does mechanical ventilation

precipitate gastro–oesophageal reflux during enteral feeding? *Archives of Disease of Childhood.* 1989; **64**, 1352–5.

161. Heldt GP. The effect of gavage feeding on the mechanics of the lung, chest wall, and diaphragm of preterm infants. *Pediatric Research.* 1988; **24**, 55–8.

162. Lucas A, Bloom R, Aynsley–Green A. Gut hormones and minimal enteral feeding. *Acta Paediatrica Scandinavica.* 1986; **75**, 719–23.

163. Aynsley–Green A, Lucas A, Lawson GR, Bloom SR. Gut hormones and regulatory peptides in relation to enteral feeding, gastroenteritis, and necrotizing enterocolitis in infancy. *Journal of Pediatrics.* 1990; **117**, S24–32.

164. Slagle TA, Gross SJ. Effect of early low–volume enteral substrate on subsequent feeding tolerance in very low birth weight infants. *Journal of Pediatrics.* 1988; **113**, 526–31.

165. Dunn L, Hulman S, Weiner J, Kliegman R. Beneficial effects of early hypocaloric enteral feeding on neonatal gastrointestinal function: Preliminary report of a randomized trial. *Journal of Pediatrics.* 1988; **112**, 622–9.

166. Brown MR, Thunberg BJ, Golub L, Maniscalco WM, Cox C, Shapiro DL. Decreased cholestasis with enteral instead of intravenous protein in the very low birth weight infant. *Journal of Pediatric Gastroenterology and Nutrition.* 1989; **9**, 21–7.

167. Bisset WM, Watt J, Rivers RPA, Milla PJ. Postprandial motor response of the small intestine to enteral feeds in preterm infants. *Archives of Disease in Childhood.* 1989; **64**, 1356–61.

168. Ostertag SG, LaGamma EF, Reisen CE, Ferrentino FL. Early enteral feeding does not affect the incidence of necrotizing enterocolitis. *Pediatrics.* 1986; **77**, 275–80.

169. Davies PA. Low birthweight infants: immediate feeding recalled. *Archives of Disease in Childhood.* 1991; **66**, 551–3.

170. Haumont D, Deckelbaum RJ, Richelle M, Dahlan W, Coussaert E, Bihain BE, Carpentier YA. Plasma lipid and plasma lipoprotein concentrations in low birth weight infants given parenteral nutrition with 20% compared to 10% Intralipid. *Journal of Pediatrics.* 1989; **115**, 787–93.

171. Committee on Nutrition, American Academy of Pediatrics. Use of intravenous fat emulsions in pediatric patients. *Pediatrics.* 1981; **68**, 738–43.

172. Kazlow P, Deckelbaum RJ. Neonatal gastroenterology and nutrition. *Current Opinion in Pediatrics.* 1991; **3**, 214–19.

173. Schreiner RL, Glick MR, Nordschow CD, Gresham EL. An evaluation of methods to monitor infants receiving intravenous lipids. *Journal of Pediatrics.* 1979; **94**, 197–200.

174. Pereira GR, Fox WW, Stanley CA, Baker L, Schwart JG. Decreased oxygenation and hyperlipemia during intravenous fat infusions in premature infants. *Pediatrics.* 1980; **66**, 26–30.

175. Teague WG, Raj JU, Braun D, Berner ME, Clyman RI, Bland RD. Lung vascular effects of lipid infusion in awake lambs. *Pediatric Research.* 1987; **22**, 714–19.

176. Uauy R, Hoffmann DR. Essential fatty acid requirements for normal eye and brain development. *Seminars in Perinatology.* 1991; **15**, 449–55.

177. Freeman J, Goldmann DA, Smith NE, Sidebottom DG, Epstein MF, Platt R. Association of intravenous lipid emulsion and coagulase–negative staphylococcal bacteremia in neonatal intensive care units. *New England Journal of Medicine.* 1990; **323**, 301–8.

178. Hulman G, Levene M. Intralipid microemboli. *Archives of Disease in Childhood.* 1986; **61**, 702–3.

179. Gilbertson N, Kovar IZ, Cox DJ, Crowe L, Palmer NT. Introduction of intravenous lipid administration on the first day of life in the very low birth weight neonate. *Journal of Pediatrics.* 1991; **119**, 615–23.

180. Hammerman C, Aramburo MJ. Decreased lipid intake reduces morbidity in sick premature neonates. *Journal of Pediatrics.* 1988; **113**, 1083–8.

181. Goutail–Flaud MF, Sfez M, Berg A, Laguenie G, Couturier C, Barbotin–Larrieu F, Saint– Maurice C. Central venous catheter–related complications in newborns and infants: a 587–case survey. *Journal of Pediatric Surgery.* 1991; **26**, 645–50.

Renal failure

182. Wahlig TM, Thompson TR, Sinaiko AR. Drug use in the newborn: Effects on the kidney. *Clinics in Perinatology.* 1992; **19**, 251–63.

183. Cuevas L, Yeh TF, John EG, Cuevas D, Pildes RS. The effect of low–dose dopamine infusion on cardiopulmonary and renal status in premature newborns with respiratory distress syndrome. *American Journal of Diseases of Children.* 1991; **145**, 799–803.

184. Shaffer SE, Norman ME. Renal function and renal failure in the newborn. *Clinics in Perinatology.* 1989; **16**, 199–218.

185. John E, Klavdianou M, Vidyasagar D. Electrolyte problems in neonatal surgical patients. *Clinics in Perinatology.* 1989; **16**, 219–32.

186. Karlowicz MG, Adelman RD. Acute renal failure in the neonate. *Clinics in Perinatology.* 1992; **19**, 139–58.

Management of neurological disorders

187. Perlman JM, Tack ED, Martin T, Shackelford G, Amon E. Acute systemic organ injury in term

infants after asphyxia. *American Journal of Diseases of Children*. 1989; **143**, 617–20.

188. Perlman JM, Tack ED. Renal injury in the asphyxiated newborn infant: Relationship to neurologic outcome. *Journal of Pediatrics*. 1988; **113**, 875–9.

189. Volpe JJ, Herscovitch P, Perlman JM, Kreusser KL, Raichle ME. Positron emission tomography in the asphyxiated term newborn: parasagittal impairment of cerebral blood–flow. *Annals of Neurology*. 1985; **17**, 287–96.

190. Hill A. Current concepts of hypoxic–ischemic cerebral injury in the term newborn. *Pediatric Neurology*. 1991; **7**, 317–25.

191. Finer NN, Robertson CM, Richards RT, Pinnell LE, Peters KL. Hypoxic–ischemic encephalopathy in term neonates: Perinatal factors and outcome. *Journal of Pediatrics*. 1981, **98**, 112–17.

192. Sarnat HB, Sarnat MS. Neonatal encephalopathy following fetal distress; a clinical and electro-encephalographic study. *Archives of Neurology*. 1976; **33**, 696–705.

193. Vannucci RC. Current and potentially new management strategies for perinatal hypoxic–ischemic encephalopathy. *Pediatrics*. 1990; **85**, 961–8.

194. Goldberg RN, Moscoso P, Bauer CR, Bloom FL, Curless RG, Burke B, Bancalari E. Use of barbiturate therapy in severe perinatal asphyxia: A randomized controlled trial. *Journal of Pediatrics*. 1986; **109**, 851–6.

195. Eyre JA, Wilkinson AR. Thiopentone induced coma after severe birth asphyxia. *Archives of Disease in Childhood*. 1986; **61**, 1084–9.

196. Levene MI, Evans DH, Forde A, Archer LNJ. Value of intracranial pressure monitoring of asphyxiated newborn infants. *Developmental Medicine and Child Neurology*. 1987; **29**, 311–19.

197. Lupton BA, Hill A, Roland EH, Whitfield MF, Flodmark O. Brain swelling in the asphyxiated term newborn: Pathogenesis and outcome. *Pediatrics*. 1988; **82**, 139–46.

198. Whitelaw A. Intervention after birth asphyxia. *Archives of Disease in Childhood*. 1989; **64**, 66–8.

199. Vannucci RC. Experimental biology of cerebral hypoxia–ischemia: relation to perinatal brain damage. *Pediatric Research*. 1990; **27**, 317–26.

200. Steinlin M, Dirr R, Martin E, Boesch C, Largo RH, Fanconi S, Boltshauser E. MRI following severe perinatal asphyxia: Preliminary experience. *Pediatric Neurology*. 1991; **7**, 164–70.

201. Byrne P, Welch R, Johnson MA, Darrah J, Piper M. Serial magnetic resonance imaging in neonatal hypoxic–ischemic encephalopathy. *Journal of Pediatrics*. 1990; **117**, 694–700.

202. Nalin A, Frigieri G, Caggia P, Vezzalini S. State of the art of magnetic resonance (MR) in neonatal hypoxic–ischemic encephalopathy. *Child's Nervous System*. 1989; **5**, 350–5.

203. Hope PL, Costello AM, Cady EB, Delpy DT, Tofts PS, Chu A, Hamilton PA, Reynolds EO, Wilkie DR. Cerebral energy metabolism studied with phosphorus NMR spectroscopy in normal and birth-asphyxiated infants. *Lancet*. 1984; **2**, 366–70.

204. Azzopardi D, Wyatt JS, Cady EB, Delpy DT, Baudin J, Stewart AL, Hope PL, Hamilton PA, Reynolds EO. Prognosis of newborn infants with hypoxic–ischemic brain injury assessed by phosphorus magnetic resonance spectroscopy. *Pediatric Research*. 1989; **25**, 445–51.

205. Moorcraft J, Bolas NM, Ives NK, Sutton P, Blackledge MJ, Rajagopalan B, Hope PL, Radda GK. Spatially localized magnetic resonance spectroscopy of the brains of normal and asphyxiated newborns. *Pediatrics*. 1991; **87**, 273–82.

206. Levene MI, Fenton AC, Evans DH, Archer LNJ, Shortland DB, Gibson NA. Severe birth asphyxia and abnormal cerebral blood flow velocity. *Developmental Medicine and Child Neurology*. 1989; **31**, 427–34.

207. Pryds O, Greisen G, Lou H, Friis–Hansen B. Vasoparalysis associated with brain damage in asphyxiated term infants. *Journal of Pediatrics*. 1990; **117**, 119–25.

208. Takeuchi T, Watanabe K. The EEG evolution and neurological prognosis of perinatal hypoxia neonates. *Brain Development*. 1989; **11**, 115–20.

209. Majnemer A, Rosenblatt B, Riley PS. Prognostic significance of multimodality evoked response testing in high-risk newborns. *Pediatric Neurology*. 1990; **6**, 367–74.

210. Taylor MJ, Murphy WJ, Whyte HE. Prognostic reliability of somatosensory and visual evoked potentials of asphyxiated term infants. *Developmental Medicine and Child Neurology*. 1992; **34**, 507–15.

211. Robertson C, Finer N. Term infants with hypoxic–ischemic encephalopathy. Outcome at 3.5 years. *Developmental Medicine and Child Neurology*. 1985; **27**, 473–84.

212. Robertson CMT, Finer NN, Grace MGA. School performance of survivors of neonatal encephalopathy associated with birth asphyxia. *Journal of Pediatrics*. 1989; **114**, 753–60.

213. Legido A, Clancy RC, Berman PH. Neurologic outcome after electroencephalographically proven neonatal seizures. *Pediatrics*. 1991; **88**, 583–96.

214. Philip AGS, Allan WC, Tito AN. Intraventricular hemorrhage in preterm infants: Declining incidence in the 1980s. *Pediatrics*. 1989; **84**, 797–801.

215. Strand C, Laptook AR, Dowling S, Campbell N, Lasky RE, Wallin LA, Maravilla AM, Rosenfeld CR. Neonatal intracranial hemorrhage: I. Changing pattern in inborn low-birth-weight

infants. *Early Human Development*. 1990; **23**, 117–28.

216. Perlman JM. Intraventricular Hemorrhage. *Pediatrics*. 1989; **84**, 913–15.

217. Cooke RWI. Trends in preterm survival and incidence of cerebral hemorrhage 1980–9 *Archives of Disease in Childhood*. 1991; **66**, 403–7.

218. Volpe JJ. Brain injury in the premature infant: Is it preventable? *Pediatric Research*. 1990; **27**, S28–S33.

219. Gould SJ, Howard S, Hope PL, Reynolds EOR. Periventricular intraparenchymal cerebral hemorrhage in preterm infants: The role of venous infarction. *Journal of Pathology*. 1987; **151**, 197–202.

220. Armstrong DL, Sauls CD, Goddard-Finegold J. Neuropathologic findings in short-term survivors of intraventricular hemorrhage. *American Journal of Diseases of Children*. 1987; **141**, 617–21.

221. Perlman JM, Goodman S, Kreusser KL, Volpe JJ. Reduction in intraventricular hemorrhage by elimination of fluctuating cerebral blood-flow velocity in preterm infants with respiratory distress syndrome. *New England Journal of Medicine*. 1985; **312**, 1353–7.

222. Goldstein RF, Collins KA, Brazy JE, Narcotic sedation stabilizes arterial blood pressure fluctuations in infants with respiratory distress syndrome. *Pediatric Research*. 1988; **23**, 409A.

223. Leviton A, VanMarter L, Kuban KCK. Respiratory distress syndrome and intracranial hemorrhage: Cause or association? Inferences from surfactant clinical trials. *Pediatrics*. 1989; **84**, 915–22.

224. Volpe JJ, Intraventricular hemorrhage in the premature infant: Current concepts: Part II. *Annals of Neurology*. 1989; **25**, 109–16.

225. Horbar JD, Prevention of periventricular–intraventricular hemorrhage In: Sinclair JC, Bracken MB, (eds). *Effective Care of the Newborn Infant*. Oxford: Oxford University Press, 1992; pp. 562–89.

226. Poland RL. Vitamin E for Prevention of Perinatal Intracranial Hemorrhage. *Pediatrics*. 1990; **85**, 865–7.

227. Dykes FD, Dunbar B, Lazarra A, Ahmann PA. Posthemorrhagic hydrocephalus in high-risk preterm infants: Natural history, management, and long-term outcome. *Journal of Pediatrics*. 1989; **114**, 611–18.

228. Ventriculomegaly Trial Group. Randomized trial of early tapping in neonatal posthemorrhagic ventricular dilation. *Archives of Disease in Childhood*. 1990; **65**, 3–10.

229. Allan WC. The IVH complex of lesions: Cerebrovascular injury in the preterm infant. *Pediatric Neurology*. 1990; **8**, 529–51.

230. Papile L, Burstein J, Burstein R, Koffler H.

Incidence and evolution of subependymal and intraventricular hemorrhage: A study of infants with birth weights less than 1500 gm. *Journal of Pediatrics*. 1978; **92**, 529–34.

231. Shuman RM, Selednik LL. Periventricular leukomalacia. A one–year autopsy study. *Archives of Neurology*. 1980; **37**, 231–9.

232. van de Bor M, Walther FJ. Cerebral blood flow velocity regulation in preterm infants. *Biology of the Neonate*. 1991; **59**, 329–35.

233. Ramaekers VTh, Casaer P, Daniels H, Marchal G. Upper limits of brain blood flow autoregulation in stable infants of various conceptional age. *Early Human Development*. 1990; **24**, 249–58.

234. Nwaesei CG, Allen AC, Vincer MJ, Brown SJ, Stinson DA, Evans JR, Byrne JM. Effect of timing of cerebral ultrasonography on the prediction of later neurodevelopmental outcome in high-risk preterm infants. *Journal of Pediatrics*. 1988; **112**, 970–5.

235. Feldman HM, Scher MS, Kemp SS. Neurodevelopmental outcome of children with evidence of periventricular leukomalacia on late MRI. *Paediatric Neurology*. 1990; **6**, 296–302.

236. Guzzetta F, Shackelford GD, Volpe S, Perlman JM, Volpe JJ: Periventricular intraparenchymal echodensities in the premature newborn: critical determinant of neurological outcome. *Pediatrics*. 1986; **78**, 995–1006.

237. Leviton A, Paneth N. White matter damage in preterm newborns – an epidemiologic perspective. *Early Human Development*. 1990; **24**, 1–22.

238. Fawer CL, Diebold P, Calame A, Periventricular leukomalacia and neurodevelopmental outcome in preterm infants. *Archives of Disease in Childhood*. 1987; **62**, 30–6.

Sepsis and infection control

239. Donowitz LG. Nosocomial infection in neonatal intensive care units. *American Journal of Infection Control*. 1989; **17**, 250–7.

240. Hendricks-Munoz KD, Shapiro DL. The role of the lumbar puncture in the admission sepsis evaluation of the premature infant. *Journal of Perinatology*. 1990; **10**, 60–4.

241. Sanchez PJ, Siegel JD, Cushion NB, Threlkeld N. Significance of a positive urine group B streptococcal latex agglutination test in neonates. *Journal of Pediatrics*. 1990; **116**, 601–6.

242. Gibbs RS, Hall RT, Yow MD, McCracken GH, Nelson JD. Consensus: Perinatal prophylaxis for group B streptococcal infection. *Pediatric Infectious Disease Journal*. 1992; **11**, 179–83.

243. Manroe BL, Weinberg AG, Rosenfeld CR, Browne R. The neonatal blood count in health and disease. I. Reference values for neutrophilic cells. *Journal of Pediatrics*. 1979; **95**, 89–98.

244. Hall SL. Coagulase-negative staphylococcal infections in neonates. *Pediatric Infectious Disease Journal.* 1991; **10**, 57–67.

245. Ford-Jones EL, Mindorff CM, Langley JM, Allen U, Navas L, Patrick ML, Milner R, Gold R. Epidemiologic study of 4684 hospital-acquired infections in pediatric patients. *Pediatric Infectious Disease Journal.* 1989; **8**, 668–75.

246. Schmidt BK, Kirpalani HM, Corey M, Low DE, Philip AGS, Ford-Jones EL. Coagulase-negative staphylococci as true pathogens in newborn infants: A cohort study. *Pediatric Infectious Disease Journal.* 1987; **6**, 1026–31.

247. Patrick CC. Coagulase-negative staphylococci: Pathogens with increasing clinical significance. *Journal of Pediatrics.* 1990; **116**, 497–507.

248. Hall SL, Hall RT, Barnes WG, Riddell S. Colonization with slime-positive coagulase-negative staphylococci as a risk factor for invasive coagulase-negative staphylococci infections in neonates. *Journal of Perinatology.* 1988; **8**, 215–21.

249. Klein JO. From harmless commensal to invasive pathogen – coagulase-negative staphylococci. *New England Journal of Medicine.* 1990; **323**, 339–40.

250. St. Geme JW, Bell LM, Baumgart S, D'Angio CT, Harris MC. Distinguishing sepsis from blood culture contamination in young infants with blood cultures growing coagulase-negative staphylococci. *Pediatrics.* 1990; **86**, 157–62.

251. Phillips SE, Bradley JS. Bacteremia detected by lysis direct plating in a neonatal intensive care unit. *Journal of Clinical Microbiology.* 1990; **28**, 1–4.

252. Schwalbe RS, Stapleton JT, Gilligan PH. Emergence of vancomycin resistance in coagulase-negative staphylococci. *New England Journal of Medicine.* 1987; **316**, 927–31.

253. Baley JE. Neonatal candidiasis: The current challenge. *Clinics in Perinatology.* 1991; **18**, 263–80.

254. Kliegman RM, Clapp DW. Rational principles for immunoglobulin prophylaxis and therapy of neonatal infections. *Clinics in Perinatology.* 1991; **18**, 303–24.

255. Gross GJ, Macdonald NE, Mackenzie AMR. Neonatal rectal colonization with *Malassezia furfur. Canadian Journal of Infectious Disease.* 1992; **3**, 9–13.

256. Dankner WM, Spector SA, Fierer J, Davis CE. Malassezia fungemia in neonates and adults: Complications of hyperalimentation. *Review of Infectious Disease.* 1987; **9**, 743–53.

257. Berman LH, Stringer DA, St Onge O, Daneman A, Whyte H. An assessment of sonography in the diagnosis and management of neonatal renal candidiasis. *Clinical Radiology.* 1989; **40**, 577–81.

258. Wang EE, Frayha H, Watts J, Hammerberg O, Chernesky MA, Mahony JB, Cassell GH. Role of *Ureaplasma urealyticum* and other pathogens in the development of chronic lung disease of prematurity. *Pediatric Infectious Disease Journal.* 1988; **7**, 547–51.

259. Christensen RD, Brown MS, Hall DC, Lassiter HA, Hill HR. Effect on neutrophil kinetics and serum opsonic capacity of intravenous administration of immune globulin to neonates with clinical signs of early-onset sepsis. *Journal of Pediatrics.* 1991; **118**, 606–14.

260. Laurenti F, Ferro R, Isacchi G, Panero A, Savignoni PG, Malagnino F, Palermo D, Mandelli F, Bucci G. Polymorphonuclear leukocyte transfusion for the treatment of sepsis in the newborn infant. *Journal of Pediatrics.* 1981; **98**, 118–23.

261. Cairo MS, Rucker R, Bennetts GA, Hicks D, Worcester C, Amlie R, Johnson S, Katz J. Improved survival of newborns receiving leukocyte transfusions for sepsis. *Pediatrics.* 1984; **74**, 887–92.

262. Hume H. Pediatric Transfusions: Quality Assessment and Assurance. In: Sacher RA, Strauss RG, (eds). Pediatric Transfusion Medicine. Arlington: *American Association of Blood Banks.* 1989: pp. 55–80.

263. DePalma L, Luban NLC. Blood component therapy in the perinatal period: Guidelines and recommendations. *Seminars in Perinatology.* 1990; **14**, 403–15.

264. Piedra PA, Kasel JA, Norton HJ, Gruber WC, Garcia-Prats JA, Baker CJ. Evaluation of an intravenous immunoglobulin preparation for the prevention of viral infection among hospitalized low birth weight infants. *Pediatric Infectious Disease Journal.* 1990; **9**, 470–5.

265. Magny JF, Bremard-Oury C, Brault D, Menguy C, Voyer M, Landais P, Dehan M, Gabilan JC. Intravenous immunoglobulin therapy for prevention of infection in high-risk premature infants: Report of a multicenter, double-blind study. *Pediatrics.* 1991; **88**, 437–43.

266. Noya FJD, Baker CJ. Intravenously administered immune globulin to premature infants: A time to wait. *Journal of Pediatrics.* 1989; **115**, 969–71.

267. Roberts RL, Szelc CM, Scates SM, Boyd MT, Soderstrom KM, Davis MW. Neutropenia in an extremely premature infant treated with recombinant human granulocyte colony-stimulating factor. *American Journal of Diseases of Children.* 1991; **145**, 808–12.

268. Cloney DL, Donowitz LG. Overgown use for infection control in nurseries and neonatal intensive care units. *American Journal of Diseases of Children.* 1986; **140**, 680–3.

269. Leclair JM, Freeman J, Sullivan BF, Crowley CM, Goldmann DA. Prevention of nosocomial respiratory syncytial virus infections through compliance with glove and gown isolation precautions. *New*

England Journal of Medicine. 1987; **317**, 329–34.

270. Gold R. Current guidelines for the prevention and treatment of chickenpox. *Canadian Journal of Diagnosis.* 1991; **8** 47–63.

271. American Academy of Pediatrics: Report of the Committee on Infectious Disease. 21st Ed. *The 1991 Red Book.* Elk Grove Village. Illinois.

272. Van de Perre P, Simonon A, Msellati P, Hitimana DG, Vaira D, Bazubagia A, Van Goethem C, Stevens AM, Karita E, Sondag-Thull D, Dabis F, Lepage P. Post-natal transmission of human immunodeficiency virus type I from mother to infant. *New England Journal of Medicine.* 1991; **325**, 593–8.

273. Pizzo PA, Butler KM. In the vertical transmission of HIV, timing may be everything. *New England Journal of Medicine.* 1991; **325**, 652–4.

274. Edwards JR, Ulrich PP, Weintrub PS, Cowan MJ, Levy JA, Wara DW, Vyas GN. Polymerase chain reaction compared with concurrent viral cultures for rapid identification of Human Immune Virus infection among high-risk infants and children. *Journal of Pediatrics.* 1989; **115**, 200–3.

Ethics

275. Pellegrino ED. Ethics and the moment of clinical truth. *Journal of the American Medical Association.* 1978; **239**, 960–1.

276. Beauchamp T, Childress J. *Principles of Biomedical Ethics.* New York, Oxford University Press, 1983.

277. Gillon R. *Philosophical Medical Ethics.* Chichester, Wiley 1986.

278. Engelhardt HT Jr. *The Foundations of Bioethics.* New York, Oxford University Press, 1985.

279. Childress J. *Priorities in Biomedical Ethics.* Philadelphia, Westminster Press, 1981.

280. Sinclair JC. High technology, high costs, and very low birth-weight newborns. In: *McMillan RC, Engelhard HT Jr, SF (eds). Euthanasia and the Newborn.* Dordrecht, Holland: D. Reidel, 1987, pp. 169–89.

281. Zawacki BE. ICU Physician's Ethical Role in Distributing Scarce Resources. *Critical Care Medicine.* 1985; **13**, 57–60.

282. Stahlman MT. Ethical issues in the nursery: Priorities versus limits. *Journal of Pediatrics.* 1990; **116**, 167–70.

283. Young E, Stevenson D. Limiting treatment for extremely premature low birth weight infants (500–700g). *American Journal of Diseases of Children.* 1990; **144**, 549–52.

284. Lantos JD, Frader J. Extracorporeal membrane oxygenation and the ethics of clinical research in pediatrics. *New England Journal of Medicine.* 1990; **23**, 408–13.

285. Stahlman M. Implications of research and high technology for neonatal intensive care. *Journal of*

the *American Medical Association.* 1989; **261**, 1791.

286. Silverman WA. Human experimentation in perinatology. *Clinics in Perinatology.* 1987; **14**, 403–16.

287. Nicholson R. Ed. *Medical Research with Children: Ethics, Law, and Practice.* 1986; Oxford, Oxford University Press, 1986.

288. Caniano DA, Kanoti GA. Newborns with massive intestinal loss: Difficult choices. *New England Journal of Medicine.* 1988; **318**, 703–7.

289. Ramsey P. *Ethics at the Edges of Life.* New Haven, Yale University Press, 1978.

290. Luce JM. Ethical principles in critical care. *Journal of the American Medical Association.* 1990; **263**, 696–700.

291. Coulter DL. Neurologic uncertainty in newborn intensive care. *New England Journal of Medicine.* 1987; **316**, 840–4.

292. Fost N. Ethical issues in the treatment of critically ill newborns. *Pediatric Annals.* 1981; **10**, 383–89.

293. Mitchell C. Care of severely impaired infant raises ethical issues. *American Nurse.* 1984; **16**, 9.

294. President's Commission for the Study of Ethical Problems in Medicine and Biomedical and Behavioral Research. *Deciding to forego Life-Sustaining Treatment.* Washington, DC: Superintendent of Documents, US Government Printing Office, 1983, pp. 197–229.

295. Brandt RB. Public policy and life and death decisions regarding defective newborns. In: McMillan RC, Engelhardt HT Jr, Spicker SF. Eds. *Euthanasia and the Newborn.* 1987, Dordrecht, Holland, D. Reidel, 1987, pp. 191–208.

296. Engelhardt HT Jr. Infanticide in a post-Christian age. In: *McMillan et al.,* vide supra, pp. 81–6.

297. American Academy of Pediatrics. Joint policy statement: Principles of treatment of disabled infants. *Pediatrics.* 1984; **73**, 559–60.

298. Canadian Paediatric Society. *Treatment decisions for infants and children.* Ottawa: Canadian Pediatric Society, 1986.

299. Shaw M. When does treatment constitute a harm? In: *McMillan et al.,* vide supra, pp. 117–37

300. Shelp EA. *Born to die? Deciding the Fate of Critically-Ill Newborns.* New York: The Free Press, 1986.

301. Silverman WA. Mismatched attitudes about neonatal death. In: Silber T, Thorofare NJ, (eds). *Ethical Issues in the Treatment of Children and Adolescents.* SLACK Inc, 1983, pp. 19–29.

302. Schoeman F. Rights of children, rights of parents, and the moral basis of the family. *Ethics.* 1980; **91**, 6–19.

303. Gaylin W, Macklin R, (eds). *Who Speaks for the Child? The Problems of Proxy Consent.* New York: Plenum Press, 1982.

304. Alderson P. *Choosing for Children: Parent's Consent*

to Surgery. Oxford: Oxford University Press,1990.

305. Campbell AG, Duff RS. Deciding the care of severely malformed or dying infants. *Journal of Medical Ethics*. 1979; **5**, 65–7.

306. Harrison H. Neonatal intensive care: Parent's role in ethical decision making. *Birth*. 1986; **13**, 165–75.

307. Duff RS, Campbell AGM. Moral communities and tragic choices. In McMillan RC, Engelhardt HT Jr,.Spicker SF. (eds). *Euthanasia and the Newborn*, Dordrecht, Holland; D. Reidel, 1987, pp. 273–89.

308. Rostain AL, Bhutani VK. Ethical dilemmas of neonatal–perinatal surgery. *Clinics in Perinatology*. 1989; **16**, 275–302.

309. Miller I. The rights of the disabled versus disabled rights. *Journal of Perinatology*. 1989; **XI**, 88–9.

310. Weir RF, Bale JF. Selective non-treatment of neurological impaired neonates. *Neurologic Clinics*. 1989; **7**, 807–21.

311. Rhoden NK. Treating Baby Doe: The ethics of uncertainty? *Hastings Center Report*. 1986; **16**, 34–42.

312. Fleischman AR. Ethical issues in neonatology: A US perspective. In: Callahan D, Dunstan GR, (eds). *Biomedical Ethics: An Anglo–American dialogue*. Annals of the New York Academy of Sciences,1988: **530**, 83–91.

313. Cassady G. Time to heal? Time to die? . . . Most certainly, time to speak. *Journal of Perinatology*. 1989; **XI**, 83–5.

314. Campbell AGN, Lloyd DJ, Duffty P. Treatment dilemmas in neonatal care: Who should survive and who should decide? *Annals of the New York Academy of Sciences, Biomedical and anglo-American dialogue*. 1988, **530**, 83–91.

315. Tooley M. *Abortion and Infanticide*. Oxford: Clarendon Press, 1983.

316. Kuhse H, Singer P. *Should the baby live? The problem of handicapped infants*. New York: Oxford, 1985.

317. Brandt RB. Public policy and life and death decisions regarding defective newborns. In: *McMillan McMillan* RC, Engelhard HT Jr, SF

(eds). *Euthanasia and the Newborn*. Dordrecht, Holland: D. Reidel, 1987, pp. 191–208.

318. Magnet JE, Kluge E-HW. Withholding Treatment from Defective Newborn Children. Cowansville, Quebec: Brown Legal Publications Inc., 1987.

319. Goldworth A. Human rights in the ommission or cessation of treatment for infants. *Journal of Perinatology*. 1989; **XI**, 79–82.

320. Brody H. Contested terrain. . . In the best interests of. . . *Hastings Center Report*. 1988; **18**, 37.

321. Kraybill EN. Team medicine in the NICU: Ship or flotilla of lifeboats? In: *The Physician as Captain of the Ship: A Critical Reappraisal*. Dordrecht, Holland : D. Reidel, 1988, pp. 77–88.

322. Frader JE. Difficulties in providing intensive care. *Pediatrics*. 1979; **64**, 10–16.

323. Cassem NH, Hackett TT. Stress on the nurse and therapist in the intensive care unit and coronary-care units. *Heart Lung*. 1975; **4**, 252–9.

324. Shelp EE. Courage: A neglected virtue in the patient–physician relationship. *Social Science and Medicine*. 1984; **18**, 351–60.

325. Fleischman AB. Bioethical review committees in perinatology. *Clinics in Perinatology*. 1987; **14**, 379–93.

326. Kliegman RN, Mahowald MB, Youngner SJ. In our best interests: Experience of workings of an ethics review committee. *Journal of Pediatrics*. 1986; **108**, 178–88.

327. Leiken S. Children's hospital ethics committees. *American Journal of Diseases in Children*. 1987; **141**, 954–8.

328. Fleischman A, Murray T. Ethics Committees for Infants Doe? *Hastings Center Report 1983;* **13**, 5.

329. Fleischman AR. Neonatal ethics: Consultation for patient, parents and professionals. In: *Ethics at the Bedside*. Hanover, NH: University Press of New England, 1990, pp. 71–86.

330. Marshall RE. Complexity: leadership in an academic neonatology unit. In: Marshall RE, Kasman C, Cape LS (eds) *Coping with Caring for Sick Newborns*. Philadelphia: W.B. Saunders, 1982, pp. 91–2 and 717–52.

Appendix 1
Unusual medical conditions in the neonate with implications for the anaesthetist

Achondrogenesis:	
Parenti–Fraccaro type	Very short neck Short limbs Early death
Langer–Saldingto type	Very large head Short limbs Early death
Adrenogenital syndrome	Defect in hydrocortisone synthesis – need hydrocortisone Virilization of the female Electrolyte disturbances
Albright–Butler syndrome	Renal tubular acidosis Hypokalaemia
Analbuminaemia	Very low serum albumin Sensitive to drugs bound to albumin (e.g. curare)
Andersen's syndrome	Mid-facial hypoplasia Airway and intubation problems
Apert's syndrome	Hypertelorism Craniosynostosis May have congenital heart disease – antibiotics necessary Intubation difficulties
Arnold-Chiari syndrome	See p. 46, 175
Arthrogryposis multiplex congenita	Congenital contracture Airway problems Difficult veins
Ask–Upmark kidney	Hypertension Areas of renal hypoplasia
Ataxia telangiectasia	Abnormal movements Telangiectasia of skin Defective immunity – sterile equipment and precautions Anaemia – correct preoperatively
Barter's syndrome	Metabolic alkalosis and hypokalaemia Overproduction of prostaglandin E Poor response to noradrenaline Electrolyte abnormalities
Beckwith's syndrome (Beckwith–Wiedemann)	High birth weight Macroglossia, exomphalos – airway problems Persistent hypoglycaemia – careful monitoring
Blackfan–Diamond syndrome	Congenital hypoplastic anaemia Defect in erythropoiesis Steroid therapy

Block–Sulzberger syndrome	Ecto- and mesodermal defects Bullous skin eruptions Microcephaly Spastic paralysis
Bonnevie–Ullrich syndrome	Similar to Turner's syndrome Redundant skin of neck Congenital heart disease
Cardiofacial syndrome	Congenital heart disease Localized facial paralysis
Carpenter's syndrome	Characteristic facies Congenital heart disease – antibiotics necessary Mandibular hypoplasia – airway problems
Cat-eye syndrome	Tristomy 22 without cleft palate
Central core disease	Hypotonia Risk of malignant hyperpyrexia Poor respiratory function
Cerebrohepatorenal syndrome (Zellweger's syndrome)	Jaundice Renal failure Cardiac failure Hypotonia
Chediak–Higashi syndrome	Immunodeficiency; recurrent infections – need to use sterile techniques Thrombocytopaenia
Chotzen's syndrome	Craniosynostosis Renal abnormalities with failure Difficult intubation
Conradi–Hunerman syndrome	Chondrodysplasia Dwarfism Cataracts Difficulty with intubation Poor veins
Cri-du-chat syndrome	Odd cry Microcephaly Hypertelorism Cleft palate Cardiac anomalies
Crigler–Najjar syndrome	Congenital jaundice Glucuronyl transferase deficiency
Crouzon's disease	Craniosynostosis Hypertelorism Difficult intubation
Dandy–Walker syndrome	Hydrocephalus Posterior fossa enlargement
Diastematomyelia	See p. 173, 176
DiGeorge syndrome	Absent thymus and parathyroids Immunodeficiency; recurrent infections Stridor Cardiac anomalies

Down's syndrome (trisomy 21)	Hypotonia Mental retardation Duodenal atresia Airway problems Cardiac anomalies; often atrioventricular defects
Dysautonomia (Riley–Day syndrome)	Deficiency of dopamine-β-hydroxylase Autonomic instability Sensitivity to catecholamines Recurrent aspiration to lungs
Ebstein's anomaly	Congenital heart disease Tricuspid valve anomaly Severe dysrhythmias
Edward's syndrome (trisomy 18)	Most have heart disease Micrognathia Intubation difficulties
Ellis–van Creveld syndrome	Ectodermal defects; short extremities Congenital heart defects Poor lung function with chest abnormalities Abnormal maxilla Intubation difficulties
Epidermolysis bullosa	Bullae from minor skin trauma Some types very severe Care with face masks and intubation
Familial periodic paralysis	Weakness secondary to K^+ disturbance Care with muscle relaxants
Fanconi's anaemia	Pancytopaenic anaemia Renal malformations Radial dysplasia – absent thumbs
Focal dermal hypoplasia (Goltz syndrome)	Papillomas of mucous membranes, especially of airway
Gangliosidosis, type I	Progressive neurological respiratory failure Early death

Glycogen storage disease:
 	
Types I–VIII (Cori's types)
 	
I von Gierke's disease
 	
II Pompe's disease
III Cori's (Forbes')
  disease
	Features include:
	  Cardiac symptoms
	  Hepatic symptoms: bleeding tendency
	  Hypoglycaemia
	  Skeletal muscles affected
	  Glucose-6-phosphatase deficiency
	  Hypoglycaemia
	  Massive cardiomegaly
	  Hepatomegaly
	  Hypotonia

Goldenhar syndrome	Mandibular hypoplasia – airway problems Congenital heart disease
Gorlin–Chaudry–Moss	Craniofacial dysostosis – difficult intubation Patent ductus arteriosus
Hallerman–Streiff syndrome	Mandibular hypoplasia Microphthalmia Glaucoma
Hermansky–Pudlak syndrome	Albinism Haemorrhagic disease

Holt–Oram syndrome	Radial dysplasia Congenital heart disease
Jervell–Lange–Nielsen syndrome (cardioauditory)	Congenital deafness Cardiac conduction defects Sudden death
Jeune's syndrome (asphyxiating thoracic dystrophy)	Severe chest malformations – need mechanical ventilation Renal failure
Kasabach–Merritt syndrome	Haemangioma Thrombocytopaenia
Kleeblattschädel	Clover leaf skull Facial abnormality Intubation difficulties
Klippel–Feil syndrome	Fusion of cervical vertebrae – difficult intubation Cleft palate
Klippel–Trenaunay–Weber syndrome	Haemangioma of whole limb Cardiac failure
Kneist syndrome	Dwarfism Cleft palate Limited joint movement
Larsen's syndrome	Congenital joint dislocations Hydrocephalus Subglottic stenosis
Leopard syndrome	Hypertelorism – intubation difficulties Cognenital heart disease Pulmonary stenosis Hypospadias Kyphoscoliosis; respiratory failure later Dark spots on the skin
18-long arm deletion	Mental retardation Cleft palate Long hands Cardiac anomalies
Maple syrup urine disease	No metabolism of leucine, isoleucine and valine Hypoglycaemia Neurological damage Acidotic episodes
Meckel's syndrome	Microcephaly, micrognathia, cleft epiglottis Heart disease Renal dysplasia
Moebius' syndrome	Paralysis of VI and VII cranial nerves Micrognathia – difficult intubation Lung damage with recurrent aspiration
Mucopolysaccharidoses: types I to VII including Hurler and Hunter syndromes (gargoylism)	Intubation difficulty Cardiorespiratory failure
Myasthenia congenita	No relaxants
Myotonia dystrophica	Weakness and myotonia Cardiac arrhythmias Respiratory failure Suxamethonium causes myotonia

Nager's syndrome	Afrofacial dysostosis Cleft palate Micrognathia Gastroschisis
Nesidioblastosis	See p. 83
Noack's syndrome	Craniosynostosis – intubation difficulties Anomalies of digits
Noonan's syndrome	Micrognathia Failure to develop Cardiac anomalies Renal dysfunction
Oppenheim's disease	Amyotonia congenita
Oral-facial-digital syndrome	Cleft palate Mandibular and maxillary hypoplasia Hydrocephalus Polycystic kidneys
Patau's syndrome (trisomy 13)	Microcephaly Micrognathia Ventricular septal defect Cleft palate Abnormal haemoglobins
Pfeiffer syndrome	Hypertelorism Craniosynostosis Syndactyly Intubation difficulties
Pierre Robin syndrome	Cleft palate Micrognathia and glossoptosis – intubation difficulties Congenital heart disease
Potter's syndrome	Renal agenesis (oligohydramnios) Typical facies – low-set ears Pulmonary hypoplasia
Prader–Willi syndrome	Hypotonia Hypoglycaemia Absent reflexes Poor respiratory effort
Prune belly syndrome	Absent abdominal musculature Poor respiratory effort Renal anomalies
Radial aplasia – thrombocytopaenia	Absent radius Thrombocytopaenia Cardiac defects
Respiratory distress syndrome	See p. 11
Reye's syndrome	Liver failure Encephalopathy Respiratory failure
Ritter's disease	Toxic epidermal necrolysis Staphylococcal infection Very severe desquamation
Romano–Ward syndrome	Prolonged QT Sudden heart block

Rubella syndrome	Mental retardation Deafness Cataract Interstitial pneumonia Osteolytic trabeculation in metaphyses Cardiac anomalies, especially ventricular septal defect
Russell–Silver syndrome	Low birthweight Very large head No hydrocephalus
Scimitar syndrome	Lung hypoplasia Systemic arterial supply Venous drainage to IVC
Short arm deletion syndromes (rare chromosomal syndromes) 4P, 18q, 21q, 22q)	Typical facies Cleft palate Heart disease Poor prognosis
Smith–Lemli–Opitz syndrome	Microcephaly Skeletal anomalies with hypotonia and respiratory failure Increased susceptibility to infection
Stickler syndrome	Micrognathia Cleft palate Retinal detachment
Sturge–Weber syndrome	Vascular naevus Intracranial haemangioma
Tay–Sachs disease	Lipoidosis – infantile type Mental, motor degeneration
Treacher Collins syndrome	Micrognathia and choanal atresia – intubation difficulties Heart disease Deafness
Trisomy 22	Microcephaly Micrognathia Congenital heart disease Cleft palate
Turner's syndrome	XO females Webneck Micrognathia Congenital heart disease Renal anomaly
VATER syndrome	Vertebral anomalies Ventricular septal defect Anal atresia Tracheo-oesophageal fistula Radial dysplasia Renal anomalies
Werdnig–Hoffmann disease	Severe muscular atrophy Respiratory failure – resulting in early death
Williams syndrome (infantile hypercalcaemia syndrome)	Mental retardation Coarse hair Aortic and pulmonary stenosis Characteristic facies

Wilson–Mikity syndrome	Prematurity Severe lung disease with fibrosis and cysts (aetiology unknown)
Wiskott–Aldrich syndrome	Thrombocytopaenia Immunological deficiency Poor prognosis
Wolff–Parkinson–White syndrome	ECG shows prolonged QRS Paroxysmal tachycardia and other arrhythmias Effects accentuated by neostigmine
Wolman's disease	Failure to thrive Xanthomatous infiltration of heart, liver, etc.

Appendix 2
Guidelines for drug dosage in paediatric anaesthetic practice

All drugs are given on the basis of body weight (kg)

Premedication

Atropine 0.02 mg·kg^{-1}
                  up to 2.5 kg   0.15 mg
                  2.5–8 kg   0.2 mg   i.m. ¾ hour preoperatively

Glycopyrrolate 0.004–0.008 mg·kg^{-1}

Injection pethidine compound (Inj. Peth Co.) 0.07 ml·kg^{-1}. ¾ hour preoperatively (rarely used nowadays).

     1 ml contains: pethidine   25 mg
                            promethazine   6.25 mg
                            chlorpromazine 6.25 mg

For cardiac catheters under sedation Peth. Co. up to 0.05 ml·kg^{-1} i.m. may be given ½ hour before catheterization.

Anaesthetic agents   all are given intravenously unless stated otherwise

Thiopentone   2–4 mg·kg^{-1}

Suxamethonium   1–2 mg·kg^{-1}
                                 1 mg·kg^{-1} for intermittent use in neonates; total dose up to 25 mg

Ketamine:
     induction   2 mg·kg^{-1} i.v. (or 10 mg·kg^{-1} i.m.)
     maintenance   1 mg·kg^{-1} i.v.

Atracurium   0.5 mg·kg^{-1}; dilute to 1 mg·ml^{-1}
                                  Infusion 8μg·kg^{-1}·min

Pancuronium   0.06 mg·kg^{-1}; dilute to 0.2 mg·ml^{-1}

Tubocurarine   0.2 mg·kg^{-1}; dilute to 0.25 mg·ml^{-1}

Vecuronium   0.1 mg·kg^{-1}; dilute to 0.4 mg·ml^{-1}
                                  Infusion 1.5 μg·kg^{-1}·min^{-1}

Reversal

Atropine and neostigmine:
     atropine   0.025 mg·kg^{-1}
     neostigmine   0.05 mg·kg^{-1}

Glycopyrrolate   0.01 mg·kg^{-1}

Analgesics   intraoperative – for cardiac anaesthesia only

Morphine   0.2 mg·kg^{-1}; up to 1 mg·kg^{-1} total dose for open heart surgery

Fentanyl $2\text{–}3\ \mu\text{g·kg}^{-1}$
$10\text{–}20\ \mu\text{g·kg}^{-1}$ for cardiac surgery with postoperative ventilation.

Antibiotics   by i.m. or i.v. injection

Ampicillin	UP to 50 mg·kg^{-1}	6-hourly for severe infections
Cloxacillin	12.5 mg·kg^{-1}	6-hourly
Erythromycin	12.5 mg·kg^{-1}	8-hourly
Gentamicin	2mg·kg^{-1}	8-hourly
Metronidazole	7.5 mg·kg^{-1}	6-hourly i.v.
Penicillin	25 mg·kg^{-1}	6-hourly
Vancomycin	20 mg·kg^{-1}	by i.v. infusion over 1 hour (12 hourly)

Other drugs   by i.v. injection unless stated otherwise

Chlorpromazine   1 mg increments up to 0.5 mg.kg^{-1}

Dexamethasone   0.25 mg·kg^{-1} i.v., then 0.1 mg·kg^{-1} 6-hourly i.m. for three doses
For cerebral oedema, up to 0.5 mg·kg^{-1}

Digoxin   Total digitalizing dose: 0.05 mg·kg^{-1}
     one-third stat
     one-third 4–6 hours
     one-third 8–12 hours
Maintenance: one-tenth digitalizing dose b.d.
For premature babies, total dose: 0.03 mg·kg^{-1}

Droperidol   0.3 mg·kg^{-1}

Frusemide   1 mg·kg^{-1}, repeatable

Hydrocortisone   1 mg·kg^{-1}

Indomethacin   0.2 mg·kg^{-1}

Labetalol   0.2 mg·kg^{-1} increments up to 1 mg·kg^{-1}

Lignocaine   1 mg·kg^{-1} (maximum dose 3 mg·kg^{-1})

Mannitol   Test dose: 0.5 g·kg^{-1}

Marcain   Caudal analgesia 0.5 ml·kg^{-1} 0.25% (maximum dose 2 mg·kg^{-1})

Methoxamine   Dilution to 0.5 mg·ml^{-1}; careful increments of 0.25 mg to achieve desired result

Methylprednisolone   30 mg·kg^{-1}

Naloxone   10 μg·kg^{-1}

Phentolamin   Dilution to 1 mg·kg^{-1}; increments of 0.5 mg for desired result

Propranolol   Dilution to 0.1 mg·kg^{-1}; increments of 0.05 mg; maximum dose 0.1 mg·kg^{-1}

Prostacycline   4–20 ng·kg^{-1}.min

Prostaglandin E_1 or E_2 30 μg·kg^{-1} in 50 ml 5% dextrose 1 ml·h^{-1}

Sodium nitroprusside   3 mg·kg^{-1} in 100 ml of 5% dextrose. Do not exceed 1–1.5 mg·kg^{-1} total dose in 24 hours

Theophylline   6 mg·kg^{-1}

Tolazoline   1–2 mg·kg^{-1} over 3 minutes; then infuse the same dose hourly

Postoperative agents   Analgesia is given with caution in the neonate after individual assessment.

Analgesics

Codeine phosphate   1 mg·kg^{-1} 4–6 hourly. Do NOT give i.v. because it causes a severe fall in cardiac output

Fentanyl   Infusion   100 μg·kg^{-1} in 50 ml 5% dextrose   ⎫   To be used with
                        2 ml·hr^{-1} = 4 μg·kg^{-1} min^{-1} ⎪   great caution in
Morphine   0.2 mg·kg^{-1} i.m. or i.v.   ⎬   spontaneously
            Infusion 0.5 mg·kg^{-1} in 50 ml   ⎪   breathing babies
            5% dextrose run at 2 ml·h^{-1} ⎭

Paracetamol   10–15 mg·kg^{-1} orally or rectally 4–6 hourly

Sedatives

Phenobarbitone   1–2 mg·kg^{-1} to control seizures (4 hourly if necessary)

Diazepam   0.2 mg·kg^{-1} orally   ⎫
Syrup of chloral   30 mg·kg^{-1} orally   ⎬   or via nasogastric tube 4 hourly
Promethazine   0.5–1 mg·kg^{-1} orally   ⎪   if necessary
Tricoflos elixir   30 mg·kg^{-1} orally   ⎭

Midazolam   0.15–0.2 mg·kg^{-1}.hr infusion

Inotropic agents   DILUTIONS ONLY ARE GIVEN. The effect of administration must be monitored. The strength may be increased if fluid restriction is necessary.

Adrenaline   ⎫
Isoprenaline   ⎬   60 μg·kg^{-1} in 100 ml 5% dextrose 1 ml·hr^{-1} =
Noradrenaline   ⎭   0.01 μg·kg^{-1}.min (dose 0.01 – 0.5 μg·kg^{-1}.min)

Dobutamine   6 mg·kg^{-1} in 100 100 ml 5% dextrose
              1 ml·h^{-1} = 1 μg·kg^{-1}.min

Dopamine   6 mg·kg^{-1} in 100 ml 5% dextrose
            1 ml·h^{-1} = 1 μg·kg^{-1}.min

            At a dose not exceeding 10 μg·kg^{-1}.min
            there is little α-adrenergic activity

Enoximone   100 mg in 40 ml water
             bolus 0.5–1 mg·kg^{-1} slowly i.v.
             infusion 10–15 μg·kg^{-1}.min

Drugs used in cardiopulmonary resuscitation

Adrenaline (1:100 000)   0.1 ml·kg^{-1} into central vein

Atropine   0.03 mg·kg^{-1} i.v.

Calcium chloride (10%)   0.25 ml·kg^{-1} into central vein

Dexamethasone   0.25 mg·kg^{-1} i.v. 6 hourly

Diazepam   0.2 mg·kg^{-1} i.v.

Sodium bicarbonate (8.4%)   1 ml·kg^{-1} i.v.; then perform blood gas analysis

Appendix 3
Normal physiological values in the neonate and adult

	Neonate	Adult
Hb	18–25 gm·dl^{-1}	15 gm·dl^{-1}
Haematocrit (PCV)	50–60 per cent	45 per cent
Blood volume	70–125 ml·kg^{-1}	70ml·kg^{-1}
Extracellular fluid (percentage of body weight)	35 per cent	20 per cent
Water turnover per 24 hours (percentage of body weight)	15 per cent	9 per cent
Serum K$^+$	5–8 mmol·l^{-1}	3–5 mmol·l^{-1}
Na$^+$	136–143 mmol·l^{-1}	135–148 mmol·l^{-1}
Cl$^-$	96–107 mmol·l^{-1}	98–106 mmol·l^{-1}
HCO$^-$	20 mmol·l^{-1}	24 mmol·l^{-1}
Blood urea nitrogen	1.3–3.3 mmol·l^{-1}	6.6–8.6 mmol·l^{-1}
pH	7.35	7.40
PaCO$_2$	4.7 kPa (35 mmHg)	4.7–6.0 kPa (35–45 mmHg)
PaO$_2$	8.7–10.7 kPa (65–80 mmHg)	10.7–12.7 kPa (80–95 mmHg)
Base excess	−5	0
Total bilirubin	100 μmol·l^{-1}	2–14 μmol·l^{-1}
Total Ca^{2+}	1.48–2.68 mmol·l^{-1}	2.13–2.6 mmol·l^{-1}
Mg^{2+}	0.7–1.1 mmol·l^{-1}	0.6–1.0 mmol·l^{-1}
Phosphate	1.15–2.8 mmol·l^{-1}	1.0–1.4 mmol·l^{-1}
Glucose	2.7–3.3 mmol·l^{-1}	2.4–5.3 mmol·l^{-1}
Total proteins	46–74 gm·l^{-1}	60–80 gm·l^{-1}
Albumin	36–54 gm·l^{-1}	35–47 gm·l^{-1}
Serum osmolality	270–285 mmol·l^{-1}	270–285 mmol·l^{-1}
Urine osmolality	50–600 mmol·l^{-1}	50–1400 mmol·l^{-1}
Na$^+$	50 mmol·l^{-1}	30 mmol·l^{-1}
Specific gravity	1005–1020	1005–1035

Appendix 4
Resuscitation charts

Endotracheal Tube

Length (cm)	Int. Dia (mm)
18–21	7.5–8.0
18	7.0
17	6.5
16	6.0
15	5.5
14	5.0
13	4.5
12	4.0
	3.5
10	3.0–3.5

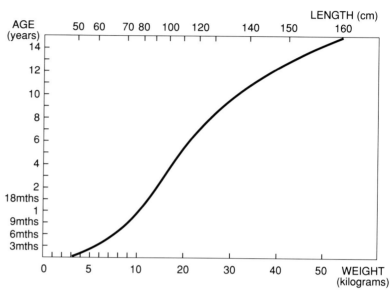

Adrenaline ml of 1:10 000	iv/et	0.5	1	2	3	4	5
Atropine mg	iv/et	0.1	0.2	0.4	0.6	0.6	0.6
Bicarbonate ml of 8.4%	iv	5	10	20	30	40	50
Calcium chloride★ mmol	iv	1	2	4	6	8	10
Diazepam mg	iv pr	1.25 2.5	2.5 5	5 10	7.5 –	10 –	10 –
Glucose ml of 50%	iv	10	20	40	60	80	100
Lignocaine mg	iv/et	5	10	20	30	40	50
Salbutamol micrograms	iv/et	25	50	100	150	200	250
Initial D.C.defibrillation joules		10	20	40	60	80	100
Initial fluid infusion in hypovolaemic shock ml		50	100	200	300	400	500

★1ml of calcium chloride 1 mmol·ml^{-1} = 1.5 ml of calcium chloride 10%
= 4.5 ml of calcium gluconate 10%

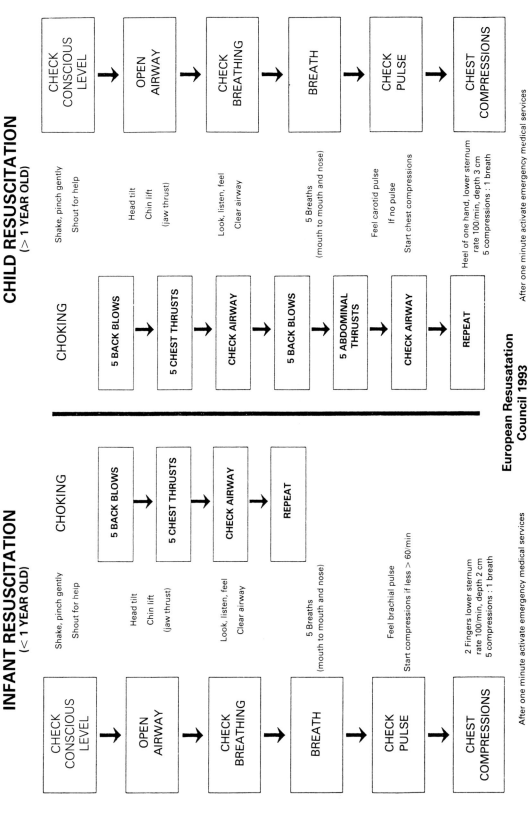

CHILD RESUSCITATION
(> 1 YEAR OLD)

CHECK CONSCIOUS LEVEL → OPEN AIRWAY → CHECK BREATHING → BREATH → CHECK PULSE → CHEST COMPRESSIONS

Shake, pinch gently
Shout for help

Head tilt
Chin lift
(jaw thrust)

Look, listen, feel
Clear airway

5 Breaths
(mouth to mouth and nose)

Feel carotid pulse
If no pulse
Start chest compressions

Heel of one hand, lower sternum
rate 100/min, depth 3 cm
5 compressions : 1 breath

After one minute activate emergency medical services

CHOKING

5 BACK BLOWS → 5 CHEST THRUSTS → CHECK AIRWAY → 5 BACK BLOWS → 5 ABDOMINAL THRUSTS → CHECK AIRWAY → REPEAT

**European Resusatation
Council 1993**

INFANT RESUSCITATION
(< 1 YEAR OLD)

CHOKING

5 BACK BLOWS → 5 CHEST THRUSTS → CHECK AIRWAY → REPEAT

Shake, pinch gently
Shout for help

Head tilt
Chin lift
(jaw thrust)

Look, listen, feel
Clear airway

5 Breaths
(mouth to mouth and nose)

Feel brachial pulse
Start compressions if less > 60/min

2 Fingers lower sternum
rate 100/min, depth 2 cm
5 compressions : 1 breath

CHECK CONSCIOUS LEVEL → OPEN AIRWAY → CHECK BREATHING → BREATH → CHECK PULSE → CHEST COMPRESSIONS

After one minute activate emergency medical services

Index